T0310689

Internet of Things and Data Mining for Modern Engineering and Healthcare Applications

This book focuses on Internet of Things (IoT) and data mining for modern engineering and healthcare applications, recent technological advancements in microwave engineering and communication, and applicability of newly developed solid-state technologies in biomedical engineering and healthcare for day-to-day applications.

The reader will be able to know the recent advancements in microwave engineering, including novel techniques in microwave antenna design and various aspects of microwave propagation. This book aims to showcase various aspects of communication, networking, data mining, computational biology, bioinformatics, biostatistics and machine learning.

Day-to-day applicability of modern communication and networking technologies is a matter of prime concern. This book covers recent trends in solid-state technologies, VLSI and the applicability of modern electronic devices and biosensing devices in bioinformatics and smart healthcare. Furthermore, it showcases the modern optimization techniques in power system engineering and machine design and discusses the role of solid-state engineering in the development of modern electronic gadgets. Societal benefits of microwave technologies for smooth and hustle-free life are also majorly focused areas.

This book will be of high interest to the researchers, academicians, scientists and industrialists as well who are involved in the role of IoT for modern engineering applications.

Features:

- This book features Internet of Things (IoT) and data mining for modern engineering and healthcare applications, recent technological advancements in microwave engineering and communication, and applicability of newly developed solid-state technologies in biomedical engineering and smart healthcare technologies.
- It showcases the novel techniques in Internet of Things (IoT)-integrated microwave antenna design and various aspects of microwave communication.
- It highlights the role of Internet of Things (IoT) in various aspects of communication, networking, data mining, computational biology, bioinformatics, biostatistics and machine learning.
- It reviews the role of Internet of Things (IoT) in solid-state technologies and VLSI and the applicability of modern electronic devices in bioinformatics and healthcare.
- It highlights the role of Internet of Things (IoT) in power system engineering, optics, RF and microwave energy harvesting and smart biosensing technologies.

Chapman & Hall/CRC Internet of Things: Data-Centric Intelligent Computing, Informatics, and Communication

The role of adaptation, machine learning, computational Intelligence, and data analytics in the field of IoT Systems is becoming increasingly essential and intertwined. The capability of an intelligent system is growing depending upon various self-decision-making algorithms in IoT Devices. IoT based smart systems generate a large amount of data that cannot be processed by traditional data processing algorithms and applications. Hence, this book series involves different computational methods incorporated within the system with the help of Analytics Reasoning, learning methods, Artificial intelligence, and Sense-making in Big Data, which is most concerned in IoT-enabled environment.

This series focuses to attract researchers and practitioners who are working in Information Technology and Computer Science in the field of intelligent computing paradigm, Big Data, machine learning, Sensor data, Internet of Things, and data sciences. The main aim of the series is to make available a range of books on all aspects of learning, analytics and advanced intelligent systems and related technologies. This series will cover the theory, research, development, and applications of learning, computational analytics, data processing, machine learning algorithms, as embedded in the fields of engineering, computer science, and Information Technology.

Series Editors:

Security of Internet of Things Nodes: Challenges, Attacks, and Countermeasures
Chinmay Chakraborty, Sree Ranjani Rajendran and Muhammad Habib Ur Rehman

Cancer Prediction for Industrial IoT 4.0: A Machine Learning Perspective
Meenu Gupta, Rachna Jain, Arun Solanki and Fadi Al-Turjman

Cloud IoT Systems for Smart Agricultural Engineering
Saravanan Krishnan, J Bruce Ralphin Rose, NR Rajalakshmi, N Narayanan Prasanth

Data Science for Effective Healthcare Systems
Hari Singh, Ravindara Bhatt, Prateek Thakral and Dinesh Chander Verma

Internet of Things and Data Mining for Modern Engineering and Healthcare Applications
Ankan Bhattacharya, Bappadittya Roy, Samarendra Nath Sur, Saurav Mallik and Subhasis Dasgupta

Internet of Things and Data Mining for Modern Engineering and Healthcare Applications

Edited by
Ankan Bhattacharya, Bappadittya Roy,
Samarendra Nath Sur, Saurav Mallik
and Subhasis Dasgupta

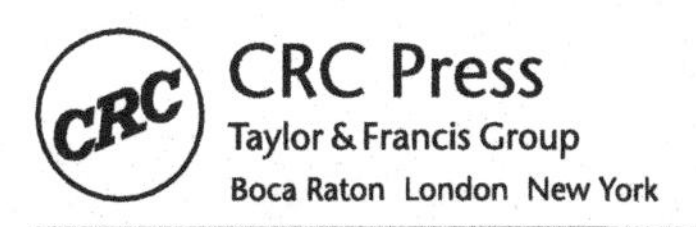

CRC Press is an imprint of the
Taylor & Francis Group, an **informa** business
A CHAPMAN & HALL BOOK

First edition published 2023
by CRC Press
6000 Broken Sound Parkway NW, Suite 300, Boca Raton, FL 33487-2742

and by CRC Press
4 Park Square, Milton Park, Abingdon, Oxon, OX14 4RN

CRC Press is an imprint of Taylor & Francis Group, LLC

Library of Congress Cataloging-in-Publication Data

Names: Bhattacharya, Ankan, editor.
Title: Internet of things and data mining for modern engineering and healthcare applications / edited by Ankan Bhattacharya, Bappadittya Roy, Samarendra Nath Sur, Saurav Mallik, Subhasis Dasgupta.
Description: First edition. | Boca Raton : Chapman & Hall/CRC Press, 2023. | Series: Chapman & Hall/CRC internet of things: data-centric intelligent computing, informatics, and communication | Includes bibliographical references and index. | Summary: "Internet of Things and Data Mining for Modern Engineering and Healthcare Applications aims to focus on the Internet of Things (IoT) and Data Mining for Modern Engineering and Healthcare Applications. It also focuses on recent technological advancements in Microwave Engineering, Communication and applicability of newly developed solid-state technologies in bio-medical engineering and healthcare. Emerging technologies and cutting-edge research in Microwave Engineering and related technologies have also been considered"-- Provided by publisher.
Identifiers: LCCN 2022009417 (print) | LCCN 2022009418 (ebook) | ISBN 9781032108544 (hardback) | ISBN 9781032323275 (paperback) | ISBN 9781003217398 (ebook)
Subjects: LCSH: Biomedical engineering. | Internet of things. | Medical informatics. | Data mining.
Classification: LCC R856 .I454 2023 (print) | LCC R856 (ebook) | DDC 610.285--dc23/eng/20220610
LC record available at https://lccn.loc.gov/2022009417
LC ebook record available at https://lccn.loc.gov/2022009418

ISBN: 9781032108544 (hbk)
ISBN: 9781032323275 (pbk)
ISBN: 9781003217398 (ebk)

DOI: [10.1201/9781003217398]

Typeset in Times
by Deanta Global Publishing Services, Chennai, India

Contents

Preface

This book focuses on Internet of Things (IoT) and data mining for modern engineering and healthcare applications, recent technological advancements in microwave engineering and communication, and applicability of newly developed solid-state technologies in biomedical engineering and healthcare. It also focuses on emerging technologies and cutting-edge research in microwave engineering and related fields.

Microwave engineering includes recent advancements and novel techniques in microwave antenna design and various aspects of microwave propagation. Starting from single/multiband antennas, this book showcases various design and performance aspects of wideband to super wideband antennas, including MIMOs for wireless communication, in various portable wireless devices.

This book highlights numerous aspects of communication, networking, data mining, computational biology, bioinformatics, biostatistics and machine learning. Also, applications of artificial intelligence and machine learning in design and optimization processes have been included.

This book covers recent trends in solid-state technologies, VLSI and the applicability of modern electronic devices in bioinformatics and smart healthcare.

Furthermore, this book discusses modern optimization techniques in power system engineering, machine design, vehicular technologies and related arena. Overall, this book showcases the cutting-edge researches by academicians, researchers and scientists in the areas of engineering and technology, including environment and healthcare.

Preface

Editor biographies

Dr. Ankan Bhattacharya

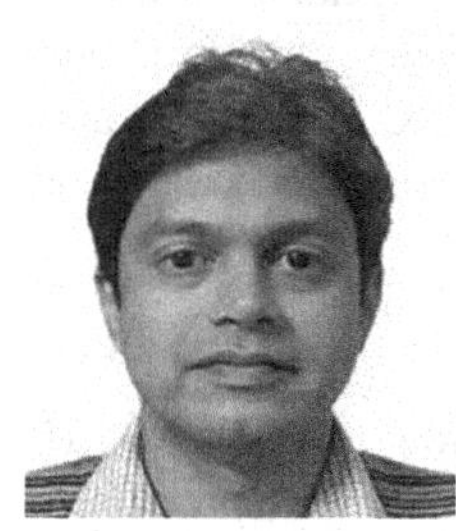

Ankan Bhattacharya obtained B.Tech. and M.Tech. degrees in electronics and communication engineering from the West Bengal University of Technology, Kolkata, India. He completed his Ph.D. from the National Institute of Technology, Durgapur, India. He is the author of several research papers which have been published in many reputed journals and conferences at national and international levels. Dr. Bhattacharya is a life-member of Forum of Scientists, Engineers and Technologists (FOSET), member of Institution of Engineers India (IEI) and member of International Association of Engineers (IAENG). His areas of research are antenna engineering, computational electromagnetics, electronic circuits and systems, signal processing, microwave devices and wireless communication technologies. He is also an editor as well as a reviewer of many reputed national and international journals. Dr. Bhattacharya is the Series Editor of *Modern Aspects of Computing, Devices and Communication Engineering*, Chapman and Hall/CRC, Routledge, Taylor & Francis Group. He has organized and participated in many national and international conferences, seminars, workshops and webinars. Dr. Bhattacharya has been active in delivering invited talks and has also been a part of many national and international conferences as coordinator, session chair, technical committee member etc. Presently, he is associated with Mallabhum Institute of Technology, Bishnupur, India, as an assistant professor in Electronics and Communication Engineering Department. Dr. Bhattacharya has been appointed as a guest editor of *SN Applied Sciences*, a multi-disciplinary, peer-reviewed journal of Springer Nature. He has also been inducted into the editorial board of *Circuits and Systems Journal* by Scientific Research Publishing (SCIRP).

Dr. Bappadittya Roy

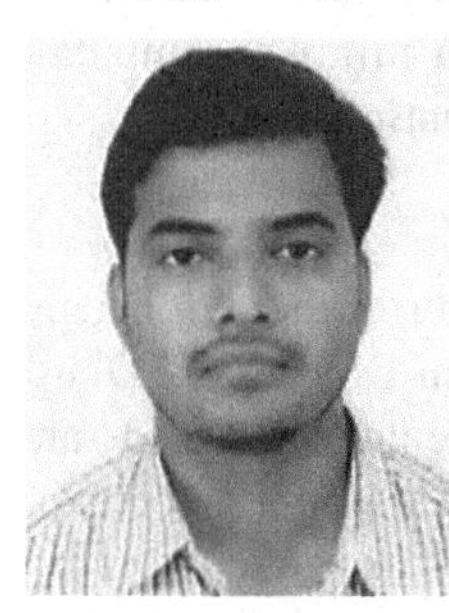

Bappadittya Roy obtained his Ph.D. in electronics and communication engineering from the National Institute of Technology, Durgapur, India. He is presently associated with VIT-AP University, Amaravati, India, as a senior assistant professor in the School of Electronics Engineering. He is a member of Institute of Electrical and Electronics Engineers (IEEE). He has received many national and international travel grants and has travelled abroad for seminars, conferences and workshops. He has published several articles in reputed journals and conferences. His research areas are microstrip antennas, fractal antennas and mobile communication. He is the general co-chair of the AISP 22 IEEE conference. He is also a reviewer of many national and international journal submissions.

Dr. Samarendra Nath Sur

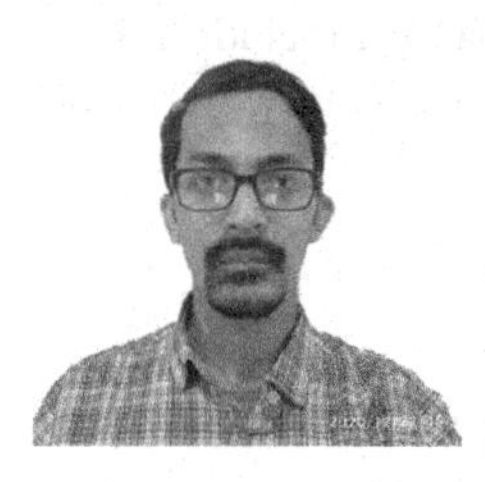

Samarendra Nath Sur was born in Hooghly, West Bengal, India, in 1984. He received B.Sc degree in Physics (Hons.) from the University of Burdwan in 2007. He received M.Sc degree in Electronics Science from Jadavpur University in 2007 and M.Tech degree in Digital Electronics and Advanced Communication from Sikkim Manipal University in 2012 and Ph.D degree in MIMO signal processing from National Institute of Technology (NIT), Durgapur. Since 2008, he has been associated with the Sikkim Manipal Institute of Technology, India, where he is currently an assistant professor in the Department of Electronics & Communication Engineering. His current research interests include Broadband Wireless Communication (MIMO and Spread Spectrum Technology), Advanced Digital Signal Processing, and Remote Sensing, Radar Image/Signal Processing (Soft Computing).

He is a Member of the Institute of Electrical and Electronics Engineers (IEEE), IEEE-IoT, IEEE Signal Processing Society, Institution of Engineers (India) (IEI) and International Association of Engineers (IAENG). He has published more than 55 SCI/Scopus indexed international journal and conference papers. He is the recipient of the University Medal and Dr. S.C. Mukherjee Memorial Gold Centered Silver Medal from Jadavpur University in 2007. He is also a regular reviewer of repute journals, namely IEEE, Springer, Elsevier, Taylor and Francis, IET, Wiley etc. He is currently editing several books with Springer Nature, Elsevier, and Routledge & CRC Press. He is also serving as Guest editor for topical collection/special issues of the journal like Springer Nature and Hindawi.

Dr. Saurav Mallik

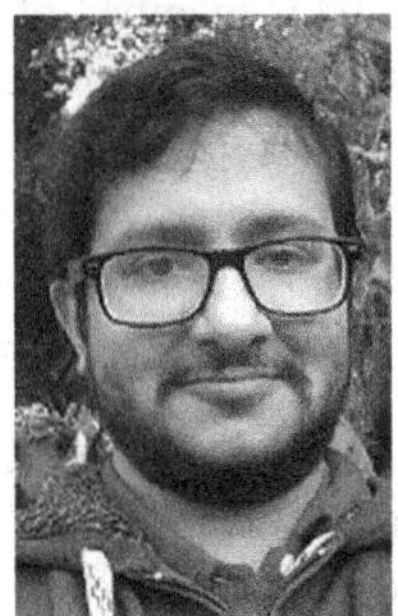

Saurav Mallik is currently working as a postdoctoral fellow at Harvard T.H. Chan School of Public Health, Boston, Massachusetts. He has previously worked at the University of Texas Health Science Center, Houston, Texas, and the University of Miami Miller School of Medicine, Miami, Florida, as a postdoctoral fellow. He obtained his Ph.D. from Jadavpur University, Kolkata, India, while his Ph.D. works was carried out at Machine Intelligence Unit, Indian Statistical Institute, Kolkata, India, as a junior research fellow and visiting scientist. He received the Award of Research Associateship from the Council of Scientific and Industrial Research (CSIR), Govt. of India. He was also the recipient of the "Emerging Researcher In Bioinformatics" award from Bioclues and BIRD Award Steering Committee, India (http://bioclues.org/). He received Travel Grant Award for International Conference on Intelligent Biology and Medicine (ICIBM) in Los Angeles, California. Dr. Mallik has more than 60 research papers in different peer-reviewed international journals having high impact factors, conferences and book chapters. Currently, he is working as an active member of the Institute of Electrical and Electronics Engineers (IEEE), USA, and American Association for Cancer Research (AACR), USA, and a life-member of a well-known non-profit organization "Bioinformatics CLUb for Experimenting Scientists" (BIOCLUES), India (http://bioclues.org/). His research interests include data mining, computational biology, bioinformatics, machine learning/deep learning and cloud computing.

Dr. Subhasis Dasgupta

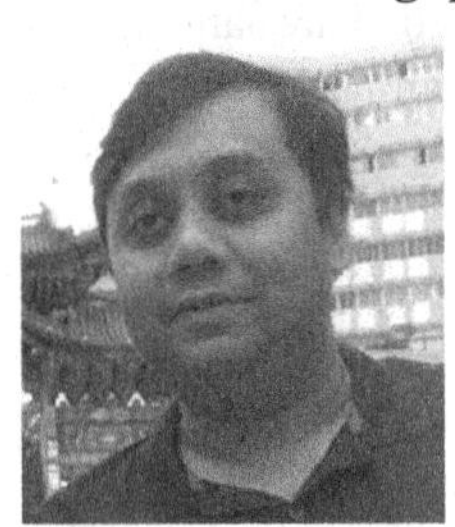

Subhasis Dasgupta is a data and computational researcher in the San Diego Supercomputer Center at the University of California San Diego (UCSD) as well as a lecturer in the UCSD Rady School of Management. He holds an additional appointment as an assistant scientist at UCSD. Dasgupta was previously a researcher at the Indian Statistical Institute as well as a systems engineer, director and founder of Kaavo India and its first US employee. Kaavo was ranked as a top-25 cloud vendor by *InformationWeek* in 2008–2009. Earlier, he worked for a Canadian startup company, DataInfoCom Inc., as a software engineer that served many Fortune-500 companies, including Dell and Microsoft. His primary research interests include database, mixed model data, access control, machine learning applications on large data and ontology engineering.

Contributors

K.R. Gokul Anand (Dr. Mahalingam College of Engineering and Technology, Pollachi, Tamilnadu, India)

Aurobinda Bag (Department of Electrical and Electronics Engineering, Madanapalle Institute of Technology and Science, Angallu, Madanapalle, India)

Debabrata Bej (Department of Electronics and Communication Engineering, National Institute of Technology Durgapur, West Bengal, India)

K. Bhaskar (Rajalakshmi Engineering College, Chennai, Tamil Nadu, India)

Ankan Bhattacharya (Department of Electronics and Communication Engineering, Mallabhum Institute of Technology, Bishnupur, West Bengal, India)

Anup Kumar Bhattacharjee (Department of Electronics and Communication Engineering, National Institute of Technology Durgapur, West Bengal, India)

Ayona Chakraborty (Electronics and Telecommunications Engineering Department, Jadavpur University, Kolkata, West Bengal, India)

Samik Chakraborty (Electronics and Communication Engineering Department, Dream Institute of Technology, Kolkata, West Bengal, India)

Ujjal Chakraborty (Department of Electronics and Communication Engineering, National Institute of Technology Silchar, Assam, India)

Soham Chattopadhyay (Department of Electrical Engineering, Jadavpur University, Kolkata, West Bengal, India)

Debika Das (Department of Electronics and Communication Engineering, National Institute of Technology Silchar, Assam, India)

Jaya Das (Department of Computer Science and Engineering, Maulana Abul Kalam Azad University of Technology, Kolkata, West Bengal, India)

Sima Das (Department of Computer Science and Engineering, Maulana Abul Kalam Azad University of Technology, Kolkata, West Bengal, India)

Arnab De (Department of Electronics and Communication Engineering, K. K. Group of Institutions, Dhanbad, Jharkhand, India)

S. Geetha (Dr. M.G.R. Educational and Research Institute, Chennai, Tamil Nadu, India)

Debarati Ghosh (Department of Electronics and Communication Engineering, National Institute of Technology Silchar, Assam, India)

Raghunath Ghosh (Department of Information Technology, Jadavpur University, Kolkata, West Bengal, India)

Sayanti Ghosh (Department of Electronics and Communication Engineering, National Institute of Technology Durgapur, West Bengal, India)

H. Sathiya Girija (Dr. Mahalingam College of Engineering and Technology, Pollachi, Tamilnadu, India)

K. Gomathi (Dr. M.G.R. Educational and Research Institute, Chennai, Tamil Nadu, India)

M. R. Harika (Department of Electrical and Electronics Engineering, Madanapalle Institute of Technology and Science, Madanapalle, Andhra Pradesh, India)

Ann Roseela Jayaprakash (Dr. M.G.R. Educational and Research Institute, Chennai, Tamil Nadu, India)

N. Kanimozhi (A.V.C. College of Engineering, Mayiladuthurai, Tamilnadu, India)

S. Kavitha (Dr. Mahalingam College of Engineering and Technology, Pollachi, Tamil Nadu, India)

Omer Koksal (Yasamkent Mah. Cankaya, ASELSAN Research Center, Ankara, Turkey)

B. Arun Kumar (Department of Electrical and Electronics Engineering, Madanapalle Institute of Technology and Science, Madanapalle, Andhra Pradesh, India)

Kalluri Vinay Kumar (Department of Electrical and Electronics Engineering, Madanapalle Institute of Technology and Science, Madanapalle, Andhra Pradesh, India)

Sumit Kundu (Department of Electronics and Communication Engineering, National Institute of Technology Durgapur, West Bengal, India)

Soufian Lakrit (Applied Mathematics and Information Systems Laboratory, EST of Nador, Mohammed First University Oujda, Nador, Morocco)

Somayya Madakam (Ben Gurion University of the Negev, Beer Sheva (ISRAEL), Sami Shamoon College of Engineering, Ashdod, Israel)

Ashis Kumar Mal (Department of Electronics and Communication Engineering, National Institute of Technology Durgapur, West Bengal, India)

Kaushik Mazumdar (Department of Electronics and Communication Engineering, IIT Dhanbad, Jharkhand, India)

Vinaytosh Mishra (QT and OM Area, FORE School of Management, New Delhi, India)

Subrata Modak (Department of Computer Science and Engineering, Maryland Institute of Technology and Management, Galudih, Jharkhand, India)

T. Nalini (Dr. M.G.R. Educational and Research Institute, Chennai, Tamil Nadu, India)

Arnab Nandi (Department of Electronics and Communication Engineering, National Institute of Technology Silchar, Assam, India)

Souvik Pal (Department of Computer Science and Engineering, Sister Nivedita University, Kolkata, West Bengal, India)

Devendra Pandey (Central Institute for Subtropical Horticulture, Lucknow, Uttar Pradesh, India)

Himanshu Pandey (Dr. Y.S. Parmar University of Horticulture and Forestry, Nauni, Himachal Pradesh, India)

Parth Sarathi Panigrahy (Department of Electrical and Electronics Engineering, Madanapalle Institute of Technology and Science, Madanapalle, Andhra Pradesh, India)

Bibhuti Bhushan Pati (Department of Electrical Engineering, Veer Surendra Sai University of Technology, Burla, Odisha, India)

T. Poornima (Amrita Vishwa Vidyapeetham, Coimbatore, Tamil Nadu, India)

B. Sai Reddy (Department of Electrical and Electronics Engineering, Madanapalle Institute of Technology and Science, Madanapalle, Andhra Pradesh, India)

Arijit Bardhan Roy (Department of Electrical and Electronics Engineering, Madanapalle Institute of Technology and Science, Madanapalle, Chittoor, Andhra Pradesh, India)

Bappadittya Roy (School of Electronics Engineering, VIT-AP University, Amaravati, Andhra Pradesh, India)

Sanjay Dhar Roy (Department of Electronics and Communication Engineering, National Institute of Technology Durgapur, West Bengal, India)

Moumita Saha (Department of Botany, Shri Gnanambica Degree College, Madanapalle, Andhra Pradesh, India)

L.R. Sassykova (Al-Farabi Kazakh National University, Almaty, Kazakhstan)

S. Sendilvelan (Dr. M.G.R. Educational and Research Institute, Chennai, Tamil Nadu, India)

Almamun Sheikh (Control and Instrumentation Section, Durgapur Projects Ltd., Durgapur, West Bengal, India)

Raed M. Shubair (Department of Electrical and Computer Engineering, New York University (NYU) Abu Dhabi, Abu Dhabi, United Arab Emirates)

Devendra Singh (Motilal Nehru National Institute of Technology Allahabad, Uttar Pradesh, India)

Pawan Kumar Singh (Department of Information Technology, Jadavpur University, Kolkata, West Bengal, India)

Virendra Singh (Maulana Azad Medical College, New Delhi, India)

K.M. Vijaylaxmi (Department of Electronics and Communication Engineering, NIT Durgapur, West Bengal, India)

Dinesh Yadav (Department of Electronics and Communication Engineering, Manipal University Jaipur, Rajasthan, India)

1 The Role of IoT in Healthcare Services

An Extensive Review

Devendra Singh, Himanshu Pandey, Virendra Singh, and Devendra Pandey

CONTENTS

1.1 INTRODUCTION

The increasing percentage of elderly residents worldwide has brought about numerous emerging challenges and problems in medical service, which needs a long-term assurance of human and medical resources [1]. In the mid 20th century, a comparatively new topic, medical rehabilitation, was introduced into the healthcare sector. Later, this new subject of medical rehabilitation was incorporated as a new therapy branch that focused on curing or alleviating mental as well as physical dysfunctions by re-constructing or treating disabilities. Medical rehabilitation (MR) has been

DOI: 10.1201/9781003217398-1

considered an effective as well as an efficient way to improve the mental and physical functions of various types of sufferers. On the other hand, the promotion of medical rehabilitation applications on a broader scale faces several hindrances. First of all, most rehabilitation treatments require intensive and long-term treatment. Second, they require an additional assistive facility to arrange easy or smooth accessibility of rehabilitation facility for patients. And finally, because of the rapidly increasing older population in the society, the availability of rehabilitation services is becoming comparatively scarcer. On the other hand, technologies like Internet of Things (IoT) can be a promising system that can be adopted to intelligentize the health service systems to deal with the aforesaid problems. In recent times, utilizing the technologies such as IoT for rehabilitation purposes has become highly popular following the introduction of several new concepts like Smart City and Smarter Earth [2]. IBM in the year 2008 proposed the concept of "Smarter Earth/Planet" with the initial aim of dealing with the requirements of real-time detecting, effective exchange of data, better productivity, decreased energy consumption and increased company efficiency. By following the above concept, a similar idea of Smart City was introduced later. Internet of things permits universal connectivity, wherein various cities' resources and public facilities are flawlessly networked. Thus, universal connections can be established between human beings or things, or both. Radio frequency identification (RFID) tags, PDAs, and sensors were made pervasive in IoT to obtain real-time information and to support different activities in decision-making [3].

Because of the smarter insight from Internet of Things, different smart cities can improve their performance of business infrastructure as well as various public services in such a way that real-time information can be easily collected and effectively analyzed, emergent and quick actions can be recognized and responded to timely and quickly, and cities' resources can be controlled and managed properly. In the case of medical services, like medical rehabilitation (MR), an Internet of Things (IoT) based technique makes it very much possible to offer one-stop services conveniently to even inhabitants of remote localities. On the other hand, in on-site conventional rehabilitation, medical services at local hospitals, as well as each and every resource related to rehabilitation, were shared with the people via a smart rehabilitation program so that convenient, smooth, and flexible treatment can be provided to the patients [4]. Thus, the maximum use of different rehabilitation resources can be availed, and it was expected that the Internet of Things-based smart technology would become an irreplaceable and very crucial system in the current medical systems. In recent times, various improvements were made in general healthcare, security and interoperability, healthcare control, and monitoring and inspecting drug interaction [5]. These abovementioned achievements of the internet of the things-based medical system have demonstrated its effectiveness, accuracy, and promising future. In spite of the ongoing success, technical problems and ambiguity will still be there with regard to the scientific establishment, quickness, and the management of big raw data and its analysis. With the aim of exploring the IoT abilities in healthcare services, many organizations, as well as researchers, are keen to develop and expand the Internet of Things-based systems for medical uses [4]. Some applications of IoT in healthcare include real-time reporting and monitoring of the patients, quick interactions with patients in remote areas by using a mobile app, easy collection of data for researchers etc. This chapter provides a detailed description of the advancement and history of IoT-based medical systems. And it also provides systematic information regarding the smart devices and technologies in IoT.

1.2 THE ORIGIN AND DEVELOPMENT OF IOT IN HEALTHCARE

Ashton and Brock were the ones who first proposed the term "IoT" (Internet of Things) and who created and started the Auto-Identification (AutoID) Center at MIT. The term "auto-identification" may denote any kind of identification (ID) system for numerous applications, like reduction in errors, efficiency enhancement, and automation. Later, in the year 2003, the AutoID Center launched the relevant electronic product code (EPC) network at its executive meeting [6]. Using this technology, movement of objects or people from one location to another location can be traced. The electronic product code network enables humans to visualize the promising future of the Internet of Things model as a universal mainstream marketable means, where microchips are networked and form the Internet of Things [7].

The development of RIFD technology clearly specifies that the IoT will successfully come out from the research laboratory and will lead the new information technology (IT) era in both industry and academy. In 2002, a report published by National Science Foundation (NSF) on convergent machinery was concentrated on the amalgamation of nanotechnology with communication and information technology to vividly improve countries' productivity as well as individuals' life quality [6]. The first report of ITU in 2005 suggests combining IoT with technologies in sensors, wireless networks, nanotechnologies, object identifications, and embedded systems to connect different objects worldwide, so that the objects can be sensed, controlled, and tagged over the internet [8].

Internet of Things commonly contains a set of systems to assist the interaction and communication between a wide variety of connected appliances and devices. IoT-supported firm systems were successfully established for numerous applications like medical services, public transportations services, as well as the environment and industrial services [8]. Interestingly, a huge interest exists in the case of developing nations as well; e.g., in the year 2009, IoT National Study Center was established, and later a speech was delivered by the former premier of China in which the main focus was to encourage research and development (R&D) of Internet of Things (IoT). Since then, more than 90 cities in China have started designing their plans in the direction of developing smart cities in China, and multiple Chinese big firms, like China Telecom, China Mobile, and China Unicom, have started connecting their big business strictly with the execution of smart cities plans in China [6].

1.3 IoT IN HEALTHCARE

Recently these IoT-supported smart rehabilitation services were introduced in the healthcare sector to alleviate or reduce the problem of limited resources because of the increasing elderly population [9]. A medical system based on IoT will join each and every available resource as a network so that healthcare activities like diagnosing, remote surgeries, and monitoring over the internet can be performed with ease [4]. In the IoT-supported rehabilitation centres, the entire structure has been devoted to extending the medical services from the clinics and societies to families. Technology like Wireless Fidelity (Wi-Fi) is commonly and widely used for the process of integration and exchange of data with the control system; the interface is considered to be one of the network managers. It is a system that connects to all of the available medical resources in the community, such as hospitals, equipment, doctors, ambulance services, nurses, and rehabilitation centres for ill persons. And the server is equipped with a single central database. The proxy server agent is mainly responsible for the analysis of data, consolidation, the identification of critical events, as well as the development of rehabilitation objectives. All of this is connected to the internet, supported as part of the programme, and based on RFID technology [10]. An automatically selected tray dispenser has been designed for rehabilitation, with solutions based on a set of definite requirements of each individual patient. The paradigm of the Internet of Things mainly comprises three parts, the first one is Master, the second one is Server, and the third part is Things. The first part, i.e., Master, consists of patients, doctors, and nurses who will have their own special permissions to access the authorized system with the help of the end-user devices like tablets, personal computers, or smartphones. The second part, Server, represents the central or main part of the complete medical system. It is also responsible for creating a receipt and prescription, analyzing data, managing database and knowledge base, and building subsystems. And the third and last part, Things, is only valid for physical items (including those of patients and person resources) which are connected by a WAN, SMS, or multimedia technology [10]. The proposed structure's effectiveness has been confirmed by a variety of innovative applications of exoskeletons [10, 11].

1.4 ENABLING IDENTIFICATION TECHNOLOGY OF IoT

Currently, the systems (including software as well as hardware) for sensing, decision-making activities, and communication have become gradually more affordable and versatile. Further, to promote the inventions of human beings in many IoT-based applications, supporting technologies are crucial. An IoT network can be composed of many nodes and all nodes are able to collect information. Each authorized node is able to access information regardless of where it is positioned. In order to attain this aim, you will need to effectively trace and recognize the websites [12]. The identification is intended to include a unique identifier (UID) of the object so that the exchange of information via this node will be clear and uninterrupted. In the system, every resource, like a rehabilitation facility, hospital, physician, or registered nurse, is directly linked with the digital ID. Accordingly, the association amongst the different subjects can be readily defined in the digital domain, which allows acquiring things in the online system to be found quickly without any errors. Numerous standards for the identification were already recommended [10, 12]. In recent times, a rising necessity for IoT is noticed in order to provide many identifiers for a particular subject and also accommodate the variations of identifiers. However, properly working smart devices of an individual are generally supported by actuators and sensors, which will be separately addressed. Throughout the product lifecycle, several components in a single device with unique identifiers can be changed [10, 12].

Thus, there is an urgent requirement in order to accommodate the deviations of identities in order to sustain the integrity of the individual's smartphones even when it is configured again. A record of configuration changes is important for keeping devices working, checking failures, and tracking items. Further, the IoT deployment will require the latest technologies firstly in order to trace the subjects on the basis of a universal ID scheme, secondly to manage the identities carefully by using the advanced and recent systems of encryption/encoding, repository management, and authentication, and thirdly to provide universal directory search and Internet of Things facilities under different UID schemes [12].

1.5 LOCATION AND COMMUNICATION TECHNOLOGIES

In any IoT-supported medical subsystem, communication technologies are the major components that support the infrastructure networking and are divided into short- (near-) and long- (far-) distance technology. But, due to the fact that the long- (far-) distance technology is mostly associated with conventional means of communication such as the internet and smartphones, this chapter will focus only on the short-range technologies. While in maximum circumstances, short (near) distance type of communication depends upon the wireless technology, such as Wi-Fi, Bluetooth, UWB, RFID, IrDA, ZigBee.

1.5.1 Location Technologies

The RTLS location system is used to keep track of and to determine the exact location of the moving thing. In medical applications, this RTLS system is used to securely monitor the process of patient treatment and assist with the configuration of the system of healthcare based on the distribution of the present resources. On the other side, the GPS is among the most crucial RTLS systems, which is a satellite-supported navigation system that is generally used to determine the location of subjects in all-weather situations, as much as the endless lines of sight that can be obtained from four or more than four satellites. For the health care industry, the satellite positioning system could be used for detecting the location of the registered doctors, patients, ambulances, and nurses. It is also worth noting that accessibility to a few systems, such as GPS and the Chinese BDS (Beidou System) in an enclosed area is usually poor due to their design that hinders the transmission of the signals from the satellite.

Meanwhile, the GPS is not sufficient to create an effective operational system of health care; thus, to overcome this problem, and to improve the precision and accuracy of the services, GPS along with the LPSs (Local Positioning Systems) is used. The record is determined by the position of an object on the basis of measurements of radio frequency signals between the subjects and a list of previously used consumers [11]. The aforesaid near-field communication systems are necessary for implementing the local positioning systems, e.g., a UWB radio, which has a very fine resolution, allows the receiver to accurately estimate the time of arrival [11]. Thus, UWB can be a perfect technology for precise positioning on the basis of radio signals. Scientists also calculated that the location of the UWB is based on the difference in the time of arrival (TDOA). On the basis of the measured time-of-arrival (ToA), an internal GPS system can be implemented [13]. Further, for implementing an internal positioning system, high-bandwidth communication in combination with the BDS or GPS offers a lot of options for the development of smart networks.

1.5.2 Short- (Near-) Distance Communication Technologies

All of these aforesaid technologies will help for the transmission of information over a short (near) distance. Because of the dissimilarity between the safety standard and the operating radio frequency, these technologies' characteristics will also differ with respect to the operating distance, transmission speeds, maintenance and installation costs, energy consumption, and allowed number of nodes. Bluetooth wireless communication technology was originally developed by the Ericsson Company as a substitute for a fixed data transfer (wired RS-232) in the year 1994. One of the biggest benefits of the Bluetooth technology is its clinical, environmental applications due to its low-rays that are less injurious to humans. In the present medical system, passive tags of RFID are used for tracking medical assets or for obtaining information concerning the condition of the patient. Wireless Fidelity (Wi-Fi) is among the most widespread methods of operating over short distances, thanks to the implementation of a local area network (LAN). And according to the Wi-Fi Alliance, if a wireless LAN product is according to the IEEE 802.11 standards, then it can be in the Wi-Fi category. At the moment, a local area network based on Wi-Fi is available in maximum hospitals. Infrared Data Association (IrDA) development project was set up by a group of 50 most prominent firms in the year 1993. Infrared Data Association (IrDA) is generally used to control remote devices.

Further, if the transmission of the information shall be protected physically, and line of sight (LOS) and a low BER can be guaranteed, then optical wireless communication may be a good decision. However, the low data transfer rate is still the main IrDA weakness. UWB was first proposed by Scholz and colleagues [14].

The main benefits of UWB are its very low power consumption and high bandwidth. High-speed transfer of data UWB can facilitate direct wireless medical monitoring without a PC. ZigBee-supported communication is in compliance with the IEEE 802.15 norms. It provides a safe communication and low data rate, as well as a long battery life [11, 13]. It also plays an analogous role to RFID in gathering health data for the Internet of Things-supported medical applications. In addition, the transmission of data using visible light, like LEDs, can be thought of as a means of communication. However, it is still in the development phase.

1.6 SENSOR TECHNOLOGY

The sensor technology is of paramount importance to obtaining many of the patient's physiological parameters so that the registered physician can correctly diagnose the disease and prescribe treatment. In addition, the new generation of sensor technology directly allows constant acquisition of information from the patients, contributing to the improvement in the treatment results and reducing the cost of health care. This section of the chapter discusses a number of examples of how to gather the data of the devices in an IoT-supported medical system, as shown in Figure 1.1.

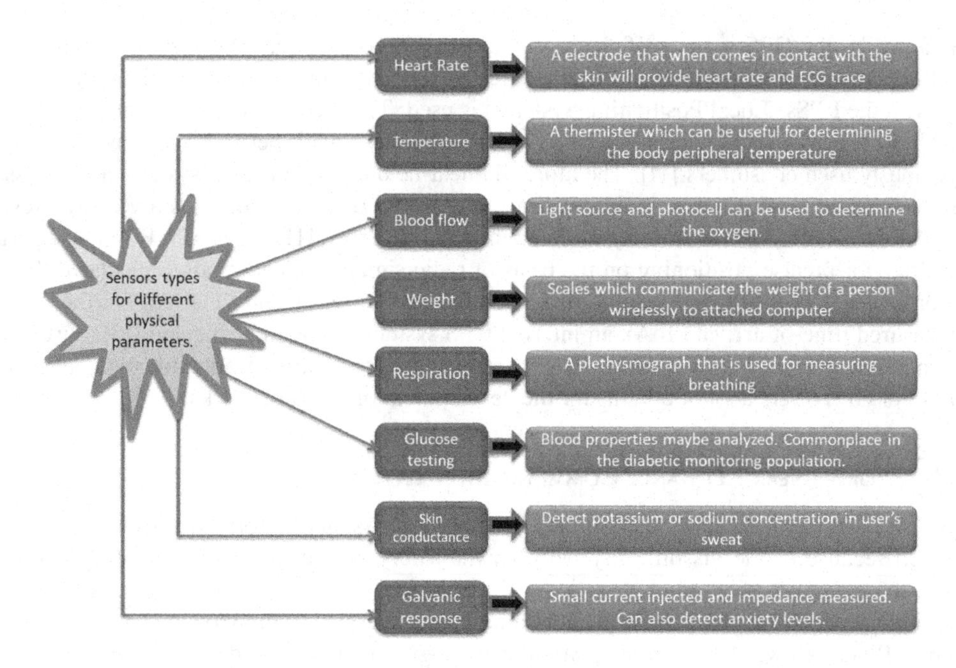

FIGURE 1.1 A systematic presentation showing various sensors types for distant physical indices.

In the year 1970, the pulse oximeter was invented and has grown to become one of the most commonly and widely used diagnostic tools [4]. The two very important health indicators, SpO_2 (blood oxygen saturation) and HR (heart rate), can be obtained reliably by using a pulse oximeter. By default, the digital signal processing (DSP) techniques will be used in order to calculate the pulse rate and oxygen saturation from the light transmission waveform. The motion sensor is a complex device consisting of many different sensors, e.g., devices like gyroscopes and accelerometers are frequently used for motion analysis [15]. A three-axis accelerometer can detect the direction and movement of each body segment, and a gyroscope is used to measure angular velocity.

And interestingly, the combination of these two can accurately determine the dynamic pose of the human limb. EMG electrodes collect statistical data related to the action potential (AP) generated by the excited muscles in the body. The EMG signal can be used on a large scale for the assessment of muscle fatigue, to predict muscular contraction, and also to identify the motion patterns in rehabilitation. Furthermore, all the data collected on the patient's health status can be converted into a digital format and immediately shared online. The use of wireless sensors has significantly simplified the data collection process and made it possible for the ill person to wear the portable sensors for extended time periods and without massive data [4, 8].

1.7 SERVICE-ORIENTED ARCHITECTURE

The IoT-dependent healthcare structure involves different nodes, which might be up to thousands or millions. Nowadays, the networking system in the computer application area should be able to exchange and make use of information; for that purpose, the SOA provides an excellent alternative and potential source [16, 17]. The SOA system is based on the proper separate functioning of individual devices that are delineated by the proposed set of interfaces. The linking system among different devices can be reorganized rapidly to execute the recent task for different services on requirement. SOA is very important and useful as it is based on a modular design, integration of various diverse applications, interoperable systems, and software reutilization. The service-oriented architecture includes an interoperation function that is based on XML, SOAP, WSDL, and UDDI [16].

Consequently, SOA has the advantage over other platforms in terms of interoperability and its functionality in various programming languages. Many scientists across the globe are involved in the exploration of the SOA application system in relation to e-Healthcare services. For example, various studies have suggested the use of SOA to design, carry out, and manage the facilities in a distributed medical health-related system. These studies have also demonstrated the use of E-Health Monitoring System (EHMS), where SOA provides a platform to organize, identify, incorporate, execute, control, and evoke e-health services. Later the important features and constituents of services-oriented architecture supported by the system are also described. In particular, the difficulties in executing service-oriented architecture at a massive scale in the distribution of the health care sector were investigated from the point of view of cost-effectiveness and riskiness [16].

1.8 HEALTHCARE SYSTEMS AND DEVICES

Currently, different types of IoT-supported medical equipment and systems have become widely available in the market. These devices proved useful in examining patients, retaining close contact with doctors, accelerating the process of recovery etc.

1.9 SMART HEALTHCARE SYSTEM

An advanced health support structure basically involves the use of sophisticated sensors, a distant server, and a highly developed networking system. It has the ability to provide multi-dimensional surveillance and essential treatment proposals. It is a prerequisite to have an advanced health support system based on necessity within a community or which can even be utilized throughout the world. Several advanced systems with wider scopes and applications are described in this book chapter. Body Media scientists started to carry out investigations on wearable devices in 1998. From that point, Body Media started creating wearable monitoring devices. The company is involved in the development of a human physiological database and making it publicly available along with the data modelling techniques. The modelling approach designed by Body Media has been effectively utilized in much further clinical research. The result obtained was evident to prove excellent dependency and authenticity. The average absolute percentage disparity of calories intake by an individual each day was less than 10 per cent. Google Health provides individual health records. It was first initiated in the year 2008. This platform was designed to provide assistance to Google users for voluntarily sharing their health records with health support system service providers. As soon as the process of data feeding is done, Google Health provides the individual with the entire set of complete health records, health-related diseases, and help in determining reaction among the allergies and drugs. To expand its area, Google Health collaborated with different corporations that provide telehealthcare services and helped their customers empower and systematize their health reports and data online. The incorporation of interdisciplinary approaches such as a hospital-based establishment system (ES) has been suggested, and exceptional advances in this area have been achieved [18]. Meanwhile, the experimentation related to major technology has been highlighted, which is characterized by the nurse-administered decision approach [6], potential management of problems, and mechanical processing outcome, etc., which all have laid a stable basis for the progress of good healthcare services [16].

1.10 ADVANCED MEDICAL EQUIPMENT

Advanced healthcare equipment or devices usually incorporate sensor-based techniques supported by IoT that facilitates medical care services provided to patients. Few such examples of these types of systems include Withings equipment and Nike+ FuelBand.

1.10.1 Withings Equipment

This equipment is a cordless frame provided with a Wi-Fi connection. It is generally utilized to measure fat percentage, the content of muscle mass, and the index of a user's body mass. The gathered information can be directly transferred to the company's website with the help of a Wi-Fi facility. It is also accessible with the help of Health 2.0 service packages like Google Health. As a result of its excellent execution, it has gained importance in the field of the tech press. The corporations also supply blood pressure measuring instruments. Correspondingly to the body scale, it can function by connecting it with an iPhone, Ipad, or iPod Touch, and the data is recorded through transmission with the help of Wi-Fi [16].

1.10.2 Other Usable Devices

Video examination of unhealthy persons is also necessary to impart better medical facilities to patients. Internet protocol (IP) camera has been utilized at a wider scale for monitoring purposes in various fields related to the health care sector. An IP camera generally transmits and acquires information with the help of a networking system. Therefore, it has the capability to examine unhealthy persons in real time based on video conferencing between doctors and patients whenever required [4]. Other movable gadgets, such as smartwatches, phones, and tablets, provide support for communication purposes in the medical sector with the help of internet services.

1.11 APPLICATION OF METHODOLOGIES AND STRATEGIES

Efficient approaches and techniques play a pivotal role in the Internet of Things-based medical sector for enhancing the ability and efficiency of the systems. The fundamental problems such as the immediate feedback capability and vulnerability to avoid risks in relation to intelligence that is strongly associated with the restoration of quality data. Risk-preventing intelligence is important because a minute error may be responsible for a severely deleterious effect on the human health system. Immediate response capability relates to the system's ability to deal with emergency health care services. Furthermore, competent system services deal with proper restoration of a system using big data analysis and demand for a well-established structured process, and a systematic and smart information management system. Therefore, fundamental challenges include resource allocation, information management, big data analysis, and advanced technology for developing and creating a telehealth care service and tele-restoration subsystem. The important rehabilitation subsystem is based on medical services. At the time of rehabilitation, the maximum of data available is based on initial findings that may be useful for future investigation. Derived from the medical data analyzed, the information generated is gathered continuously. The big data analysis and its understanding provide the basis for medical and health care treatment, as shown in Figure 1.2.

The various aspects related to the health care sector are discussed under different subheadings.

1.11.1 Resource Management

Management of resources involves the process related to tracking, detection, and verification. For medical care services, data allocation is important for a properly operating system and is highly useful, as it provides the basis for later treatment, rehabilitation, and identification.

1.11.2 Tracking

It is the process that provides solutions for the problem related to lack of "visibility" on the specific areas, the state of victim, physicians, medical tools and apparatus, or other beneficial facilities because the visualization issue paves the way for ambiguity in current healthcare services. If the

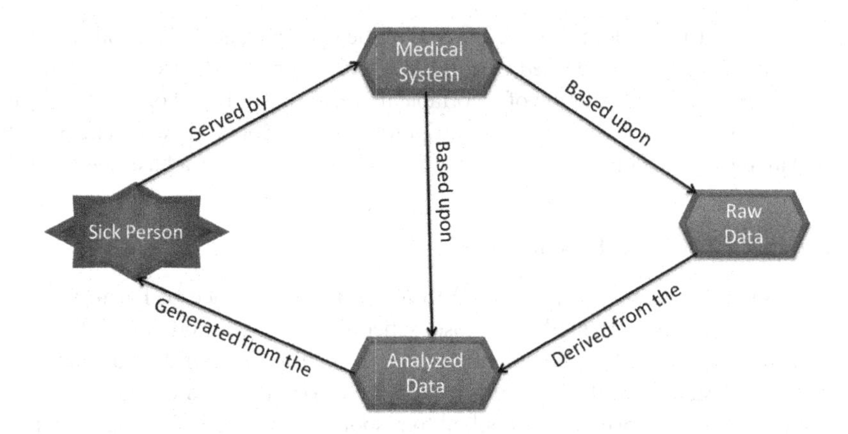

FIGURE 1.2 The diagrammatic representation of the relations between the crucial methodologies in the Internet of Things-based rehabilitation system.

state of medical equipment is not examined in real-time, its everyday functioning could be lost. Moreover, the disorganized movement of patients would lead to emergency health care services. In all situations, the major purpose of tracking services is to determine the locations of individuals or objects in real time. Later a real-time tracking network for a hospital's medical setting using Wi-Fi signals was also introduced. The network took the help of radio signalling from broadcasting points to trace the positions of the labelled assets. The resolving power of positioning was more than 1.5 m.

Furthermore, the precise records related to tracking data were accessible for future purposes. The ultra-badge positioning system [19] is an alternate system that is commonly applicable in different hospitals. It is a 3D label to locate the deceased person's position. If an unhealthy individual is in a particular zone where there is a chance that a patient can fall, the system instantly alarms the medical workers. Researchers have also structured the position technique with video inspection methodology and broadcasting multimedia information systems to enhance the medical services for elderly people. Marco et al. [20] devised a locating system that involved the application of ultrasound having a multiple-cell range for a medical purpose. Comparisons are mentioned in Table 1.1.

1.11.3 Sensing

These techniques are related to the patient and act as both empowering methodology and useful technology in IoT-based medical care services and systems. The equipment is produced to detect patients' wellbeing and to provide real-time data on their health [4]. The utility subject includes various telemedicine service systems, tracking systems, and health care alarming systems. Innovative

TABLE 1.1
A Comparison Between the Studies on Tracing Technology

Communication Technology	Purpose	Features
ZUPS	Monitoring and alarm for disabled and aged peoples	Economical, easy, and simple extension and calibration
Video surveillance and RFID	Supporting quick monitoring as well as analysis	Easy and simple-to-use
Wi-Fi	Tracking a crowded and busy healthcare atmosphere	Wireless network, generating and reporting the complete logs of assets status

researches have been carried out in this sector. One of the examples is MobiHealth which is known to be one of the initial systems that embed wearable devices in portable devices like smartphones and smartwatches. Alarm Net is an example of a portable medical sensor based on a networking system. It imparts both physiological observation and position tracking. Mobile ECG is a device applied for measuring and analysing ECG for patients having smartphones acting as a base station [16].

1.11.4 Authentication and Identification

Reorganization and identification are essential to minimize the chance of harmful errors to diseased persons, like inappropriate medicine, dose, schedule of drug, or process. For nursing attendants, authentication is generally applied to allow the availability of restricted data and to increase employee morale by listening to the sufferer's privacy concerns. For medical care sources, identification and authentication are principally applied to respond to the needs for safety approaches and prevent the loss of important equipment and devices.

1.11.5 Data Management

The medical care sector is now empowered by advanced information, so the acquirement, development, collection, and reutilization of medical care knowledge in the advanced system are important to improve efficiency. Amongst the different types of information management systems, an ontology may provide encouraging results that allow comfortable exchange and reutilization of current information [21]. This idea has excellent benefit in equipping well-organized domain information of rehabilitation engineering so that mining of data from the different databases can be executed with distinct hierarchical relations without any uncertainty. Therefore, ontology assists the concurrent knowledge among medical personnel to discover suitable therapy and corresponding sources. Moreover, the utilization of the ontology facilitates information exchange in terms that knowledge with the equivalent structure substantially enhances the opportunity for information reprocesses.

Fan et al. [12] suggested two different types of ontologies: localized ontology and disease ontology. The disease ontology is useful for comparing points of view and serves to find out one or more comparable cases in the databank. One can advance with a similar medication approach employed for the previous cases to manage the recent case. The resource ontology validates health resources comprising both individual resources and substantial resources, for example, rehabilitation robots and CPM. It supports the medical system to select suitable resources rapidly based on the cure needed to be obtained by the disease ontology. So, when used in rehabilitation systems, ontology assists in performing two major objectives. Firstly, ontological information organization allows more systematic and precise reasoning. Secondly, ontology contributes well to organize a specific area of information on rehabilitation engineering, empowering easy information exchange and utilization. An extremely organized ontology determines the relationship among different expressions in the rehabilitation glossary, which are useful in diagnosing and characterizing the diseases.

1.11.6 Management of Big Information

The execution of IoT-supported medical care systems depends upon the huge data collected from medical centres, rehabilitation centres, hospitals, and asylums. The information gathered from these places is updated instantaneously, and the information transfer may occur altogether between hundreds of things. Theoretically, every available data should be kept in the database. Despite low storage cost, storage of large data requires a substantial amount of money, thus a costly affair. Hereby, extremely effective smart algorithms should be generated to eliminate redundant data. Big data analysis also provides an opportunity to mine the data and knowledge from the database. The information-based data mining system can be incorporated to help the doctors in the assignment of diseases. Though, it is very complicated for a computer to differentiate important data from a big dataset. Till now, efficient data mining approaches for medical care information devices are still missing due to the complex and specific medical centres related to hospitals. As an important part of IoT, Cloud Computing is becoming popular in terms of academic and industrial purposes [22]. It serves as an advanced platform for networking and sharing a pool of configurable computing sources. Different applications of Cloud Computing can be observed in different sectors. For example, two diverse types of advanced data mining systems can be effectively developed for vehicular information cloud services in the IoT-based environment [23]. Since it is important for medical care services to have open access to information at a specific time and ubiquitously, a number of researches have been performed in the medical care sector [16]. A source supported by data retrieval technology, namely UDA-Internet of Things, can be created to obtain and process Internet of Things-based information universally and has proven effective in a cloud and smartphone computing process, from which both healthcare workers and managers will be benefitted [24]. To cope with scattered and diverse data environments, an Internet of Things-based information storage structure incorporating a database management system can be developed for cloud computing technology [25]. The cloud computing technique specifies standard dimensions and matrix to aggregate service quality, and researches [22] have been performed to generate a standard model which will be utilized to depict, quantify, and correlate the quality of the benefactors, thus attaining a mutual agreement.

1.12 METHODS FOR BUILDING AND DESIGNING TELEREHABILITATION AND TELEHEALTH SUBSYSTEM

Telecare services mainly focus on providing the best health-associated services and suggestions remotely with the help of internet facilities [26], the scope of which is useful for the timely diagnosis of diseases and their cure. Telehealth care services can be carried out in four different modes: (1) store and forward telecare services where multimedia data, namely audio, video, and images, are gathered and saved at a particular place and then can be transferred from one position to another whenever required; (2) real-time telecare, in this model patients and healthcare workers, communicate with each other through telephonic service or via by video-conference; (3) remote patient inspection where individual produce the sensed and monitored information at one side, and the physician identify the cause and suggest the necessary medication at another side; and (4) remote training where profound care is delivered to suffers over the networking system, generally for those with an acute severe condition. Internet of Things can be widely applied to grant beneficial assistance to the aged or person suffering from severe diseases at homes or specific sites. Later, a prototype model for distant medical care services was also presented [27]. It has utilized the technology related to smartphones, sensors, Web services, and Internet Protocol video cam for data retrieval and interaction. Researchers also devised multi-modal system interfaces to provide tele-home medical care [28]. As supported by statistics from the WSD platform provided by the health department of the United Kingdom, telecare model service can decrease the unneeded refuse of medical sources substantially.

1.13 CHALLENGES/SHORTCOMINGS OF IOT APPLICABILITY IN HEALTHCARE

There are two major challenges; firstly, the bulk volume of data generated in healthcare is one of the toughest tasks to manage. The concept of utilizing IoT will surely increase the requirement for data stockpiling. The huge amount of information generated by IoT gadgets and devices may probably cause an unanticipated problem if the organizations are unprepared to handle it properly. Secondly, the outdated Infrastructure will hamper the healthcare industry/sectors.

1.14 CONCLUSION AND FUTURE DEVELOPMENT

It is concluded that the rapidly progressing knowledge and developing IoT techniques have paved the way for the greater possibility for emerging medical care information models. However, difficulties still exist in attaining safe and efficient telemedical care services. Some defined sectors for future progress are documented in following ways: (1) Self-education and self-development. Facing enormous data and a high level of difficulty, IoT itself cannot contribute to the rehabilitation care system or to creating medical sources. Proper and efficient treatments must be available depending upon major factors like immediate identification of the patient's disease and providing proper rehabilitation treatments on the basis of disease identification. Even with identical symptoms, the state of the sufferer varies from one to another. All the elements have to be considered in order to provide efficient medical treatment. A computer-based system that is merely supported by data acquired with the help of sensors helps to keep previous records of former cases, whereas self-learning technology can actively and intelligently identify the disease and help in providing proper treatments. Some self-learning algorithms, for example, Genetic Algorithm (GA), Ant-Colony Optimization (ACO), and Simulated Annealing (SA), can be utilized to investigate data and mining information.

Topology and ontology supported by advanced algorithms have shown their significance in the determination of optimum solutions for a huge-scale model. In the process of the creation of wearable equipment, the problem of how to accomplish unobtrusiveness still holds a huge obstruction because proper convenience is a major interest. The requirement for incorporation of different types of sensors into one system, like PATHS and LiveNet, opposes the problem of unobtrusiveness. Different researches carried out on multifunctional sensors with lighter substances like carbon fibre, or mainly fabric, may be very advantageous in the upcoming time. Another problem faced in sensor-based equipment is the power source, and the solution to this problem is to use rechargeable cells. Although regular recharging may be tedious generally for the aged, it may also lead to suspension of the service.

A large group of researchers have assisted in developing and standardizing IoT-based techniques like the AutoID Laboratory have been multiplied all across the globe. The regularization of the Internet of Things was chiefly affected by the inputs from the different machine-groups of the European Telecommunications Standards Institute (ETSI) and from some Internet Engineering Task Force (IETF) working communities. It is needed to incorporate all of the budding ideas as a general solution for the reference and normalization of future web services. Based on the results from the CERP-IoT model [11], future web services will be extensions of the present networking system, either in portable form or firmly fixed. The normalization will be helpful for future use of IoT-supported healthcare models. The essential requirement for utilizing an IoT-based model is utility and protection for individuals. For Internet of Things (IoT) based services, information gathering, data mining, and furnishing are all prerequisites based on Internet facility is necessary and easy to use. Therefore, a chance for improper data collection is always there. The privacy of the individual must be assured to avoid illegal diagnoses and tracking. From this point of view, the maximum level of autonomy and knowledge of the tools and studies related to the health care sector may lead to substantial objections related to privacy issues.

Furthermore, IoT-supported systems are significantly useful because of two factors: (1) most of the interaction occurs through wireless mode;, (2) generally, components of IoT are known for low power and low computing capacity. So they can barely be applied to complicated schemes. It can be observed that the data mining and storage of a large number of things in a medical care model generally leads to numerous safety issues. To avoid the unethical application of private data and allow their proper use, in-depth knowledge is required in the field of dynamic trust, safety, and privacy execution. With the concluding remark, we prognosticate that an acceptable advanced rehabilitation model will ultimately emerge.

ABBREVIATIONS

EPC Electronic Product Code
GPS Global Positioning Systems
ID Identification
IrDA Infrared Data Association
IT Information technology
IoT Internet of Things
LAN Local area network
LPS Local Positioning System
MR Medical rehabilitation
RFID Radio frequency identification
UID unique identifier
Wi-Fi Wireless Fidelity

REFERENCES

1. Paré, G., Moqadem, K., Pineau, G., and St-Hilaire, C., 2010. Clinical effects of home telemonitoring in the context of diabetes, asthma, heart failure and hypertension: A systematic review. *Journal of Medical Internet Research, 12*(2), e21.
2. Dohler, M., Ratti, C., Paraszczak, J., and Falconer, G., 2013. Smart cities. *IEEE Communications Magazine, 51*(6), 70–71.
3. Le Gall, F., Chevillard, S. V., Gluhak, A., and Xueli, Z., 2013. Benchmarking Internet of things deployments in smart cities. 2013 27th International Conference on Advanced Information Networking and Applications Workshops, pp. 1319–2132, doi: 10.1109/WAINA.2013.230.
4. Aghdam, Z. N., Rahmani, A. M., and Hosseinzadeh, M., 2021. The role of the Internet of things in healthcare: Future trends and challenges. *Computer Methods and Programs in Biomedicine, 199*, 105903.
5. Feki, M. A., Kawsar, F., Boussard, M., and Trappeniers, L., 2013. The Internet of Things: The next technological revolution. *Computer, 46*(2), 24–25.
6. Roco, M. C. and Bainbridge, W. S. *Converging Technologies for Improving Human Performance: Nanotechnology, Biotechnology, Information Technology and Cognitive Science.* 2002. National Stroke Foundation.
7. Weisman, R., 2004. The Internet of Things: Start-ups jump into next big thing: Tiny networked chips. *The Boston Globe.*
8. Kelly, J. T., Campbell, K. L., Gong, E., and Scuffham, P., 2020. The Internet of Things: Impact and implications for health care delivery. *Journal of Medical Internet Research, 22*(11), e20135.
9. Rohokale, V. M., Prasad, N. R., and Prasad, R., 2011. A cooperative Internet of Things (IoT) for rural healthcare monitoring and control. In *Proceedings of the 2nd International Conference on Wireless Communication, Vehicular Technology, Information Theory and Aerospace and Electronic Systems Technology (Wireless VITAE)*, IEEE Publications, pp. 1–6.
10. Yin, Y. H., and Chen, X., 2012. Bioelectrochemical control mechanism with variable-frequency regulation for skeletal muscle contraction - Biomechanics of skeletal muscle based on the working mechanism of myosin motors (II). *Science in China (Series E), 55*(8), 2115–2125.
11. Sadat, S., Fardis, M., Geran, F., Dadashzadeh, G., Hojjat, N., and Roshandel, M., 2006. A compact microstrip square-ring slot antenna for UWB applications. In *2006* IEEE Antennas and Propagation Society International Symposium, IEEE Publications, Institute of Electrical and Electronics Engineers, pp. 4629–4632.
12. Fan, Y. J., Yin, Y. H., Xu, D. L., Zeng, Y., and Wu, F., 2014. IoT-based smart rehabilitation system. *IEEE Transactions on Industrial Informatics, 10*(2), 1568–1577.
13. Young, D. P., Keller, C. M., Bliss, D. W., and K. W., 2003. Forsythe ultra-wideband (uwb) transmitter location using time difference of arrival (TDOA) techniques. In *Proceedings of the Conference Record of the Thirty-Seventh Asilomar Conference on Signals, Systems and Computers, 2*, IEEE Publications, pp. 1225–1229.

14. Win, M. Z., and Scholtz, R. A., 2000. Ultra-wide bandwidth time-hopping spread-spectrum impulse radio for wireless multiple-access communications. *IEEE Transactions on Communications*, *48*(4), 679–689.
15. Abdulqader, T., Saatchi, R., and Elphick, H., 2021. Respiration measurement in a simulated setting incorporating the Internet of Things. *Technologies*, *9*(2), 30.
16. Yin, Y., Zeng, Y., Chen, X., and Fan, Y., 2016. The Internet of Things in healthcare: An overview. *Journal of Industrial Information Integration*, *1*, 3–13.
17. Erl, T., 2005. *Service-Oriented Architecture: Concepts, Technology, and Design*. Pearson Education India.
18. Fradinho, J. M. D. S., 2014. Towards high performing hospital enterprise systems: an empirical and literature based design framework. *Enterprise Information Systems*, *8*(3), 355–390.
19. Hori, T., and Nishida, Y., 2005. Ultrasonic sensors for the elderly and caregivers in a nursing home. In *Proceedings of the* Seventh *International Conference on Enterprise Information Systems*, SciTePress, pp. 110–115.
20. Marco, A., Casas, R., Falco, J., Gracia, H., Artigas, J., and Roy, A., 2008. Location-based services for elderly and disabled people. *Computer Communications*, *31*(6), 1055–1066.
21. Chandrasekaran, B., Josephson, J. R., and Benjamins R. V., 1999. What are ontologies and why do we need them? *IEEE Intelligent Systems*, *14*(1), 20–26.
22. Zheng, X., Martin, P., Brohman, K., and Xu, D. L., 2014. CLOUDQUAL: A quality model for cloud services. *IEEE Transactions on Industrial Informatics*, *10*(2), 1527–1536.
23. He, W., Yan, G., and Xu, L., 2014. Developing vehicular data cloud services in the IoT environment. *IEEE Transactions on Industrial Informatics*, *10*(2), 1587–1595.
24. Xu, B., Xu, L. D., Cai, H., Xie, C., Hu, J., and Bu, F., 2014. Ubiquitous data accessing method in IoT-based information system for emergency medical services. *IEEE Transactions on Industrial Informatics*, *10*(2), 1578–1586.
25. Jiang, L., Xu, L. D., Cai, H., Jiang, Z., Bu, F., and Xu, B., 2014. An IoT oriented data storage framework in cloud computing platform. *IEEE Transactions on Industrial Informatics*, *10*(2), 1443–1451.
26. Nguyen, H. Q., Carrieri-Kohlman, V., Rankin, S. H., Slaughter, R., and Stulbarg, M. S., 2005. Is Internet-based support for dyspnea self-management in patients with chronic obstructive pulmonary disease possible? Results of a pilot study. *Heart Lung*, *34*, 51–72.
27. Leijdekkers, P., Gay, V., and Lawrence, E., 2007. Smart homecare system for health tele–monitoring. In *Proceedings of the* First *International Conference on the Digital Society*, IEEE, January, p. 3.
28. Lisettia, C., Nasoza, F., LeRougeb, C., Ozyera, O., and Alvarezc, K., 2003. Developing multimodal intelligent affective interfaces for tele-home health care. *International Journal of Human-Computer Studies*, *59*(1), 245–255.

2 Smart Healthcare and IoT Technologies

Academic and Service Provider Review

Vinaytosh Mishra and Somayya Madakam

CONTENTS

2.1 INTRODUCTION

As rightly said by our ancestors, "Health Is Wealth"; among all assets, health is one of the most important factors for human survival. Therefore, maintaining good health throughout our lives is essential for a long and happy life. However, human life faces many dangers, including manmade disasters, natural calamities, and even unexpected pandemic diseases like COVID-19. The five-letter word "COVID-19" was given by medical scientists to a deadly virus that caused chaos throughout the world (Madakam and Revulagadda, 2021). From the last months of 2019 onwards, the entire world has faced the pathogen irrespective of age, sex, tribe, and economic status. It affected a large number of people across the world, wherein patients were treated in hospitals, and many even lost their lives. Hence, international health bodies, national bureaucracies, medical practitioners, nurses, and volunteers laboured a lot and continued working to resolve this issue. However, creating a resistance to the Coronavirus pandemic was a great challenge for the techies, developers, physicians, pharmacists, and even regular people.

In light of this, many clinical trials is working together to get rid of this pandemic situation. Hence, there is an urgent need for technocrats, software developers, and mechatronics producers to develop healthcare-related products and services by planning carefully, designing properly, developing the right solution, testing with six sigma quality level, and deploying and demonstrating healthcare solutions. That is why Smart Healthcare is becoming one of the buzzwords on everybody's lips across the world. Much work has already been done on Smart Healthcare. Many academicians, researchers, and graduate- and post-graduate-level students and corporate people are doing

DOI: 10.1201/9781003217398-2

research and publishing innovative Smart Healthcare manuscripts with renowned publishers like Springer, SAGE, Emerald, Taylor & Francis, and Oxford, to name a few. There has been an explosion of publications in PubMed databases since COVID-2019 started that explore its characteristics, healthcare needs, treatment solutions, patient care, and post-treatment mechanisms. Much literature has already been produced in the form of books, book chapters, journal articles, annual reports, white papers etc. A study by Oueida et al. (2019) explored healthcare systems in medical sectors that attend to the health of entire populations and highlighted the need to change those healthcare systems from traditional services to smart health delivery. A series of seminars, webinars, and online discussions are being organized by different industries and academic institutions to make the public more aware of Smart Healthcare solutions that use advanced technologies. Existing communication technologies are unable to fulfil the complex and dynamic needs that are put on communication networks by diverse Smart Healthcare applications (Ahad et al., 2019). A growing world population, along with rising numbers of elderly people, is causing a rapid increase in healthcare costs. Technologies (e.g. Internet-of-Things, Edge-of-Things, and Cloud-of-Things) in healthcare systems are going through a transformation where health monitoring of people is possible without hospitalization (Uddin, 2019). The healthcare domain has emerged as one of the most preferred use cases of Internet-of-Things (IoT) and its related technologies. However, widespread adoption is still a distant dream (Tripathi et al., 2020). This shows that there is an urgent need to develop Smart Healthcare solutions that use advanced technology to improve human life. That is why many multinational companies that develop Smart Healthcare solutions for better patient care are mushrooming, including ESO (2004), Headspace (2010), Kyruus (2010), Wellframe (2011), and Medely (2015), among others. In addition to those just mentioned, here are some of the new-age innovators of the healthcare industry that are harnessing powerful technologies to develop healthcare products and services that benefit patients: CONTUS, OSP Labs, Pattem Digital Technologies, Mindbowser, HQSoftware Lab, Mobiloitte, Biz4Intellia, Amar InfoTech, Bridgera, and KORE Wireless.

2.2 METHODOLOGY

The research methodology is a systematic process in any kind of qualitative or quantitative research. It could be experimental, survey, ethnography, focused group discussions, in-depth interviews, action research etc.; the researchers need to adopt the right research methodology. The methodology plays an important role in any kind of research investigation and manuscript writing. This study attempts to understand the phenomena based on secondary data. Therefore, the authors retrieved data from the web of science database using keywords like "IoT", "Internet of Things", "Healthcare", "Smart Healthcare", and "'Body Area Networks" to understand the phenomena in a crystal clear way. However, our major focus was on articles about Smart Healthcare using IoT. Hence, the authors are limited to this phrase and those types of articles. The documents were searched from the dates 1-4-2021 to 31-08-2021. The articles were from different publishers like SAGE, Emerald, Springer, Taylor & Francis, and Elsevier. We also got many articles from the PubMed database.

2.2.1 Web of Science – Analytics

There were a total of 2656 search results on the Web of Science database for research manuscripts on Smart Healthcare within the date range 2001 to 26/6/2021. Among these publications, the term "Smart Healthcare" was found 50644 times, an average of 19.07 per manuscript, with an h-index of 97. The articles are indexed in SCI-Expanded, SSCI, and A&HCI. Moreover, some of the research manuscripts titles are (1) "A Survey on Wearable Sensor-Based Systems for Health Monitoring and Prognosis"; (2) "Wearable Sensors for Human Activity Monitoring: A Review"; (3) How Smartphones Are Changing the Face of Mobile and Participatory Healthcare: An Overview, with an Example from Ecaalyx"; (4) Stimulus-Responsive Hydrogels: Theory, Modern Advances, and Applications"; (5) Smart Wearable Systems: Current Status and Future Challenges"; (6) Unobtrusive

Sensing and Wearable Devices for Health Informatics; (7) "Fiber-Based Generator for Wearable Electronics and Mobile Medication"; (8) "An IoT-Aware Architecture for Smart Healthcare Systems"; (9) "Healthcare Data Gateways: Found Healthcare Intelligence on Blockchain with Novel Privacy Risk Control"; and (10) "A Review on Recent Advances in Doppler Radar Sensors for Noncontact Healthcare Monitoring". These are just a few of the articles exploring Smart Healthcare.

Below are the recorded research areas, as shown in Figure 2.1 (tree map), for the 2656 articles, including Computer Science (1105), 41.604%; Engineering (1037), 39.044%; Telecommunication (656), 24.699%; Chemistry (341), 12.839 %; Materials Science (294),

11.069%; Instruments Instrumentation (251), 9.450%; Science Technology other topics (243), 9.149%; Physics (197), 7.417%; Health Care Sciences Services (195), 7.342%; Medical Informatics (182), 6.852%; Public Environmental Occupational Health (70), 2.636%; General Internal Medicine (64), 2.410%; Environmental Sciences Ecology (51), 1.920%; Pharmacology Pharmacy (47), 1.770%; Mathematical Computational Biology (46), 1.732%; Automation Control Systems (39), 1.468%; Business Economics (37), 1.393%; Operations Research Management Science (33), 1.242%; Electrochemistry (31), 1.167%; Information Science Library Science (30), 1.130%; Research Experimental Medicine (30), 1.130%; Energy Fuels (27), 1.017%. Seventy-five research areas' value(s) are not mentioned here. This tree map shows that the Smart Healthcare phenomenon is interdisciplinary; hence, it can be applied in many disciplines. That means this phenomenon has a sea of applications in our daily life.

The next section discusses the countrywide publications on Smart Healthcare; Figure 2.2 also depicts the same. From January to June 2021, the United States leads with 579 publications followed by the People's Republic of China with 532, India with 359, and South Korea with 296. Moreover, England (247), Saudi Arabia (185), Australia (140), Pakistan (140), Italy (134), Canada (124), Taiwan (119), and Spain (102) are also contributing significantly to research. Countries like France (72), Germany (68), Singapore (68), Portugal (58), Brazil (55), Malaysia (55), and Egypt (51) are making huge investments, conducting research and exploring Smart Healthcare solutions to the external world. However, Iran (49), Japan (48), Sweden (45) and other countries are putting efforts into Smart Healthcare technologies for better hospital services.

The following section (Figure 2.3) discusses the Smart Healthcare work started in the year 2001 as per the Web of Science database; we found numerous publications: 2001 (1); 2002 (2); 2003 (2);

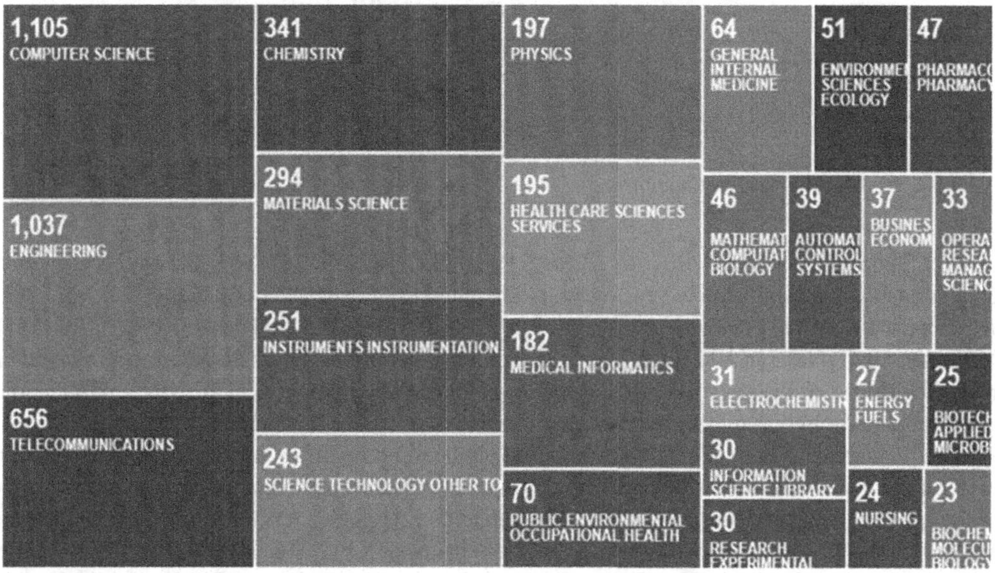

FIGURE 2.1 Research areas – tree map.

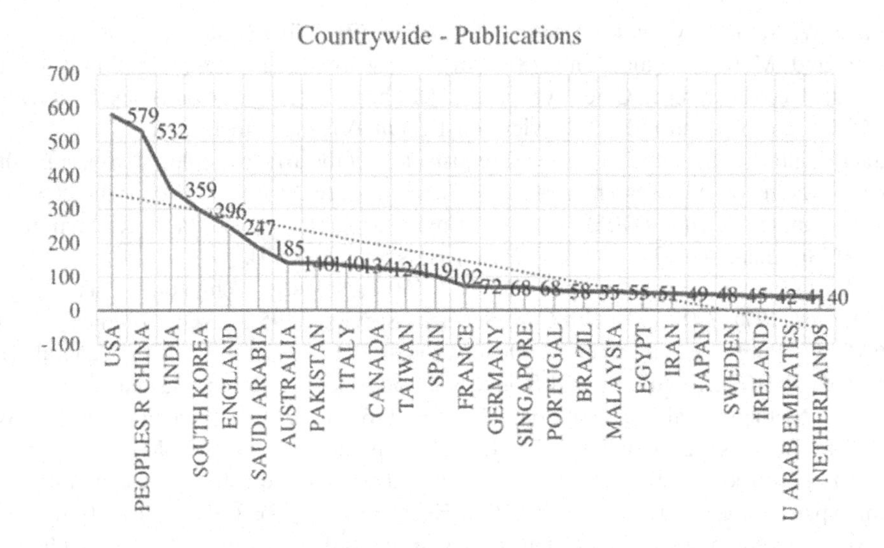

FIGURE 2.2 Countrywide – publications.

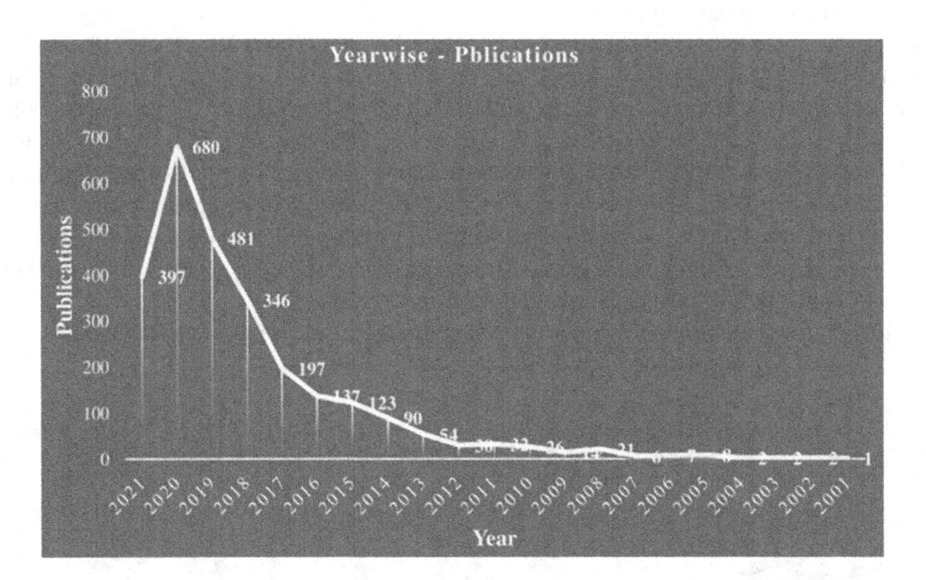

FIGURE 2.3 The year-wise publications.

2004 (2); 2005 (8); 2006 (7); 2007 (6); 2008 (21); 2009 (14); 2010 (26). This shows the growth of publications is increasing slowly year by year. The number of articles continued to rise from 2011 till 2021: 2011 (32); 2012 (30); 2013 (54); 2014 (90); 2015 (123); 2016 (137); 2017 (197); 2018 (346); 2019 (481); 2020 (680); and 2021 (397). In the coming years, more publications are yet to come on Smart Healthcare, as we are still in mid of the year. This kind of exponential growth in publications shows an increase in research by academicians and researchers in this field.

Figure 2.4 (spider graph) depicts the number of publications by different authors in different journals. Here papers from the authors with more than ten research publications have been taken into consideration. These are Kumar N. (29); Muhammad G. (21); Kim J. (19); Kumari S. (19); Hossain M.S. (17); I X (17); Chen M. (16); Lee S. (16); Rodrigues J.J.P.C. (16); Das A.K. (15); Mohanty S.P. (15); Yang J. (15); Zhang Y. (15); Sood S.K. (14); Kim D. (13); Kumar R. (13); Park J.H. (13); Chung K. (12); Hassan M.M. (12); Kumar S. (12); Lee J. (12); Khan M.K. (11); Ray P.P. (11); and

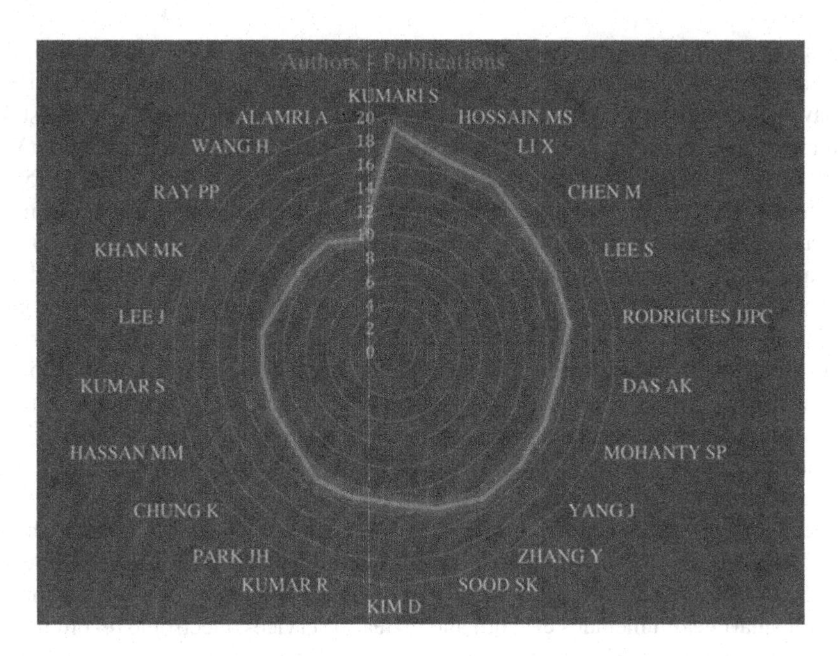

FIGURE 2.4 Authors – publications.

Wang H. (11). Many authors have not been listed here but have contributed research papers on Smart Healthcare. The next section details the literature, which is found in many journals, books, annual reports, blogs etc.

2.2.2 Academic Background

Man always strives for a better life in comparison to the present existing life. In this way, he is always intent on conducting research and innovating different tools and technologies to enhance quality of service, which leads to improved quality of life. Above all, good health is an important parameter of quality of life. Other parameters include sound economic conditions, good psychological state, physical security, etc. as per the past academic literature. Hence, it is of paramount importance that humans take care of their health. However, recently, we all have experienced a tough time due to the outbreak of coronavirus (COVID-19) which has put further strain on human life and healthcare systems. Moreover, a rapidly ageing population and the dramatic increase in the cost of in-hospital healthcare have led to the recognition of the importance of efficient healthcare systems (Nia et al., 2015). Therefore, Smart Healthcare Systems (SHSs) are being considered as a solution to current challenges in healthcare (Scott et al., 2020).

A study states that a blessing in disguise has been an increased adoption of digital technologies in healthcare during the pandemic, especially telemedicine (Mishra, 2020). Moreover, the advances in ICTs are shaping the paradigm in healthcare and their adoption provides new opportunities as well as discloses novel and unforeseen application scenarios (Aceto et al., 2018). A cost-effective and sustainable healthcare information system relies on the ability to collect, process, and transform healthcare data into information, knowledge, and action (Demirkan, 2013). The perceived benefits of these technologies along with ease of use are the most common factors for their adoption in different fields. Issues related to design, technical concerns, familiarity with technologies, and time are the most important factors cited in the literature (Gagnon et al., 2012). Therefore, in-depth research is needed to understand the specific socio-technical factors shaping digital innovations in healthcare (Habran et al., 2018). However, now with the help of global corporate structure and information technology (IT/ITeS), advanced manufacturing companies across the globe are planning, designing, manufacturing, supplying, and deploying different kinds of Internet of Things (IoT) technologies and solutions in both personal and official processes. In the past decade, there have been encouraging developments in the utilization of Internet of Things. Internet of Things-enabled solutions have been spurring the advent of novel and fascinating applications for the past few years. Among others, mainly radio frequency identification (RFID), wireless sensor network (WSN), and smart mobile technologies are leading this evolutionary trend (Catarinucci et al., 2015). We have witnessed an increased use of digital technologies like mobile apps in contact tracing and continuous monitoring of the patients during the pandemic outbreak. Technologies like continuous glucose monitoring and insulin pumps are increasingly being used over the past two decades and their adoption is expected to increase in coming years as their cost is falling and people are becoming more technophilic. Also, the market for wearable technologies such as fitness watches has significantly increased in recent years. These devices can communicate with the caregiver and help in customizing treatment plans. These wearable and assistive technologies are generating massive amounts of data. If we analyse this data, we can not only increase quality of care but also individualize the care provided to a patient. Needless to say, sensors will shape the future of medicine, being termed "precision medicine".

Smart Healthcare Systems are being considered as solutions to several current challenges in healthcare (26Scott et al., 2020). Smart Healthcare is defined as the use of advanced technologies to improve the diagnosis of disease and treatment of patients, and thus quality of life for them. The key concept of smart health includes eHealth and mHealth services, electronic record management, smart home services, and intelligent and connected medical devices. The terms "smart health" and "digital health" have been interchangeably used in much literature (Lupton, 2014). Smart Healthcare can promote interaction between all parties in the healthcare field, ensure that participants get the services they need, help the parties make informed decisions, and facilitate the rational allocation of resources (Tian et al., 2019). However, the use of smart health is not very well developed, and its potential has been little exploited. There are many reasons for the limited diffusion of these digital health technologies and knowledge: opportunities for training and ethical and privacy issues to name a few (Gjellebæk et al., 2020).

Smart Healthcare not only means adopting new products and technologies for diagnosis and treatment but also includes a greater exchange of information among the parties, a more active role for patients during treatment, and, finally, better management of clinical data. Smart Healthcare Systems need a wide range of technology to be implemented properly (Haque et al., 2021). In the past decade, there have been encouraging developments in the utilization of Internet of Things (IoT) in healthcare. IoT can be defined as a network of devices interacting with each other via machine-to-machine (M2M) communications, enabling collection and exchange of data. These technologies enable automation in healthcare and are being hailed as the driver of the fourth revolution in healthcare also termed "Healthcare 4.0" (Islam et al., 2015; Yuehong et al., 2016). These technologies include computing processes, in which each object uses sensors, micro-controllers, and transceivers for enabling communication among connected devices. Suitable protocol stacks help these devices in interacting with each other and communicating with the users (Kodali et al., 2015). Medical IoT (m-IoT) aggregates analyses and communicates synchronous medical information to the cloud, thus making it possible to collect, store, and analyse this voluminous data in various forms to get useful insights. Karjagi and Jindal (2021) explain the following four steps of the IoT implementation in the healthcare system: (1) deployment of interconnected devices; (2) data aggregation and pre-processing; (3) storage of data in the cloud, and; (4) data analysis for effective decision-making. These four steps are summarized in Figure 2.5. Thus, m-IoT enables continuous and ubiquitous communication among connected medical devices so that they can help in improving the quality of care. Each of these devices is powered by batteries and hence it is of utmost importance that power consumption is minimized to prolong the life of healthcare systems. Thus, IoT-based medical devices are improving the quality of care with regular monitoring and reducing the cost of care with increased efficiency. Considering their usefulness, IoT-enabled medical solutions are increasingly being used in recent years (Catarinucci et al., 2015). Some of the major advantages of IoT in healthcare are (1)

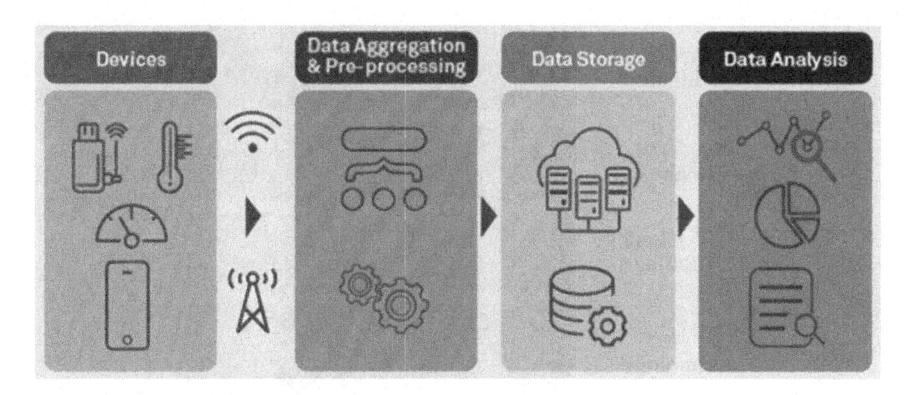

FIGURE 2.5 The four stages of IoT solutions. *Source*: Authors.

cost reduction through real-time monitoring; (2) improved treatment and diagnostics; (3) proactive treatment; (4) drug and equipment management; and (5) reduced errors, waste, and system costs.

Internet of Things enables data collection technologies like wireless body area networks (WBAN) and wireless sensor networks (WSN) which are increasingly being used for collecting, storing, and processing patient-centric data. Accurate information and real-time data sharing have helped increase the quality of emergency medical care (Edoh, 2019). Also, Anderson and Knickman (2001) in their research article envisaged the increased usefulness of IoT in chronic illness. As continuous monitoring is an essential component in the management of various diseases such as diabetes and other metabolic disorders, IoT-based solutions are immensely helpful (Longva and Haddara, 2019). Internet of Things is also useful in providing information and monitoring during pandemics like COVID-19. It can be used to provide an automated and transparent treatment process to tackle the pandemic situation (Singh et al., 2020). In their seminal paper highlighted the importance of IoT-based application in contact tracing to avoid spreading infectious diseases. To realise the full potential of IoT in healthcare, it needs to overcome some apparent challenges, including security, privacy, wearability, and low-power consumption (Baker et al., 2017). There is a need for a Smart Healthcare System (SHS) that makes the healthcare system smarter in order to protect data and maintain the privacy of patients. An SHS contains several IoT devices, sensors, and mobile nodes that collect data from the patient's body and store it remotely (Singh and Chatterjee, 2021). In addition, there is a need for research at the intersection of healthcare, data analytics, wireless communication, embedded systems, and information security. With the rapid change in the landscape of healthcare, it is imperative to review the recent applications of IoT in healthcare. Smart Healthcare may reduce the need for frequent visits to physicians for regular health check-ups. Wearable sensors generate enormous data, which need to be stored securely as well processed for extraction of information (Saif et al., 2021).

2.3 CASES

This section discusses the use cases of technologies in Smart Healthcare.

2.3.1 Case 1: Watson Health

International Business Machines (IBM) Watson Health is a division of IBM, headquartered in New York. It enables organizations to solve important challenges for stakeholders by offering a data-driven solution and real results. According to information available on their website, they use smart technologies for solving problems in healthcare (Figure 2.6).

They claim that their healthcare consulting clients have an average return on investment (RoI) of 10:1. Watson Health's natural language processing (NLP), hypothesis generation, and evidence-based learning capabilities contribute to clinical decision support systems. In 2011, IBM entered a

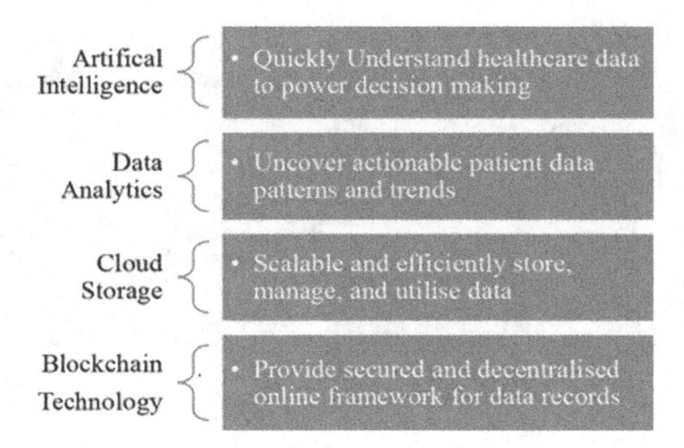

FIGURE 2.6 Watson Health's smart technologies. *Source*: Authors.

partnership with Cleveland Clinic to utilize Watson Health for augmenting medical professionals' expertise in treating patients. Recently, IBM and Manipal Hospital in India announced the use of Watson Health for the oncology department. It is believed that it will be carrying the knowledge base of 1000 cancer specialists and will be a game-changer in cancer treatment. Watson Health has other non-clinical use cases like compensation management, inventory management, preventive maintenance, theft detection, and fraud detection to name a few. Moreover, Watson Health can help in delivering efficient healthcare and significantly improved quality of care.

2.3.2 Case 2: Verily

Google recently renamed its company Google Lifesciences to Verily. Verily is Google's ambitious attempt to foray into the trillion dollars healthcare industry. Verily marks Alphabet's official entry into the field of Smart Healthcare using the Internet of Things to gain insight into patients' health. The healthcare industry is facing the dual challenge of cost and quality worldwide. This tech giant aims to solve these perennial problems with Smart Healthcare technologies. The firm will look to collect data from sensors, fitness bands, smartwatches equipped with monitors, and other IoT devices and analyse this data using Google's AI capabilities to detect the pattern, which could lead to a proactive treatment or individualized care. The company has already done its "Baseline Study" to find out what constitutes a healthy human being in order to analyse the deviation from this state. The company has developed smart contact lenses that help in the identification of glaucoma. Verily, in collaboration with Vanderbilt University Medical Center and the Broad Institute of Massachusetts Institute of Technology (MIT) and Harvard, built the data research and support centre to organize the multi-modal and complex data sets collected. Verily in association with American Heart Association (AHA) and AstraZeneca has come up with a research initiative "One Brave Idea". This initiative aims to uncover new approaches to prevent and treat coronary heart diseases (CHDs). It also has notable research initiatives like Parkinson's Progressive Markers Initiative, Immune Profiler, and analysis of risk factors of Multiple Sclerosis (MS). Google have developed a machine learning (ML) algorithm to make it easier to screen various diseases such as diabetes retinopathy (DR) and diabetic macular edema (DME). Google conducted a clinical research programme in association with Aravind Eye Hospital in Madurai, with a focus on India, a country being termed "the diabetes capital of the world" (Kasumi and Virmani, 2021).

The ML based process for DR and DME screening is shown in Figure 2.7.

2.3.3 Case 3: Intel Healthcare and Life Sciences

Smart Healthcare can help to enrich the life of every person across the globe. Technologies like artificial intelligence (AI), robotics, and the Internet of Things are making healthcare and life sciences

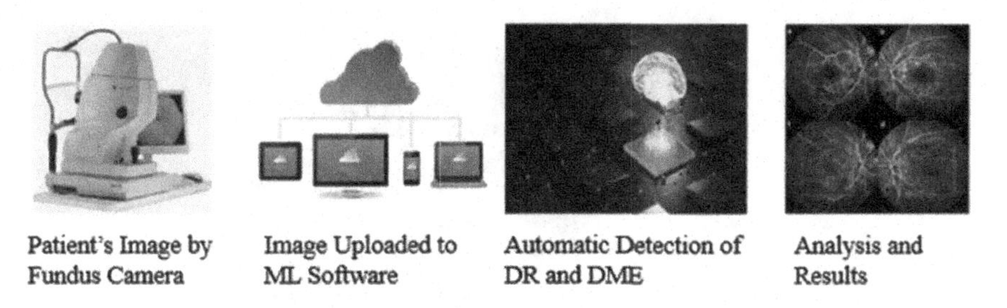

FIGURE 2.7 Steps for machine learning screening works at the hospital in Madurai. *Source*: Authors.

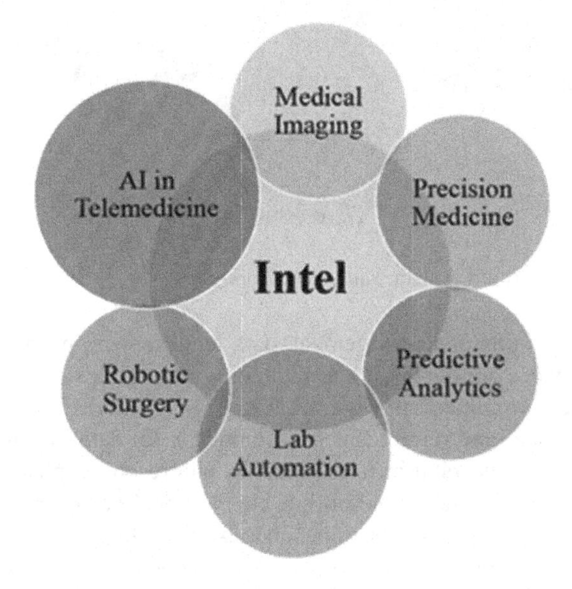

FIGURE 2.8 Use cases of IBM healthcare technologies. *Source*: Authors.

more connected, personalized, and intelligent. M/s. Intel is a tech giant that has envisioned the use of technologies in making healthcare smarter. It has invested profoundly in its healthcare and life sciences division. Its technologies have applications in medical imaging and disinfecting hospital premises. Intel has collaborated with the Broad Institute of MIT and Harvard to provide the impetus for their genomics research. Technological advancements in recent years have made it possible to practise precision medicine. With the help of Intel's healthcare technologies, clinicians use a combination of genomic data, health records, lab tests, and other patient data to customize their care. In a nutshell, Intel healthcare technologies are efficient enough to enable care providers to focus more on the human side of care delivery. Some of the use cases of Intel's healthcare technologies are listed in Figure 2.8.

2.3.4 Case 4: Lumiata

Intel's venture capital arm Intel Capital has heavily invested in a Smart Healthcare start-up named Lumiata. It is reshaping the healthcare enterprise at a large scale through the application of AI, bringing predictive power within the reach of business leaders and data science teams. Its data science productivity tools and pre-trained models comprise a scalable platform, purpose-built for healthcare, and generated from more than 120 million patient records, in-depth clinical knowledge, and Lumiata's proprietary disease codes. The platform offered by the company enables users to run their customized predictive model for various use cases. The company offers services and consulting in clinical as well as allied healthcare areas, actuarial and underwriting, care and disease

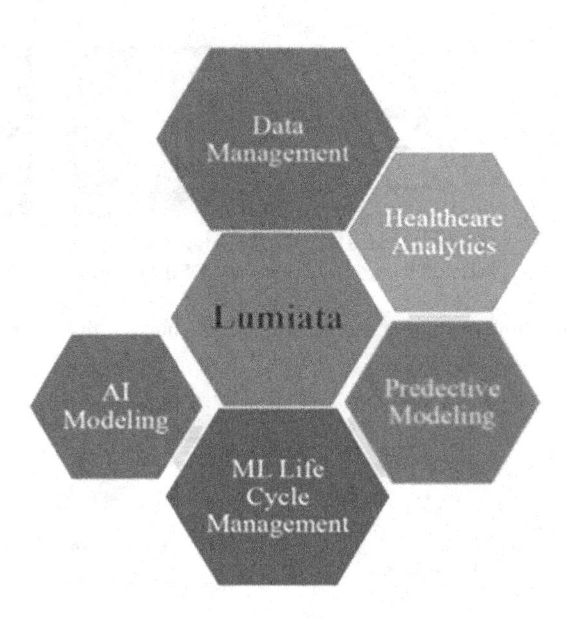

FIGURE 2.9 Service offerings of Lumiata. *Source*: Authors.

management, COVID planning and management, data management, payment integrity, and telemedicine. These all services are deployed and monitored through a single solution. The services offered by Lumiata are summarized in Figure 2.9, i.e. (1) AI modelling (using supervised, unsupervised, semi-supervised, and reinforcement techniques); (2) data management (huge amount of healthcare data relating to hospital infrastructure, human resource, pharmaceutical, in and out patient data and operations, treatments and billing, etc.); (3) healthcare analytics (patient data collection, data cleaning, feature selection, training, and testing and generating model); (4) predictive modelling (predicting the output results and their associated costs in the future for better treatment); and (5) machine learning-life cycle management (technological management right with the hospital information system designing, developing and testing, deploying advanced technologies in the premises, and providing maintenance).

2.4 DISCUSSION

Healthcare systems are facing unprecedented challenges such as the outbreak of infectious diseases, increased prevalence of chronic disease, shortage of doctors and clinicians, lack of timely medicines, ageing population, rising costs, etc. Hence, Healthcare systems worldwide should focus on better individualized care, improved population health, and lower healthcare cost. That means addressing these issues requires the use of smart health technologies that make healthcare more intelligent, distributed, and personalized. These advanced technologies like IoT smart devices, Edge (Fog) computing, artificial intelligence, and computer vision are shaping the landscape of the future of healthcare. Moreover, applied technologies like medical imaging (MI), bedside telemetry, and natural language processing (NLP) are augmenting the work of clinicians and hence enabling them to focus more on the human side of care. Among all, the Internet of Things technologies have been immensely used in healthcare. Internet of Things-enabled devices have made remote monitoring of patients possible and have many applications in managing chronic diseases and providing geriatric care. For example, a closed-loop system having a continuous glucose monitoring system (CGMS) and insulin pump can act as an artificial pancreas for a diabetes patient having insulin resistance and are a boon for Type-2 Diabetes Mellitus patients. IoT-enabled devices can generate an alarm in case of hypoglycaemia and save the life of a diabetic patient. IoT-enabled devices are used for performance monitoring of critical medical equipment and raise alarm or notify the care provider when preventive maintenance is required. Bluetooth-enabled proximity tracking apps have also been found very helpful in contact tracing during the recent outbreak of COVID-19 disease. Besides this, IoT also has other non-clinical applications such as hospital environment monitoring through closed-circuit television (CCTV)/internet protocol (IP) camera, inventory management, and theft detection round the clock.

IBM, Google, Intel, Microsoft, and many more tech giants have realized the potential of Smart Healthcare and are actively working on future technologies to overcome the challenges faced by the healthcare industry. Venture capitalist Intel Capital has envisaged the growth of Smart Healthcare in near future and invested in Smart Healthcare start-ups such as Lumiata. Another area where technology companies are seeing potential is telemedicine. The COVID-19 pandemic has increased the acceptance of telemedicine services. Telemedicine coupled with haptics, body sensors, and new protocols can bring telehealth one echelon up in near future. However, due to several technological reasons, Smart Healthcare technologies deployment on hospital premises, such as hospital information systems (HIS), has been challenging at present. Moreover, privacy and security are some of the concerns in the use of connected healthcare technologies relating to patients' confidential data, including demographic and chronic disease physiognomies. Hence, the HIS should be installed with various malware and fraud detection software, including antivirus and firewalls from reliable sources like Symantec, Dr. Solomon, Trend Micro, and Kaspersky. In addition, the government should come up with standard processes and regulations for the deployment of these technologies in order to ensure cybersecurity in these concerned areas. The European Union has started framing General Data Protection Regulation (GDPR) for securing citizen data. If managed appropriately, Smart Healthcare can introduce many new opportunities in patient care, which will ultimately lead to quality of life.

2.5 CONCLUSION

This chapter discussed the Smart Healthcare phenomenon using advanced technologies. We know that healthcare deals with patients, diseases, medicines, doctors, nurses, treatments, and its associated health information systems. The current healthcare systems are not self-sufficient and not fully deployed with advanced technologies to bring operational efficiency to the entire medicinal treatments. Hence, information technology (IT/ITeS) service providers are involved in research and development (R&D) to develop more advanced technologies for better assistance to hospitals and in patient care. Internet of Things involves new technologies that are used to connect to physical things or objects using intelligence-embedded technologies to identify, automate, monitor, and control. There is an ocean of applications of the Internet of Things that we are experiencing in our daily life, including the services in the healthcare sector. Sensors, actuators, Wi-Fi (Wireless Fidelity), Bluetooth, ZigBee, microcontrollers (Raspberry Pi and Arduino), radio frequency identification (RFID, active, passive, and semi-passive), barcodes, electronic product code (EPC), quick response (QR) codes, web 3.0, enterprise resource planning (ERP), geographic information systems (Arc GIS), cloud storage, and geographic position systems (GPS) are some of the information technologies currently being using in hospitals and remote patient care. The healthcare sector is the first to use IoT technologies at a wider level, including x-ray, CT scanning, stethoscope, and other healthcare devices for the check-up of body parameters. Internet of Things is heavily used for monitoring the remote patient, heart rate, glucose, hand hygiene, depression, and mood. Moreover, Parkinson's disease monitoring includes connected inhalers and ingestible sensors to name some more IoT applications in healthcare. IoT devices are very useful in various hospital fields, including tagging with sensors, GIS and GPS for tracking the real-time location of medical equipment like wheelchairs, defibrillators, nebulizers, oxygen pumps, and other monitoring equipment. Besides, the body area network (BAN) is also one of the upcoming healthcare technology wherein Smart Healthcare devices will be embedded into the human body based on the functionality of BAN to sense human body parameters like sweating and temperature, and logs of patient's medical data, which will be shared to analysts. Furthermore, the increasing use of wireless networks and the constant miniaturization of electrical devices has empowered the development of wireless body area networks (WBANs) (Latré et al., 2011). There are many smarter care solutions available in the market like home care, old age, antenatal care, and chronic patients. Hence, the best way to get rid of pandemic situations like corona-wave 1 is to adopt the Internet of Things in all the fields of the healthcare sector so that quality services can be provided 24/7 for quality of life.

This book chapter also explored the existing academic literature on Smart Healthcare and IoT's basic definitions, connotations, and technologies. So finally, we understood that Smart Healthcare is nothing but the provision of health-related services provided by IoT devices and its sister technologies for patient care in a better way. Web of Science analysis on academic literature gives some statistics on publications related to these phenomena while categorizing them by author, country, year, and other search terms. Moreover, the discussed cases are better explanations of the deployment of Smart Healthcare in different industries across the globe. From this book chapter, we can also understand that there is a need for planning, designing, developing, and deploying IoT healthcare technologies in all healthcare fields on a wider scale for Smart Healthcare Systems to provide quality of life to all human beings. Let us welcome Smart Healthcare in a bigger way in our daily life to face any kind of pandemic situation in the future. Therefore, simply understand the principle:

"Smart Healthcare = Healthcare + Internet of Things"

IoT-enabled healthcare has many advantages but it comes with its own challenges. The biggest challenge associated with Smart Healthcare is security and privacy of data. IoT devices can pose a threat to users' security and privacy. The second daunting challenge is inter-realm authentication and interoperability issues. In addition, there is a shortage of skilled human resources for managing Smart Healthcare operations. If these challenges are addressed satisfactorily, Smart Healthcare can solve many perennial problems associated with traditional healthcare.

REFERENCES

Aceto, G., Persico, V. and Pescapé, A., 2018. The role of Information and Communication Technologies in healthcare: taxonomies, perspectives, and challenges. *Journal of Network and Computer Applications, 107*, pp.125–154.

Ahad, A., Tahir, M. and Yau, K.L.A., 2019. 5G-based smart healthcare network: architecture, taxonomy, challenges and future research directions. *IEEE Access, 7*, pp.100747–100762.

Anderson, G. and Knickman, J.R., 2001. Changing the chronic care system to meet people's needs. *Health Affairs, 20*(6), pp.146–160.

Baker, S.B., Xiang, W. and Atkinson, I., 2017. Internet of things for smart healthcare: technologies, challenges, and opportunities. *IEEE Access, 5*, pp.26521–26544.

Catarinucci, L., De Donno, D., Mainetti, L., Palano, L., Patrono, L., Stefanizzi, M.L. and Tarricone, L., 2015. An IoT-aware architecture for smart healthcare systems. *IEEE Internet of Things Journal*, 2(6), pp.515–526.

Demirkan, H., 2013. A smart healthcare systems framework. *It Professional, 15*(5), pp.38–45.

Edoh, T., 2019. Internet of things in emergency medical care and services. In H. Farhadi (Ed.),*Medical Internet of Things (m-IoT)-Enabling Technologies and Emerging Applications.* London: IntechOpen. 10.5772/intechopen.76974

Gagnon, M.P., Desmartis, M., Labrecque, M., Car, J., Pagliari, C., Pluye, P., Frémont, P., Gagnon, J., Tremblay, N. and Légaré, F., 2012. Systematic review of factors influencing the adoption of information and communication technologies by healthcare professionals. *Journal of Medical Systems, 36*(1), pp.241–277.

Gjellebæk, C., Svensson, A., Bjørkquist, C., Fladeby, N. and Grundén, K., 2020. Management challenges for future digitalization of healthcare services. *Futures, 124*, p.102636.

Habran, E., Saulpic, O. and Zarlowski, P., 2018. Digitalisation in healthcare: an analysis of projects proposed by practitioners. *British Journal of Healthcare Management, 24*(3), pp.150–155.

Haque, A.B., Muniat, A., Ullah, P.R. and Mushsharat, S., 2021, February. An automated approach towards smart healthcare with blockchain and smart contracts. In *2021 International Conference on Computing, Communication, and Intelligent Systems (ICCCIS)* (pp.250–255). IEEE.

Islam, S.R., Kwak, D., Kabir, M.H., Hossain, M. and Kwak, K.S., 2015. The internet of things for health care: a comprehensive survey. *IEEE Access*, *3*, pp.678–708.

Karjagi, R. and Jindal, M. What IoT can do for healthcare? Assessed on June 4, 2021. https://www.wipro.com/business-process/what-can-iot-do-for-healthcare-/

Kodali, R.K., Swamy, G. and Lakshmi, B., 2015, December. An implementation of IoT for healthcare. In *2015 IEEE Recent Advances in Intelligent Computational Systems (RAICS)* (pp.411–416). IEEE.

Latré, B., Braem, B., Moerman, I., Blondia, C. and Demeester, P., 2011. A survey on wireless body area networks. *Wireless Networks*, *17*(1), pp.1–18.

Longva, A.M. and Haddara, M., 2019. How can iot improve the life-quality of diabetes patients? In *MATEC Web of Conferences* (Vol. 292, p.03016). EDP Sciences.

Lupton, D., 2014. Critical perspectives on digital health technologies. *Sociology Compass*, *8*(12), pp.1344–1359.

Madakam, S. and Revulagadda, R.K., 2021. Software engineering analytics—the need of post COVID-19 business: an academic review. In Patnaik, S., Tajeddini, K., Jain, V. (eds), *Computational Management. Modeling and Optimization in Science and Technologies*, Vol 18. Springer, Cham. https://doi.org/10.1007/978-3-030-72929-5_11.

Mishra, V., 2020. Factors affecting the adoption of telemedicine during COVID-19. *Indian Journal of Public Health*, *64*(6), p.234.

Nia, A.M., Sur-Kolay, S., Raghunathan, A. and Jha, N.K., 2015. Physiological information leakage: a new frontier in health information security. *IEEE Transactions on Emerging Topics in Computing*, *4*(3), pp.321–334.

Oueida, S., Aloqaily, M. and Ionescu, S., 2019. A smart healthcare reward model for resource allocation in smart city. *Multimedia Tools and Applications*, *78*(17), pp.24573–24594.

Saif, S., Datta, D., Saha, A., Biswas, S. and Chowdhury, C., 2021. Data science and AI in IoT based smart healthcare: issues, challenges and case study. In *Enabling AI Applications in Data Science* (pp. 415–439). Springer.

Scott, B.K., Miller, G.T., Fonda, S.J., Yeaw, R.E., Gaudaen, J.C., Pavliscsak, H.H., Quinn, M.T. and Pamplin, J.C., 2020. Advanced digital health technologies for COVID-19 and future emergencies. *Telemedicine and e-Health*, *26*(10), pp.1226–1233.

Singh, A. and Chatterjee, K., 2021. Securing smart healthcare system with edge computing. *Computers & Security*, 108, C (Sep 2021): 102353.

Singh, R.P., Javaid, M., Haleem, A. and Suman, R., 2020. Internet of Things (IoT) applications to fight against COVID-19 pandemic. *Diabetes & Metabolic Syndrome: Clinical Research & Reviews*, *14*(4), pp.521–524.

Tian, S., Yang, W., Le Grange, J.M., Wang, P., Huang, W. and Ye, Z., 2019. Smart healthcare: making medical care more intelligent. *Global Health Journal*, *3*(3), pp.62–65.

Tripathi, G., Ahad, M.A. and Paiva, S. (2020, March). S2HS-A blockchain based approach for smart healthcare system. In *Healthcare* (Vol. 8, No. 1, p.100391). Elsevier.

Uddin, M.Z., 2019. A wearable sensor-based activity prediction system to facilitate edge computing in smart healthcare system. *Journal of Parallel and Distributed Computing*, *123*, pp.46–53.

Widner, K. and Virmani, S. New milestones in helping prevent eye disease with Verily. Assessed on June 4, 2021. https://www.blog.google/technology/health/new-milestones-helping-prevent-eye-disease-verily/

Yuehong, Y.I.N., Zeng, Y., Chen, X. and Fan, Y., 2016. The Internet of Things in healthcare: an overview. *Journal of Industrial Information Integration*, *1*, pp.3–13.

3 Recognizing Human Activities of Daily Living Using Mobile Sensors for Health monitoring

Raghunath Ghosh, Soham Chattopadhyay and Pawan Kumar Singh

CONTENTS

3.1 INTRODUCTION

Nowadays human activity recognition (HAR) has become an indispensable part of the health monitoring system. Unhealthy human daily activities may lead to many incurable diseases [1]. Predicting these types of activities at an early stage by using a health monitoring system will be beneficial for human beings and here research on HAR plays a very important role in accurate recognition of daily-life activities. HAR by using electronic devices cropped up in the late 1990s [2]. As technology progressed, the demand for HAR and data capture methodologies increased [3, 4]. HAR can be performed from various sources of input data like still images of human activities [5], videos [6], or time-series data from sensor-based time-like devices. In our work, we consider time-series smartphone sensor data. In today's world, getting sensor data is not very difficult as sensor-based smartphone devices or IoT devices are affordable to most people. According to Statista [7], currently the number of subscriptions to smartphones worldwide exceeds six billion and is forecast to further increase by several hundred million in the next few years, which indicates that more data from accelerometer and gyroscope will be available. Like smartphone utilization, the evolution in the internet of things (IoT) technology has empowered medical devices to make real-time analysis that was not achievable for doctors a few years ago [8]. Different sensor-based wearables (e.g. watch, wristband and shoes) and IoT devices aid patients and healthcare professionals to identify human activity remotely which helps healthcare professionals to deal with various health issues in a more effective way. So the data from various devices can be used for human activity recognition (HAR). A recent study shows sensors like accelerometer and gyroscope give illuminating information to identify human activities [4, 9, 10, 11].

The sensor data for HAR is highly dynamic and may vary from one person to another. To predict the activity from the dynamic data is the main aim of HAR. The HAR encompasses two types:

DOI: 10.1201/9781003217398-3

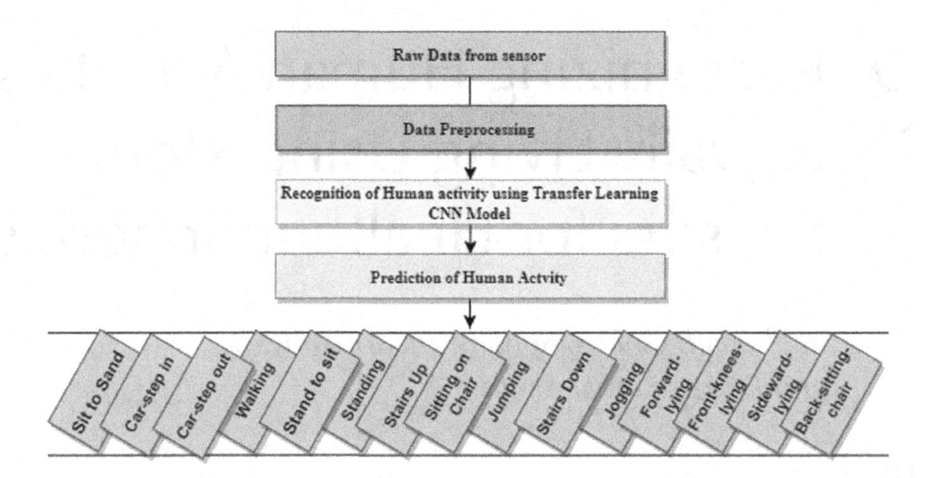

FIGURE 3.1 Overall architecture of proposed model.

transition actions and *basic actions.* There are moderately few studies on the transition movement from walking to standing, standing to sitting, and so on in the research of human activity recognition due to the low incidence and short duration of the transition movement. Anyhow, the research on transitional movement plays a key role in human activity recognition. Transition action recognition cannot be ignored to enhance the activity recognition rate. A different variety of basic actions in frequent alterations was known as transition action. The precise division of the transition action can precisely split the streaming data to a certain range and ultimately enhance the recognition rate. On top of that, the activity identification procedures based on traditional patterns have fallibility like manual feature extraction. With the implementation and progress of deep learning in different fields [12–16] [1], the deep learning model also shows great advantages in the field of HRA [17]. In our work, we train three widely used convolutional neural network (CNN)-based models using transfer learning. Transfer learning is a kind of supervised learning context, where the input remains the same but the target output can be of some other nature [18]. The main aims of this work are summarized as follows:

- To read accelerometer and gyroscope sensors data and transform it to an image to train deep learning models. The "MobiAct v2" is a publicly available dataset, used in the experiment. The dataset contains the gyroscope, orientation and accelerometer sensors of a smartphone of 11 activities of daily living (ADL) Activity, 4 types of FALL.
- To train three different CNN transfer learning models with the transformed heat map images and recognize the activities.

  Figure 3.1 describes the overall architecture of our proposed work. Details on the model and experimental results are mentioned in subsequent sections of the chapter.

This work is structurally arranged as follows: In section 3.2, a brief literature analysis to highlight previous work on sensor-based data is given, and in section 3.3, our proposed model architecture has been discussed. Experimental results and analysis are mentioned in section 3.4. Finally, section 3.5 (conclusion part) covers the overall summary of our work and future work.

3.2 LITERATURE ANALYSIS

HAR is one of the emerging researches that have become popular in the past decade and that play an important role in interpersonal relations and human-to-human interaction. As a result, human–computer interaction (HCI), healthcare applications, robotics and video surveillance systems (VSS) for human behaviour classification require a multiple-activity recognition system. Human activities, such as "standing", "sitting" and "walking" emerge very common in daily life, known as ADLs. In this chapter, we are performing ADLs and fall recognition on inertial data with transfer learning techniques. The two main queries come in HAR, "What is the activity?" and "How to process the source data?". To answer these questions, different researchers follow various techniques, and some snippets of previous work are mentioned here.

In the beginning, Bayatet al. [19] proposed a smartphone-based recognition system. When the user kept the smartphone in his/her hand, in that system application of a low-pass filter (LPF) and a combination of LogitBoost, Multilayer Perceptron and Support Vector Machine (SVM) classifiers, an overall accuracy of 91.15% was obtained. Similarly Anjumet al. [20], Zheng et al. [21], Saputri et al. [22] proposed different HAR classification approaches by carrying the smartphone in various positions mentioned in Table 3.1.

Post reviewing the previous works mentioned in Table 3.1, C. Chatzakiet al. [25] observed common issues in the dataset like differentiation in smartphone positions, the kinds of activities addressed and sampling frequency, along with the relatively small number of subjects. They developed a MobiAct dataset to handle these issues. Some of the existing research on the MobiAct dataset is mentioned here.

C. Chatzakiet al. [25] proposed an optimized feature set (OFS) feature selection and classification scheme to recognize human activities in the MobiAct dataset. To achieve the desired goal, they had done analysis comprehensively on the dataset to find the best features. They achieved 99.9% accuracy on six common ADLs only. Later, they extended their work [26] and experimented on the MobiAct 2.0 dataset where 12 ADLs and 4 falls had been considered. They were able to achieve 97.1% accuracy, It has been noticed that the accuracy of fall activities was low (Fall: Forward-lying accuracy was 68.8%). Similarly, Paul Compagnonet al. [27] suggested an approach to identify the activity by using the Gated Recurrent Units (GRU) and inertial sequences method on the MobiAct dataset. They are able to achieve around 87.4% accuracy on ADL and 91.1% on fall. Later, they [28] presented an approach for personalized ADL classification based on matching networks combined with sequence-to-sequence pre-training (SSMN) where the model can be trained with just one from one example. But they achieve 90% three-way accuracy and twelve-way accuracy in fall detection by using the MobiAct dataset. In both approaches of Paul Compagnon et al., it has been observed that the accuracy is lower on the MobiAct v2 dataset. By using the CNN model, Hongkaiet al. [29] used a hybrid multisensor multi-modal data from MobiAct v2.0 which includes the optimal tensor model to use as the input to the CNN. They achieved 97.66% of accuracy on 11 ADL activities. They did not consider fall activity during their excrement. Like Hongkai et al., Mohammad Mehedi Hassan et al. [30] suggested a hybrid model (CNN-LSTM) to build on a mobile-enabled fall detection (MEFD) framework on the MobiAct dataset. They have achieved 97% and 96.75 % for their experiments 1 and 2, respectively. But the proposed model did not classify all activities and was only able to detect falls. E. Ramanujamet al. [31] presented an automatic fall detection system using

TABLE 3.1
Research Data Collection Process

Research	Smartphone Position	Sampling Frequency	Activities
Bayat et al. [19]	Hand of the user	100 Hz	RUN, SWL,FWL, ADN, STU,STN
Anjum et al. [20]	Various positions	15 Hz	RUN, STN,STU, BIK, STC, DRI,INA
Zheng et al. [21]	Freely in pocket	100 Hz	SIT, STD,WAL, RUN
Siirtola et al. [23]	5 smartphones at various position	40 Hz	WAL,RUN, BIK,DRI,SIT/STD
Buber et al. [24]	Mobile kept at front pocket	20 Hz	WAL,JOG, STN,STU, SIT,JUM, BIK
Saputri et al. [22]	Mobile kept at front pocket	50 Hz	WAL, RUN,STN,STU,HOP

the MobiAct dataset. They achieved using machine learning algorithms J48, k-Nearest Neighbor (KNN) and achieved 96.73% accuracy. Similarly, Di Pietro et al. [32] proposed a new neural network (NN) model named as MIxedhiSTory Recurrent Neural Networks (MIST) which they tested on MobiAct V2, among others. They split users into fixed train, validation and test groups and executed the same experiment 50 times and kept the five best results. Their proposed model needs less computation and produces better results than LSTM. Moreover, Mukherjee et al. have developed EnsemConvNet [4] for the same task. Another GCN-based approach was also used for the HAR task [33]. Das et al. [17] proposed a multi-modal HAR model called MMHAR-EnsemNet and achieved state-of-the-art results. Visual HAR is another interesting task. Guha et al. [34] have come up with a feature selection model named CGA for the mentioned task. Additionally, [6], [5] are deep learning and transfer learning based approaches for various HAR tasks.

After reviewing the previous works, it was observed that HAR accuracy reduced on combining data from both ADL and falls. Our proposed model considers both 11 ADLs and 4 falls by using the CNN model to achieve benchmark accuracy on the MobiAct v2 dataset. HRA using CNNs is a cutting-edge technology as, for recognition tasks, it is significant to detect temporal correlations within the input data, and this can be handled using CNNs. Three widely used CNNs based models – VGG 11[35], GoogLeNet[36], and ResNet[37] – are used in this work.

3.3 PROPOSED MODEL

In the proposed work, three different transfer learning CNN models are used, and based on the model's output, different daily life human activities have been predicted. The overall architecture snippet is shown in Figure 3.2.

The MobiAct dataset consists of accelerometer and gyroscope sensors' data recordings of body movements of different volunteers performing activities and the raw data recorded into a ".txt" file. The raw data are transformed into Heatmap to feed into the CNN model. A heatmap is a graphical presentation where each value of a matrix is represented as colours. In data pre-processing, five seconds activity window data is taken. If an activity is performed for more than five seconds, it splits the data into multiple datasets of five seconds intervals. At the time of the split, if any dataset contains less than five seconds of data, then that data will be ignored to maintain the same time window. During data splitting, we observe that a number of accelerometer and gyroscope sensors value records in that interval are not the same. Padding logic is also applied to make both the counts same. Less number of records dataset is being padded with the average value.

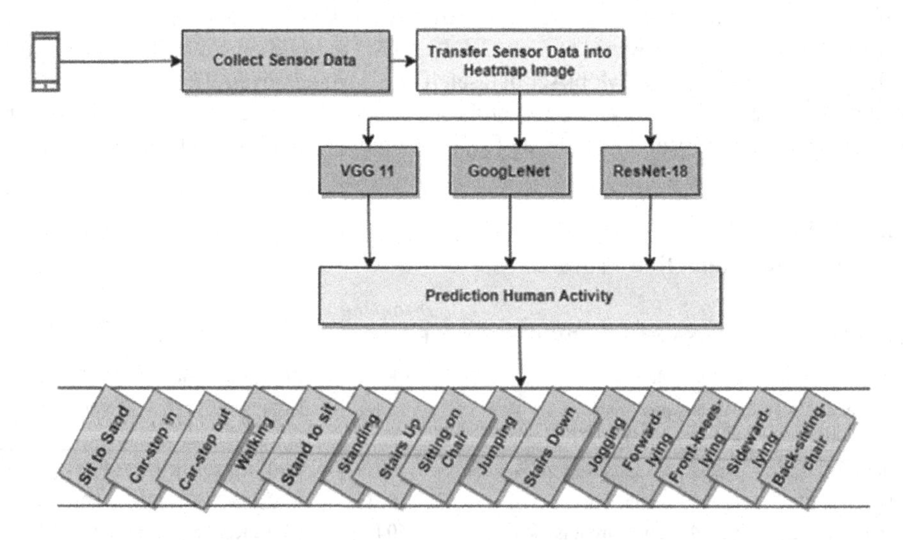

FIGURE 3.2 Proposed model architecture.

Example:

If the total number of accelerometer records is less than the total number of gyroscope records, the accelerometer dataset is padded with the average accelerometer of the window dataset, making the dataset same as that of the gyroscope records. The same thing applied if the number of gyroscope records is less than the number of accelerometer records.

$$\text{Padded Average Value} = (\text{Summation value within the window})/(\text{Number of records within the window}) \quad (3.1)$$

We used the Seaborn Python library [38] to generate a 1600x800 pixel .JPG HeatMap image file. In HeatMap, *X*-axis contains time and *Y*-axis accelerometer sensor X, Y, Z (*acc_x, acc_y, acc_z*), gyroscope sensor X, Y, Z (*gyro_x, gyro_y, gyro_z*). Sample images of all activities are shown in Figure 3.3.

Those images are sent as input to three different types of CNN models,

- Residual network model (ResNet)
- GoogleNet
- VGG 11

Residual networks[37] was introduced by Microsoft Research Asia, it is one of the most popular deep neural networks models in the image processing and recognition area. This model overcomes the vanishing / exploding gradients problem of previous multiple deep neural networks by introducing a feedforward network with a shortcut connection. As shown in Figure 3.4, the identity connection comes from the input and goes to the end of the residual block. Thus, a shortcut connection is introduced to add the input "*a*" to the output after a few weight layers. So, the output will be:

$$U(a) = G(a) + a \quad (3.2)$$

Due to this feature, this model is used to produce a very good classification accuracy without enhancing the model complexity. There are multiple residual network models available based on the number of neural network layers like ResNet-18, ResNet-34, ResNet-50, ResNet-101, ResNet-110, ResNet-152, ResNet-164 and ResNet-1202. The ResNet-152 model has been used in our proposed model. ResNet-152 model achieves top five errors of 3.57% in a classification task.

The GoogLeNet [36] neural network model was introduced by Google. To overcome the overfitting problem with many deep layers, this model contains multiple filters with multiple sizes which can work on the same level thus the model becomes wider rather than deeper. It follows the Hebbian Principle.

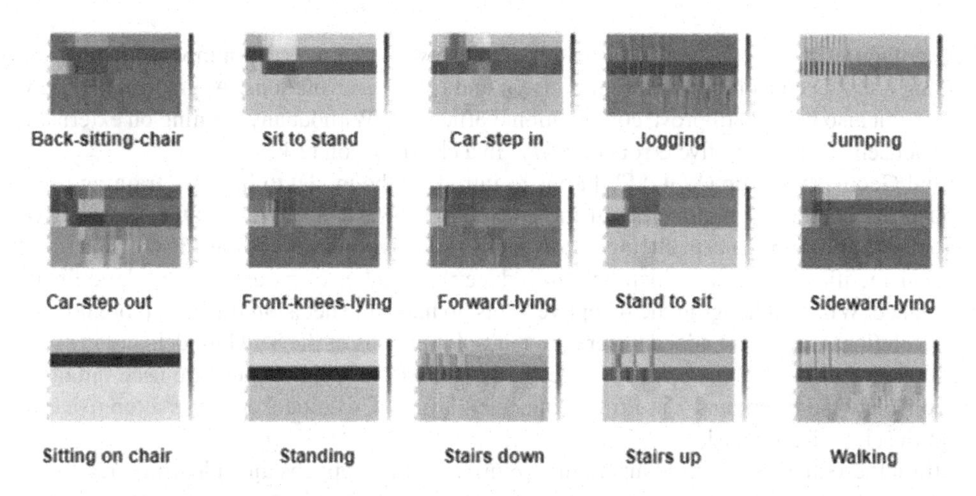

FIGURE 3.3 Sample heatmap images generated for different human activities.

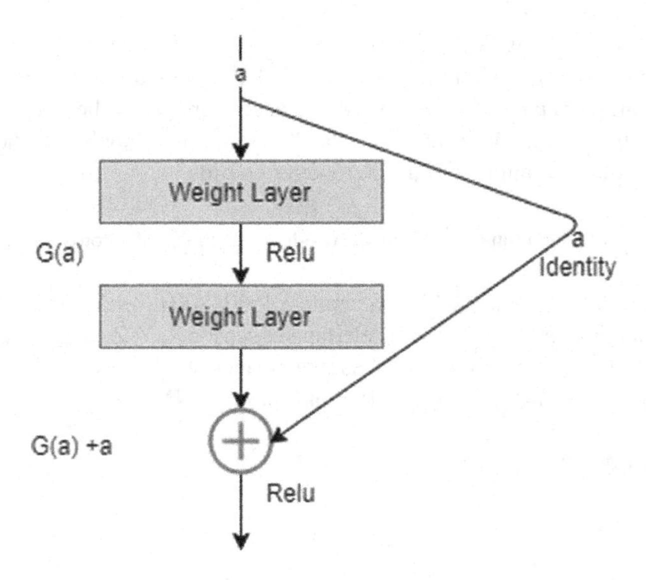

FIGURE 3.4 Residual block of residual network.

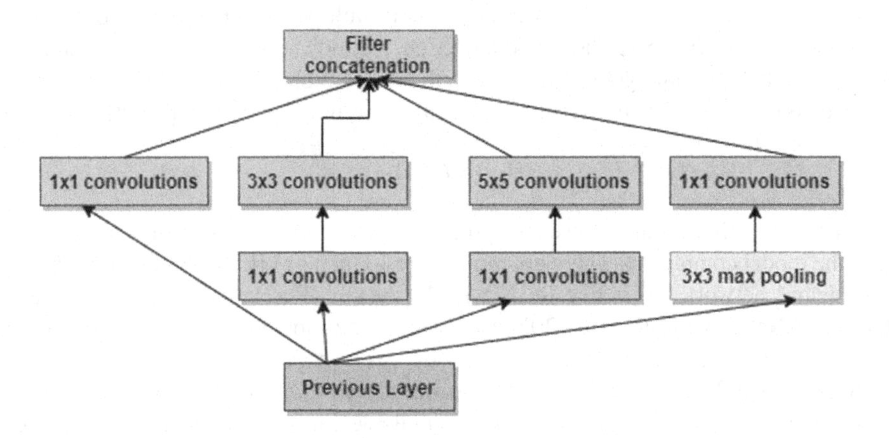

FIGURE 3.5 Building blocks of GoogleNet architecture.

As per Figure 3.5, to reduce the dimensions of the network, it limits the number of input channels by adding a (1×1) convolution before the (3×3) and (5×5) convolutions. Apart from the network dimension, it also helps to improve computational efficiency. Without any training on external data, this model achieved the top five errors of 6.67% in a classification task.

Visual Geometry Group (VGG) [35] aims to introduce the model to improve training time and to reduce the number of parameters in the convolution layers. So it substitutes TanH activation function with ReLU by encapsulating its different features for over-pooling. It contains multiple non-linear rectification layers which help to reduce the number of parameters while maintaining performance. Without changing the receptive fields, to make the decision function more non-linear, 1x1 convolutional layers are added. There are multiple versions of the VGG model, and in our comparative study, we use VGG 11. As described in Figure 3.6, 11 weight layers are used out of which 8 are convolutional layers and 3 are fully connected layers. This model achieves a top five error of 7.3% in the classification task.

To train these models, we used an Adam optimizer with 50 epochs and a learning rate of 0.001. The comparative results are presented in the subsequent section. The experimental models were tested on three parts:

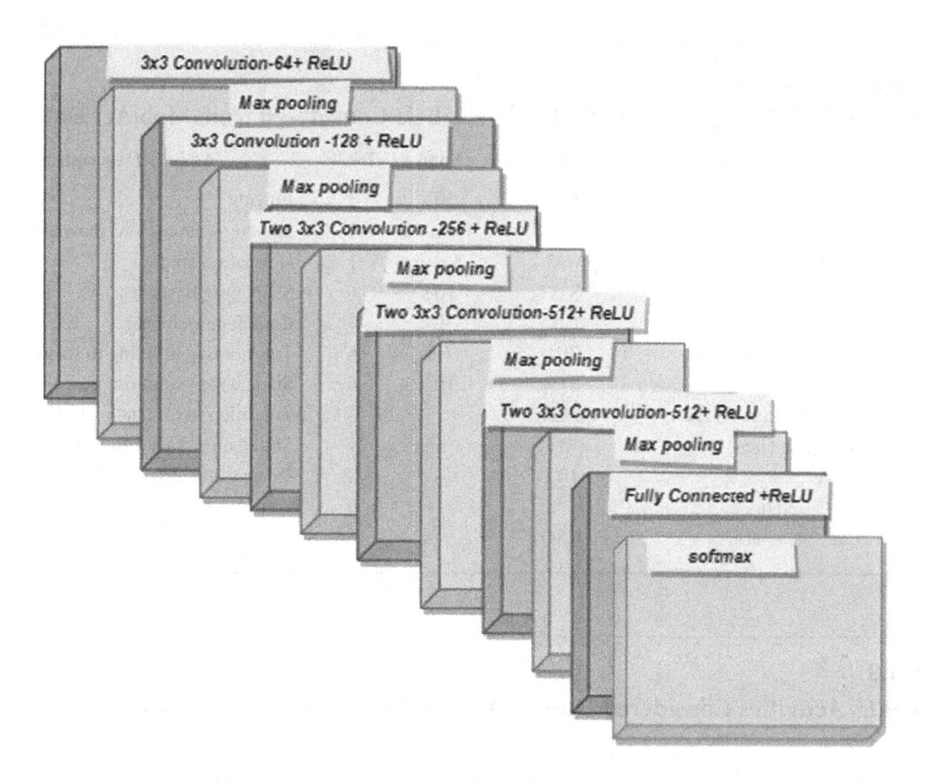

FIGURE 3.6 VGG model architecture used in the present work.

1. Combining 11 ADLs and 4 Fall
2. 11type ADLs
3. 4 type Fall

3.4 EXPERIMENTAL RESULTS AND ANALYSIS

3.4.1 Dataset Description

The v2 version of the publicly available MobiAct dataset has been used for the experiment (*available in* www.bmi.teicrete.gr). It contains data from smartphones where participants are performing various types of activities and a range of falls. Below activities data are present in the dataset:

- Four different types of falls performed by 66 participants (mentioned in Table 3.3)
- Eleven different types of activity of daily living (ADL) performed by 19 participants and nine types of ADLs performed by 59 participants (mentioned in Table 3.2)
- Five sub-scenarios which construct one scenario of daily living, which consists of a sequence of 50 activities and performed by 19 participants.

For each activity, the corresponding accelerometer and gyroscope values are saved into respective .txt files where

- the accelerometer value represents acceleration force along the x, y, z axes (including gravity)
- the gyroscope value represents the rate of rotation around the x, y, z axes (angular velocity).

The list of different activities and falls performed by participants are mentioned in Tables 3.1 and 3.2, respectively. Scenario and lying activity data were not considered in our experiment as there is no activity classification data present in the raw data file.

TABLE 3.2
Activities of Daily Living Along with Its Class Labels Considered from MobiAct Dataset

Serial No	Activity Name	Activity Code	Span	Trials	Activity Description
1	Jogging	JOG	30 s	3	Jogging
2	Standing	STD	5 min	1	Standing with devious movements
3	Walking	WAL	5 min	1	Normal walking
4	Stairs up	STU	10 s	6	Stairs up – 10 stairs
5	Jumping	JUM	30 s	3	Continuous jumping
6	Sit to stand -chair up	CHU	6 s	6	Transition from sitting to standing
7	Stairs down	STN	10 s	6	Stairs down -10 stairs
8	Stand to sit(sit on chair)	SCH	6 s	6	Transition from standing to sitting
9	Sitting on chair	SIT	1 min	1	Sitting on a chair with subtle movements
10	Lying	LYI	-	12	Taken from the lying period after a fall
11	Car – step in	CSI	6 s	6	Step in a car
12	Car – step out	CSO	6 s	6	Step out a car

TABLE 3.3
List of FALL Activities Considered During Data Collection of MobiAct Dataset

Serial No	Activity Name	Activity Code	Span	Trials	Activity Description
1	Sideward-lying	SDL	10 s	3	Fall side wards from standing, bending legs
2	Back-sitting-chair	BSC	10 s	3	Fall reverse while trying to sit on a chair
3	Front-knees-lying	FKL	10 s	3	Fall ahead from standing, first impact on knees
4	Forward-lying	FOL	10 s	3	Fall ahead from standing, use of hands to dampen fall

3.4.2 Evaluation Metrices

In this current work, we have estimated the performance of the proposed framework by using some standard evaluation criteria such as accuracy, precision, recall and f1 score. For a multi-class problem, these parameters are defined as follows:

1. Accuracy:
2. Precision:
3. Recall:
4. F1 score:

These parameters help to assess the performance more robustly. The elementary measures present in the Confusion matrix, True positive (TP), False positive (FP), True Negative (TN) and False Negative(FN) values are being used to calculate these values. Calculation methods are mentioned below using the respective equations (3.3–3.6). [39]

Accuracy:

Accuracy depicts how the model performs across all classes. It calculates the ratio of the number of correct predictions to the total number of input samples.

$$\text{Accuracy} = \frac{\text{TP} + \text{TN}}{\text{TP} + \text{TN} + \text{FP} + \text{FN}} \times 100\% \tag{3.3}$$

Precision:
This is also called a positive predictive value. It depicts the model's accuracy in classifying a sample as positive.

$$\text{Precision} = \frac{\text{TP}}{\text{TP} + \text{FP}} \tag{3.4}$$

Recall:
It is known as sensitivity. The recall depicts the model's ability to detect positive samples.

$$\text{Recall} = \frac{\text{TP}}{\text{TP} + \text{FN}} \tag{3.5}$$

F1 score:
It merges the precision and recall of the model, and is defined as the harmonic mean of the model's precision and recall.

$$\text{F1Score} = \frac{2}{\frac{1}{\text{Recall}} + \frac{1}{\text{Precision}}} \tag{3.6}$$

3.4.3 Results

The experimental model was tested on three parts:

1. Combining 11ADLs and 4Fall
2. 11 types of ADLs
3. 4 type Fall

The results values of each part are shown in Tables 3.4, 3.5 and 3.6, respectively. It can be seen that the ResNet-18 model performs better than both GoogLeNet and VGG11 models.

TABLE 3.4
Performance Results (in Terms of Four Evaluation Metrices) Produced by the Individual Models Combining ADLs and Fallon MobiAct Dataset

Models	Accuracy	Precision	Recall	F1 Score
ResNet-18	98.91	0.99	0.98	0.98
GoogLeNet	97.75	0.98	0.99	0.95
VGG11	94.49	0.95	0.97	0.93

TABLE 3.5
Performance Results (in Terms of Four Evaluation Metrices) Produced by the Individual Models on ADLs of MobiAct Dataset

Models	Accuracy	Precision	Recall	F1 Score
ResNet-18	97.73	0.97	0.96	0.97
GoogLeNet	96.61	0.95	0.96	0.96
VGG11	92.34	0.93	0.89	0.91

TABLE 3.6
Performance Results (in Terms of Four Evaluation Metrices) Produced by the Individual Models on Fall of MobiAct Dataset

Models	Accuracy	Precision	Recall	F1 Score
ResNet-18	94.41	0.91	0.94	0.94
GoogLeNet	91.10	0.92	0.92	0.92
VGG11	90.05	0.91	0.88	0.89

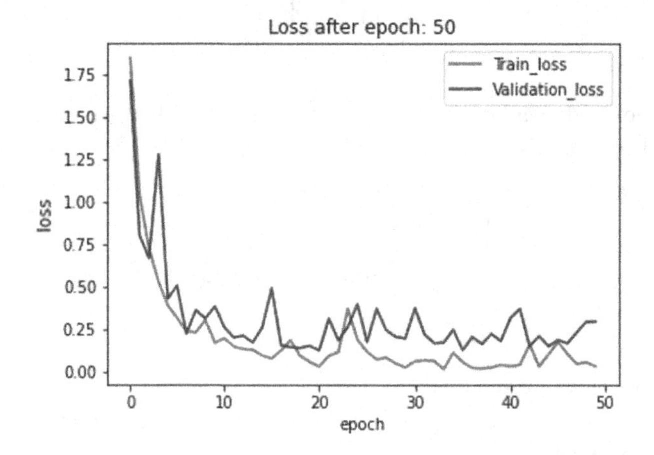

FIGURE 3.7 Loss plot of ResNet-18 model combining ADLs and Fallon MobiAct dataset.

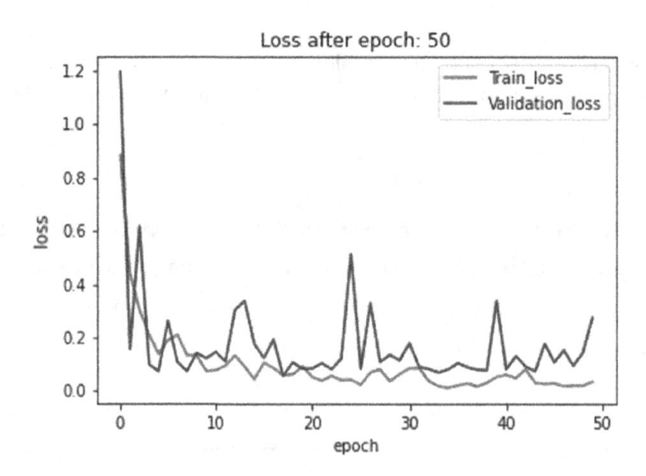

FIGURE 3.8 Loss plot of GoogLeNet model combining ADLs and fall on MobiAct dataset.

3.4.4 Loss Plots

The train and validation loss plots of the combination of ADLs and fall are shown in Figures 3.7, 3.8 and 3.9 for each respective model. As mentioned earlier, the models are trained for 50 epochs upon each dataset. From Figures 3.7, 3.8 and 3.9, we can observe that loss value decreases with respect to epoch, which means the models learn from input objects and the prediction probability increases. Among these three models, the training loss was almost in line with validation Loss in the ResNet-18 plot (Figure 3.7), and on the other hand, some certain spikes were present in both

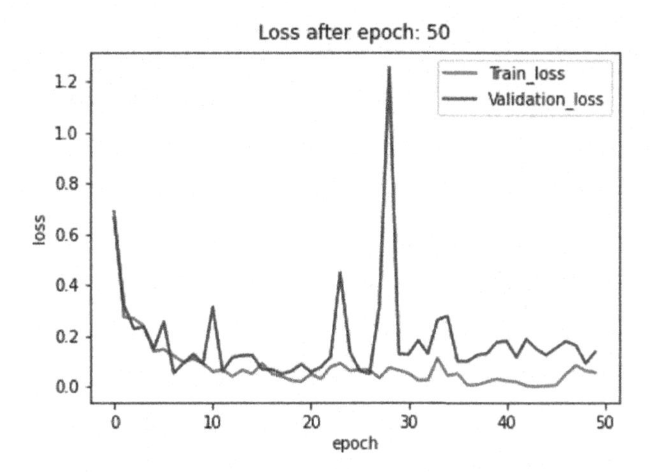

FIGURE 3.9 Loss plot of VGG11 model combining ADLs and dall on MobiAct dataset.

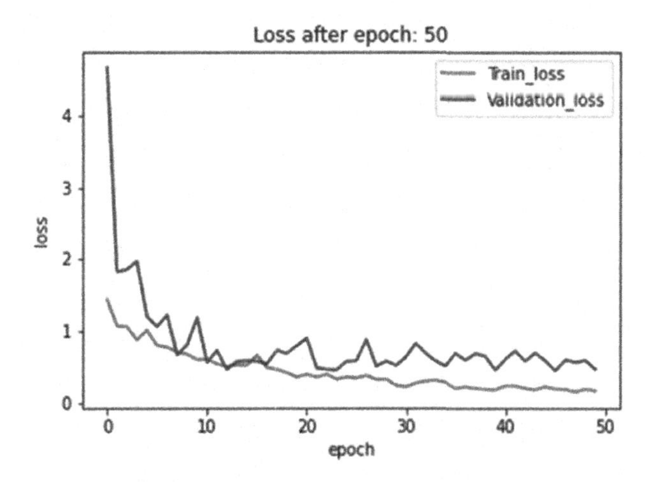

FIGURE 3.10 Loss plot of ResNet-18 model of Fallon MobiAct dataset.

GoogLeNet and VGG11. It indicates that ResNet-18 trained better than GoogLeNet and VGG11 with the experimental dataset.

The train and validation loss plots of fall are shown in Figures 3.10, 3.11 and 3.12 for each respective model. As mentioned earlier, the models are trained for 50 epochs upon each dataset. Among these three models, the training loss was almost in line with validation Loss in the VGG11 plot (Figure 3.12) and on the other hand, some certain spikes were present in both GoogLeNet and ResNet-18 models.

Similarly, the train and validation loss plots of the combination of ADLs are shown in Figure 3.13, 3.14 and 3.15 for each respective model. Out of these three models, the VGG11 plot (Figure 3.15) has less certain spikes than GoogLeNet and ResNet-18. Based on the loss plots, it can be said that, when the number of activities is less, the VGG11 model is getting trained better than both GoogLeNet and ResNet-18 models.

3.4.5 Comparison with Existing Models

Our proposed model was able to achieve 98.91% accuracy on 15 different activities present in the MobiAct V2 dataset. The comparison with previous work is illustrated in Table 3.7. It can be

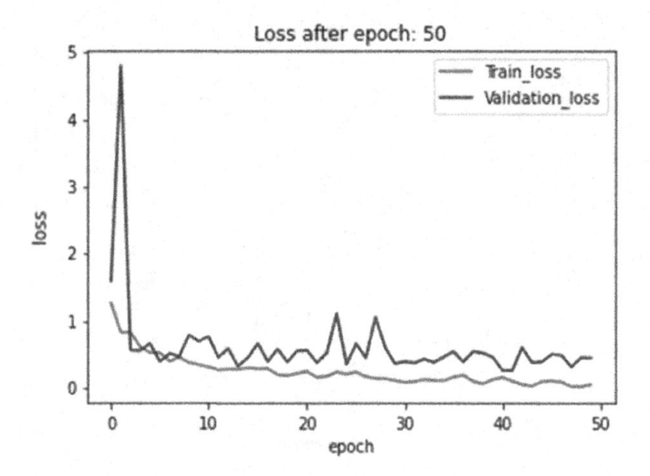

FIGURE 3.11 Loss plot of GoogLeNet model of Fallon MobiAct dataset.

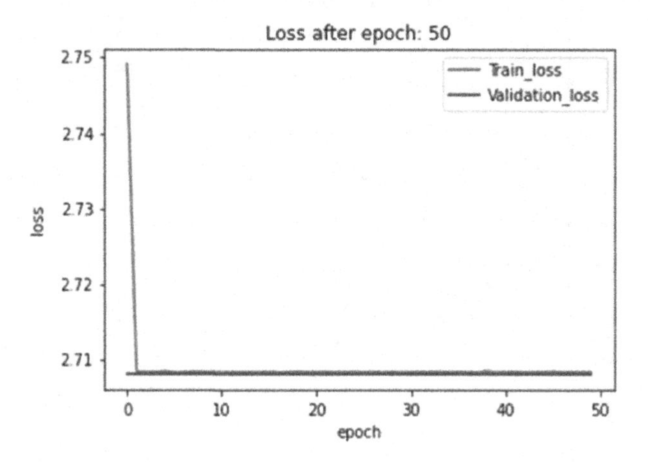

FIGURE 3.12 Loss plot of VGG11 model of Fallon MobiAct dataset.

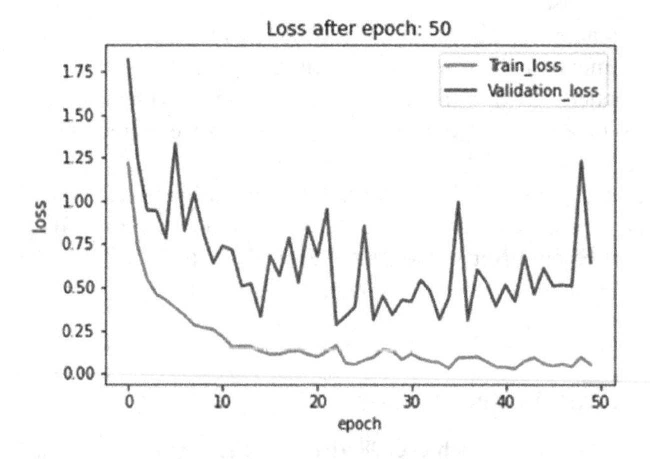

FIGURE 3.13 Loss plot of ResNet-18model of ADLs on MobiAct dataset.

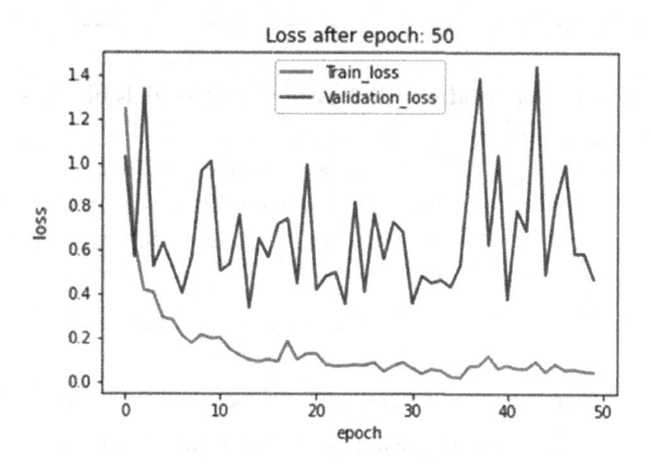

FIGURE 3.14 Loss plot of GoogLeNet model of ADLs on MobiAct dataset.

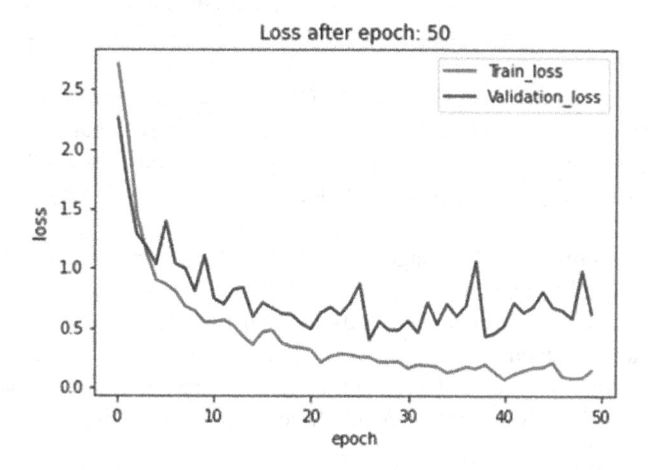

FIGURE 3.15 Loss plot of VGG11 model of ADLs on MobiAct dataset.

TABLE 3.7
Comparison of Our Proposed Model with Previous HAR Models Including Fall and ADLs

Research	Number of Activity	Type of Activities Considered	Accuracy (%)
C. Chatzaki et al. [26]	16	STD, JOG,WAL, STU,STN, JUM,SCH, CHU,CSI, SIT,CSO,LYI,FOL,BSC,SDL,FKL.	97.1
Our Proposed Model	15	STD,JOG, WAL,JUM,STN,SCH,STU,CHU,C SI,SIT,CSO,FOL,BSC,SDL,FKL,	98.91

observed from Tables 3.7, 3.8 and 3.9 that our proposed ResNet-18 model performs better than previous work.

3.5 CONCLUSION

The present work shows the use of three different types of CNN models in human activity reorganization. Based on the three model experimental result comparison, we can see that the ResNet-18

TABLE 3.8
Comparison of Our Proposed Model with Previous HAR Models of ADLs

Research	Number of Activities	Type of Activities Considered	Accuracy (%)
Hongkai et al.[29]	11	STD, JOG, STU,STN, JUM,SCH,SIT,CSI,CSO, WAL,,CHU	97.66
Our Proposed Model	11	STD,JOG, WAL,STU,STN,JUM, SCH,SIT,CSI,CSO,CHU	97.73

TABLE 3.9
Comparison of Our Proposed Model with Previous HAR Models of Falls.

Research	Number of Activities	Type of Activities Considered	Accuracy (%)
PaulCompagnon et al. [27]	4	FOL, FKL, BSC, SDL	91.1
Our Proposed Model	4	FOL,FKL,BSC,SDL	94.41

model performs better than the GoogLeNet and VGG11 models and provides better accuracy than previous benchmark on ADLs and fall of the MobiAct V2 dataset; that is, the proposed simple framework is found to very much outperform other popular methods. This is the main contribution of this paper. For further improvements in this field, we can do the following:

- Extract deep features from the images and classify them using traditional ML classifiers such as SVM, KNN and so on.
- Reduce the data frame from five seconds for real-time HAR prediction from different types of IoTs and smartphones.
- Use various optimization algorithms such as genetic algorithm and particle swarm optimizer for optimal feature set selection and dimensionality reduction.

So the proposed work provides a solid foundation for using CNN-based transfer learning for human activity reorganization. It can be integrated with different types of IoTs and smartphones which will be beneficial in various domains such as mobile apps and healthcare.

REFERENCES

1. F. Tahavori, et al., "Physical activity recognition of elderly people and people with parkinson's (PwP) during standard mobility tests using wearable sensors,". International Smart Cities Conference (ISC2), pp. 1–4, 2017, doi: 10.1109/ISC2.2017.8090858.
2. O. D. Lara and M. A. Labrador, "A survey on human activity recognition using wearable sensors," *IEEE Commun. Surv. Tutorials*, vol. 15, no. 3, pp. 1192–1209, 2013, doi: 10.1109/SURV.2012.110112.00192.
3. N. Y. Hammerla, S. Halloran, and T. Plötz, "Deep, convolutional, and recurrent models for human activity recognition using wearables," *IJCAI Int. Jt. Conf. Artif. Intell.*, vol. 2016, pp. 1533–1540, 2016.
4. D. Mukherjee, R. Mondal, P. K. Singh, R. Sarkar, and D. Bhattacharjee, "EnsemConvNet: a deep learning approach for human activity recognition using smartphone sensors for healthcare applications," *Multimed. Tools Appl.*, vol. 79, no. 41, pp. 31663–31690, 2020, doi: 10.1007/s11042-020-09537-7.
5. S. Chakraborty, R. Mondal, P. K. Singh, R. Sarkar, and D. Bhattacharjee, "Transfer learning with fine tuning for human action recognition from still images," *Multimed. Tools Appl.*, vol. 80, no. 13, pp. 20547–20578, 2021, doi: 10.1007/s11042-021-10753-y.
6. R. Mondal, D. Mukhopadhyay, S. Barua, P. K. Singh, R. Sarkar, and D. Bhattacharjee, "Chapter 14 - a study on smartphone sensor-based human activity recognition using deep learning approaches". In J. Nayak, B. Naik, D. Pelusi, and A. K. B. T.-H. of C. I. in B. E. and H. Das, (Eds.), Handbook of Computational Intelligence in Biomedical Engineering and Healthcare, Academic Press, 2021, pp. 343–369.

7. S. O'Dea, "Number of smartphone users from 2016 to 2021," *Statista*, https://www.statista.com/statistics/330695/number-of-smartphone-users-worldwide/.
8. A. Dey, S. Chattopadhyay, P. K. Singh, A. Ahmadian, M. Ferrara, and R. Sarkar, "A hybrid meta-heuristic feature selection method using golden ratio and equilibrium optimization algorithms for speech emotion recognition," *IEEE Access*, vol. 8, pp. 200953–200970, 2020, doi: 10.1109/ACCESS.2020.3035531.
9. D. Garcia-Gonzalez, D. Rivero, E. Fernandez-Blanco, and M. R. Luaces, "A public domain dataset for real-life human activity recognition using smartphone sensors," *Sensors (Switzerland)*, vol. 20, no. 8, 2020, doi: 10.3390/s20082200.
10. I. Pires, N. Garcia, N. Pombo, F. Flórez-Revuelta, and S. Spinsante, "Pattern recognition techniques for the identification of activities of daily living using mobile device accelerometer," *PeerJ Preprints*, vol. 7, e27225v2 2019.
11. W. T. D'souza and R. Kavitha, "Human activity recognition using accelerometer and gyroscope sensors," *International journal of engineering and technology*, vol. 9, no. 2017, 1171–1179, 2017, doi: 10.21817/ijet/2017/v9i2/170902134.
12. S. Chattopadhyay, L. Zary, C. Quek, and D. K. Prasad, "Motivation detection using EEG signal analysis by residual-in-residual convolutional neural network [Formula presented]," *Expert Syst. Appl.*, vol. 184, no. February, 2021, doi: 10.1016/j.eswa.2021.115548.
13. S. Chattopadhyay, A. Dey, P. K. Singh, Z. W. Geem, and R. Sarkar, "Covid-19 detection by optimizing deep residual features with improved clustering-based golden ratio optimizer," *Diagnostics*, vol. 11, no. 2, pp. 1–27, 2021, doi: 10.3390/diagnostics11020315.
14. S. Chattopadhyay and H. Basak, "Multi-scale Attention U-Net (MsAUNet): a modified U-Net architecture for scene segmentation," 2020, http://arxiv.org/abs/2009.06911.
15. S. Chattopadhyay, A. Dey, and H. Basak, "Optimizing speech emotion recognition using Manta-Ray based feature selection," no. 2, 2020, http://arxiv.org/abs/2009.08909.
16. H. Basak, S. Ghosal, M. Sarkar, M. Das, and S. Chattopadhyay, "Monocular depth estimation using encoder-decoder architecture and transfer learning from single RGB image," in *2020 IEEE 7th Uttar Pradesh Section International Conference on Electrical, Electronics and Computer Engineering (UPCON)*, pp. 1–6, 2020, doi: 10.1109/UPCON50219.2020.9376365.
17. A. Das, P. Sil, P. K. Singh, V. Bhateja, and R. Sarkar, "MMHAR-EnsemNet: a multi-modal human activity recognition model," *IEEE Sens. J.*, vol. 21, no. 10, pp. 11569–11576, 2021, doi: 10.1109/JSEN.2020.3034614.
18. B. Yoshua and C. Aaron, *Deep Learning (Adaptive Computation and Machine Learning Series)*. The MIT Press, 2016
19. A. Bayat, M. Pomplun, and D. A. Tran, "A study on human activity recognition using accelerometer data from smartphones," *Procedia Computer Science*, vol. 34, 2014, doi: 10.1016/j.procs.2014.07.009.
20. A. Anjum and M. U. Ilyas, "Activity recognition using smartphone sensors," in *2013 IEEE 10th Consumer Communications and Networking Conference (CCNC)*, pp. 914–919, 2013, doi: 10.1109/CCNC.2013.6488584.
21. L. Zheng, Y. Cai, Z. Lin, W. Tang, H. Zheng, H. Shi, B. Liao, and J. Wang, A novel activity recognition approach based on mobile phone. In J. Park, SC. Chen, JM. Gil, N. Yen (Eds.), Multimedia and Ubiquitous Engineering. Lecture Notes in Electrical Engineering, vol 308. Berlin, Heidelberg: Springer. 2014, doi: 10.1007/978-3-642-54900-7_9.
22. T. R. D. Saputri, A. M. Khan, and S. W. Lee, "User-independent activity recognition via three-stage GA-based feature selection," *Int. J. Distrib. Sens. Networks*, vol. 2014, 1–152014, doi: 10.1155/2014/706287.
23. P. Siirtola and J. Röning, *Ready-to-Use Activity Recognition for Smartphones*, pp. 59–64, 2013. doi: 10.1109/CIDM.2013.6597218.
24. E. Buber and A. Guvensan, *Discriminative Time-Domain Features for Activity Recognition on a Mobile Phone*. 2014 IEEE Ninth International Conference on Intelligent Sensors, Sensor Networks and Information Processing (ISSNIP), pp. 1–6, 2014, doi: 10.1109/ISSNIP.2014.6827651.
25. G. Vavoulas, C. Chatzaki, T. Malliotakis, M. Pediaditis, and M. Tsiknakis, "The MobiActDataset: recognition of activities of daily living using smartphones," In Proceedings of the International Conference on Information and Communication Technologies for Ageing Well and e-Health (ICT4AWE 2016), pp. 143–151. 2016, ISBN: 978-989-758-180-9.
26. C. Chatzaki, M. Pediaditis, and G. Vavoulas, Human daily activity and fall recognition using a smartphone's acceleration sensor. In Carsten Röcker, John O'Donoghue, Martina Ziefle, Markus Helfert & William Molloy (Ed.), ICT4AgeingWell (Selected Papers), Springer, pp. 100–118, 2016

27. P. Compagnon, “Personalized posture and fall classification with shallow gated recurrent units,” 2019 IEEE 32nd International Symposium on Computer-Based Medical Systems (CBMS), 2019, pp. 114–119, doi: 10.1109/CBMS.2019.00034.
28. P. Compagnon, G. Lefebvre, S. Duffner, and C. Garcia, “Learning personalized ADL recognition models from few raw data,” *Artif. Intell. Med.*, vol. 107, p. 101916, 2020, doi: https://doi.org/10.1016/j.artmed.2020.101916.
29. H. Chen, S. Mahfuz and F. Zulkernine, "Smart Phone Based Human Activity Recognition," 2019 IEEE International Conference on Bioinformatics and Biomedicine (BIBM), 2019, pp. 2525–2532, doi: 10.1109/BIBM47256.2019.8983009.
30. M. M. Hassan, A. Gumaei, G. Aloi, G. Fortino and M. Zhou, "A Smartphone-Enabled Fall Detection Framework for Elderly People in Connected Home Healthcare," in IEEE Network, vol. 33, no. 6, pp. 58–63, Nov.-Dec. 2019, doi: 10.1109/MNET.001.1900100.
31. E. Ramanujam, S. Padmavathi, G. Dharshani and M. R. R. Madhumitta, "Evaluation of Feature Extraction and Recognition for Human Activity using Smartphone based Accelerometer data," 2019 11th International Conference on Advanced Computing (ICoAC), pp. 86–89, 2019, doi: 10.1109/ICoAC48765.2019.247124.
32. R. DiPietro, C. Rupprecht, N. Navab, and G. D. Hager, “Analyzing and exploiting NARX recurrent neural networks for long-term dependencies,” Workshop track - ICLR 2018 pp. 1–14, 2017.
33. R. Mondal, D. Mukherjee, P. K. Singh, V. Bhateja, and R. Sarkar, “A new framework for smartphone sensor-based human activity recognition using graph neural network,” *IEEE Sens. J.*, vol. 21, no. 10, pp. 11461–11468, 2021, doi: 10.1109/JSEN.2020.3015726.
34. R. Guha, A. H. Khan, P. K. Singh, R. Sarkar, and D. Bhattacharjee, “CGA: a new feature selection model for visual human action recognition,” *Neural Comput. Appl.*, vol. 33, no. 10, pp. 5267–5286, 2021, doi: 10.1007/s00521-020-05297-5.
35. K. Simonyan and A. Zisserman, “Very deep convolutional networks for large-scale image recognition,” *3rd Int. Conf. Learn. Represent. ICLR 2015 - Conf. Track Proc.*, pp. 1–14, 2015.
36. C. Szegedy, W. Liu, Y. Jia, P. Sermanet, S. Reed, D. Anguelov, D. Erhan, V. Vanhoucke, A. Rabinovich “Going deeper with convolutions,” Proceedings of the IEEE Conference on Computer Vision and Pattern Recognition (CVPR), vol. 07–12 June, pp. 1–9, 2015, doi: 10.1109/CVPR.2015.7298594.
37. K. He, X. Zhang, S. Ren, and J. Sun, “Deep residual learning for image recognition,” *Proc. IEEE Comput. Soc. Conf. Comput. Vis. Pattern Recognit.*, vol. 2016 December, pp. 770–778, 2016, doi: 10.1109/CVPR.2016.90.
38. P. Lemenkova, Python libraries matplotlib, seaborn and pandas for visualization geospatial datasets generated by QGIS. *Analele Stiintifice Ale Universitatii "alexandru Ioan Cuza" Din Iasi - Seria Geografie*, vol. 64, no. 1, 13–32. 2020 https://doi.org/10.5281/zenodo.4050413.
39. M. Grandini, E. Bagli, and G. Visani, “Metrics for multi-class classification: an overview,” pp. 1–17, 2020, http://arxiv.org/abs/2008.05756.

4 Internet of Things with Machine Learning-Based Smart Cardiovascular Disease Classifier for Healthcare in Secure Platform

Sima Das, Jaya Das, Subrata Modak, and Kaushik Mazumdar

CONTENTS

4.1 INTRODUCTION

In today's epoch, different cardiac diseases and cardiopulmonary arrest are the most common problems in majority of people. Peoples are not focusing on or paying attention to their health problems because of various reasons like work pressure, stress, or indolence. Bad quality of food also raises cholesterol levels. Furthermore, lack of technology results in a delay in the diagnosis of these types of diseases [1]. Modern healthcare technologies not only abet the physicians an early diagnosis of ailment but also helps to lower the death rate [2]. The world is digitalized day by day and maximum health records are saved on online platforms. Internet of Things with machine learning techniques

DOI: 10.1201/9781003217398-4

are creating a smart intelligent platform in the world. Electronic health records and mobile health data are popularized for their efficiency. Data theft is the most challenging thing for virtual platforms. Data breach costs $380 per record according to data breach study's phenomenon cost in 2017 and 27314647 records of patients were breached according to the report of breach barometer in 2016 [3]. The main objective of a smart healthcare system is privacy and accuracy. In our previous work, the heartbeat rate of subjects was measured in three categories: normal, slow, and fast, by using a backpropagation neural network while watching a movie and the rating of the movie was sent by the user using Telegram Bot [4].

In this chapter, we focus on the gap between secure data preserving techniques for human–computer interaction. Our proposed model captures electrocardiogram signals via an intelligent IoT sensor, and by using blockchain, data can be secured in an online database platform. Data can be classified as to whether a person has suffered from cardiovascular disease or not by using machine learning techniques.

4.1.1 Introduction to Cardiovascular Disease

Cardiovascular disease (CVD) belongs to a class of diseases that concern the blood vessels or heart. CVD comprises myocardial and angina infarction (commonly known as a heart attack), also called coronary artery disease (CAD). Strokes and heart attacks are usually acute events, and these are primarily caused by a blockage that obstructs the blood flow to the heart or brain. The general reason is the deposit of fat build-up on the blood vessel's inner walls which supply the blood to the brain or heart. Strokes can occur by bleeding in the brain from blood clots or from a blood vessel. Other CVDs include heart failure (sometimes known as congestive heart failure, which occurs if blood pumping by the heart is not as good as it should), cardiomyopathy, thromboembolic disease, stroke, hypertensive heart disease, abnormal heart rhythms, rheumatic heart disease (a bacteria-caused, mainly streptococcal-induced, damage to heart valves and muscles of the heart by a fever called rheumatic fever), congenital heart disease (defects from birth that impact the natural functioning and development of the heart caused by the impairment of structure of the heart), venous thrombosis, valvular heart disease, peripheral artery disease (a blood vessels disease which is the medium to supply blood to the legs and arms), carditis, and aortic aneurysms.

Depending on the disease, the underlying mechanisms vary. Stroke, peripheral artery disease, and coronary artery disease imply atherosclerosis. This may be caused by smoking, high blood pressure, lack of exercise, obesity, diabetes mellitus, poor diet, high cholesterol of blood, and an excessive amount of alcohol consumption, among others. Prevention of CVD is possible by improving health by doing exercise and eating a healthy diet and by minimizing risk factors by avoiding alcohol intake, smoking, and tobacco use. Treating risk factors like blood lipids, diabetes, and high blood pressure is also beneficial. Treating persons having strep throat with antibiotics decreases the risk of rheumatic heart disease.

4.1.2 Introduction to Machine Learning Method for Cardiovascular Disease Classification

Cardiovascular disease is a class of coronary artery diseases (myocardial infarction angina, hypertensive heart disease, stroke, heart failure, abnormal heart disease, etc.) (Figure 4.1).

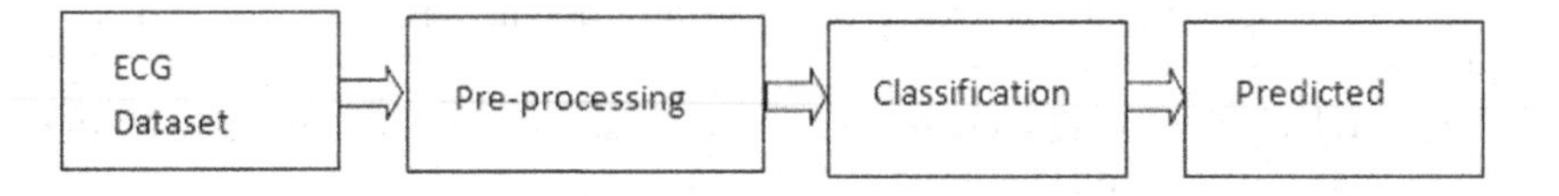

FIGURE 4.1 Generalized machine learning method for disease classification.

4.1.3 Introduction to Internet of Things in Healthcare

Internet of Things (IoT) expresses the network for physical "things" – those that are immersed with software, sensors, and other technologies for the requirement of exchanging data by connecting over the internet with other devices. The new motion of connectivity is going in the direction of connected smart homes, cars, connected wearables, connected healthcare and smart cities, and as far as smartphones and laptops. We can say that the IoT provides, in essence, a linked living. Progressively, to add intelligence to IoT devices, IoT applications employ machine learning and artificial intelligence. IoT applications on devices can be precise to more or less every industry, including healthcare. Patients' connections with doctors are limited to telephonic visits and text communications without Internet of Things. Without IoT, it becomes difficult to monitor the health of a patient regularly and continuously by hospitals or doctors and to provide recommendations to a patient properly and timely. Use of Internet of Things (IoT) empowered devices help the patients to stay healthy; remote monitoring technique help physicians to monitor patient health condition remotely. IoT has also escalated patient satisfaction and engagement because of easier and more efficient interactions of patients with doctors. Furthermore, the hospital stay length is reduced and re-admissions are prevented by patient's health remote monitoring. The Internet of Things also has a super impact on cost reduction in healthcare and on improving treatment outcomes. In delivering healthcare solutions by redefining the devices' space and people interaction, IoT is unquestionably transforming the healthcare industry worldwide. IoT has provided benefits to patients, physicians, families, hospitals and also to insurance companies, by its application.

4.1.4 Introduction of Blockchain

In the healthcare industry, a high volume of sensitive data is being generated from daily patient monitoring data, insurance policy processed records, financial truncation records, clinical research, and medical records. Online healthcare services like the electronic medical record (EMR) play a sensitive role in the healthcare industry for sharing, storing, accessing, and processing personal patient data [5, 6]. Security of such sensitive information is an important concern today as most of the patient monitoring data are coming from different Internet of Things (IoT)-based health care monitoring devices [7]. There are a number of security issues in the healthcare industry which cause theft of patient-sensitive records.

A blockchain can be thought of as a type of database. One basic difference between a blockchain and a typical database is the way the structure of the data is organized. Information collected together in a batch in blockchain is known as blocks. Blocks hold information sets. Blocks are chained onto the earlier filled block. Blocks have certain storage capacities and forming this chain of data is called "blockchain". New information follows a freshly added block, assembling into a block, which is freshly formed that once filled is attached to the chain. The aim of blockchain is to permit digital data to be distributed and recorded, but not allow them to be edited (Figure 4.2).

4.1.5 Structure of the Blockchain Technology

Hash, Timestamp, other information, and data are the main components of each block of a blockchain network. The blockchain structure is given in Figure 4.3.

- Data

In the block, the use of data depends on the specific application such as it may be the services in the blockchain network [8, 9]. For example: the bank accounts data, banking transaction of an organization, medical records of patients or data of IoT sensors. In order to make decisions, these data are used in many applications, like healthcare systems and IoT devices [10].

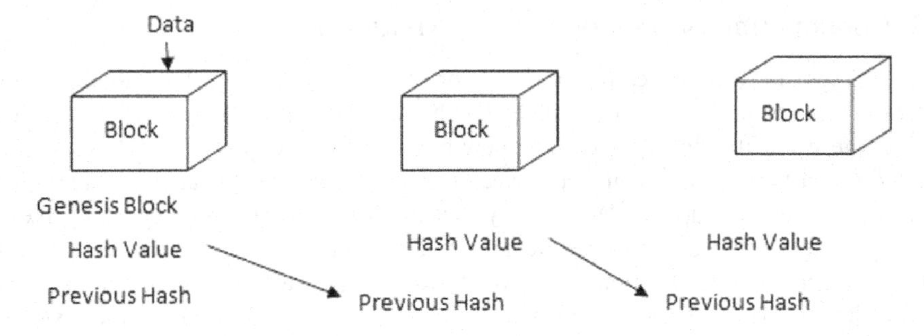

FIGURE 4.2 working principle of the blockchain.

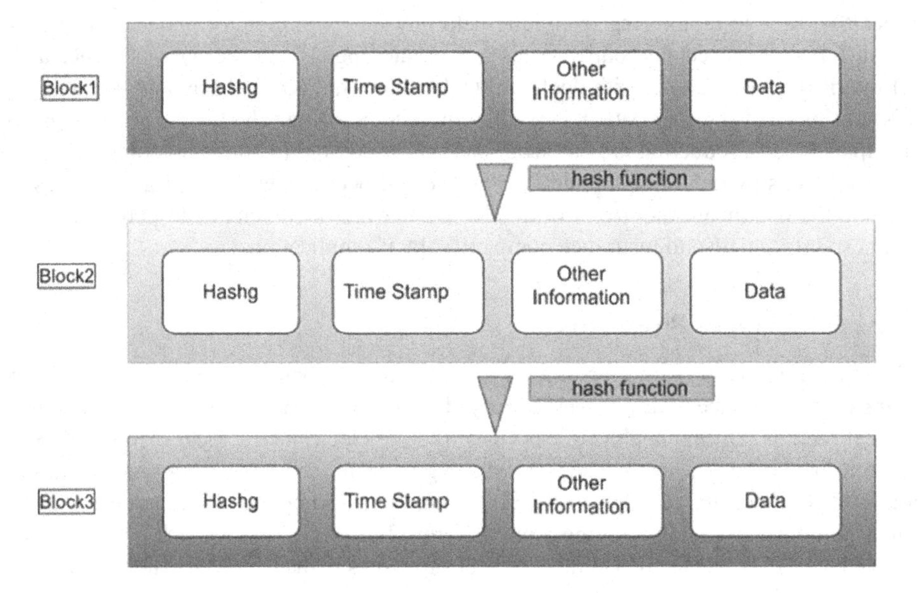

FIGURE 4.3 Structure of the blockchain.

- Hash

Hash is a special function that is most important in the blockchain. Data of a block can be of any size. The hash function is applied to the data in order to generate a unique, fixed-size hash value. The output of the hash value significantly changes if the original block data is modified [9, 11]. This hash function is performed on the data after the transactions of the block are executed, and the result is transmitted to every node [8].

- Timestamp

Timestamp is a time value that is used to indicate the change of the data in the block. The timestamp function is applied to generate the timestamp after applying the hash function when the block data is modified in the network [8, 9, 11].

- Other Information

The supplementary information is related to data that could be nBits, user-defined, and blocks signature values [8, 9, 10] (Figure 4.4).

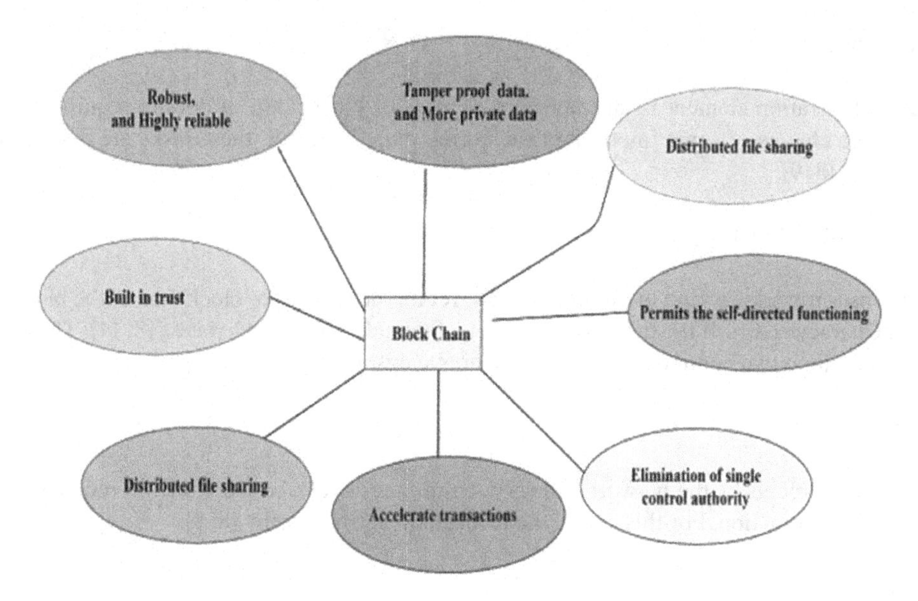

FIGURE 4.4 Advantages of blockchain technology.

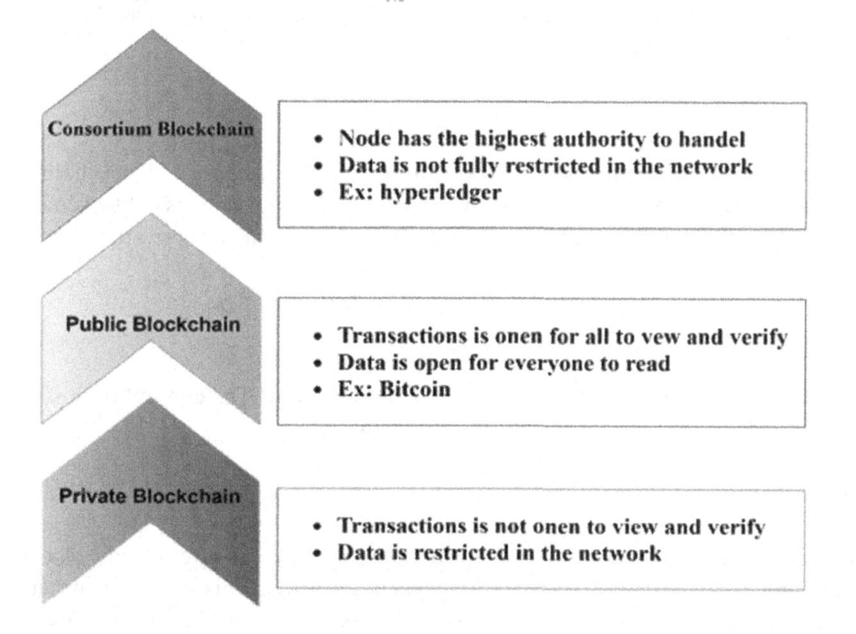

FIGURE 4.5 Taxonomy of blockchain.

4.1.6 Taxonomy of Blockchain

Mainly three types of blockchain are available in blockchain technology: private blockchain, consortium blockchain, and public blockchain [8, 9, 10, 12, 13, 14]. Figure 4.3 shows and describes the concept of each type of blockchain. The particular type of blockchain is used depending on the services and appropriate area where the Blockchain is fit for [10] (Figure 4.5).

4.1.7 Blockchain Elements

Many elements are used in blockchain to ease the particular services given by the blockchain network [8, 9].

- Decentralization

This decentralization element is an important element of blockchain. It doesn't require a central node that is a change of some important task storing data. However, these tasks are disseminated among nodes [8, 9].

- Consensus Model:

The consensus model is a kind of protocol used to retain the privacy of block data in the blockchain network. Characteristics of the protocols are safety, fault tolerance, and liveness [8, 14]. These properties are based on two contrivances, which are applicability and efficiency [8].

- Transparent

The blockchain rechecks the network in every ten minutes cycle, which works to reconcile in the middle of the transaction. For this cause, the blockchain is trustworthy [8, 9].

- Open Source

Only public blockchain technology has access rights. Everyone can set up an application or use the benefits of public blockchain [9].

- Access and Identity

The access and identity of each node of blockchain rely on the category of blockchain technology [8]. The public blockchain permits everyone to view and verify transactions of blockchain. The data is not completely confidential in the case of consortium blockchain. The private blockchain data is confidential [8, 9].

- Autonomy

The blockchain data is transmitted and modified in a secure way. The concept of this autonomy is to assure everybody's trust in the whole blockchain network [8, 9].

- Immutable

Since the data is stored and accessed in a secure way, nobody can alter or edit block data. The modification process is settled on the data in a specific process. This process is executed by the authorized person only when he has authority over the node in the blockchain network [8, 9].

- Anonymity

Trust is the big trouble that occurs between nodes. Trust problems can be solved by transferring data between known nodes in the network. That doesn't require any other information, for example, a person's details or any other information [8, 9].

The rest of the chapter includes (4.2) literature survey, (4.3) proposed work, (4.4) conclusion and future work.

4.2 LITERATURE SURVEY

Literature surveys on security in healthcare using IoT and ML techniques are as follows:

Blockchain technology is being recommended to secure the storage of medical data according to Azaria et al. [15]. The authors addressed a blockchain-based network approach to diminish the problem of the inter-portability of medical data. The main issue is that the Ethereum-based permissionless blockchain technology is employed to secure the storage of data. Dwivedi et al. [16] have introduced blockchain-based secure information exchange protocols using key distribution in supply chain management to resolve issues of tampering with product information, delayed product delivery, fraud, vital features such as decentralization, information transparency, and a trustless environment. They have addressed smart contract approaches for key distribution to all the connected people, block, and transaction validation protocols.

Stacked Denoising Autoencoders [17] and its property have been improved for the classification of arrhythmias. A vast amount of stream data is put down from remote systems for a long period. Blockchain technology is proposed to securely access data and storage from outside storage locations.

Telecare Medical Information Systems have been proposed to protect patient-sensitive data shared via the insecure public internet. The key establishment protocols and authentication protocols have been recommended to secure the transmission of medical records between the medical server and the patient party. They have mainly focused on Madhusudhan-Nayak protocols which are unable to provide anonymity and unable to achieve mutual authentication. Authors have improved the mutual authentication method using key establishment for TMIS [18].

Intelligent-based recommendations system not only enhances patient lifestyle but also reduces the periodic clinical check-up cost. System statistical data analysis helps to find more appropriate suggestive recommendations from time to time for the patient [19].

An electrocardiogram diagnostic system plays a significant role to analyse and predict cardiovascular diseases in patients. Heartbeat rhythms pattern helps to find cardiovascular disease by applying popular, well-known techniques such as classification and feature selection techniques [20, 21].

The classification process and the feature extraction process have been used to find accurate results for cardiac disease by using the algorithms such as convolutional neural network, support vector machine (SVM), principal component analysis, and fuzzy-C-mean [22, 23]. The tree-based approach is used to classify heart failure chances in Canada and tree-based computation results give highly correct results as a contrast to the convolutional-based regression tree algorithm. Logistic regression, Naïve Bayes, backpropagation, decision tree, and bagging neural network are the popular ML-based techniques for disease prediction in future.

In their study, Marshal et al. [24], they faced security challenges and analyzed important features to be taken for better security for IoT-based smart healthcare devices. The Internet of Things' enormous range of applications and benefits has enticed every industry to implement it in their environs in order to reap its benefits. The implementation of devices from various manufacturers in the Internet of Things area has also allowed threat actors to conduct a variety of assaults by putting to use vulnerabilities in these devices.

The main objective of the work by K. Matousek [25], is to protect the distributed healthcare system from risk analysis, security awareness, network protection, and application protection. The purpose of this paper is to summarize and introduce the essential security and dependability considerations for designing software systems which are distributed in healthcare. It specifies the security goal as well as the safeguarding of system assets. The importance of risk analysis is emphasized. The weaknesses and threats to the system are presented. Human security awareness is required, as are conventional security and reliability.

In their work by A. Jayanthilladevi et al. [26], Protected Healthcare Information (PHI) and HIPPA Act for electronic health records for discussing various necessities to safeguard confidentiality and privacy are discussed. The healthcare industry has seen a pattern shift as a result of the digitizing medical record, which has increased the data's complexity, diversity, and timeliness. Security breaches in healthcare databases pose a serious threat to the healthcare business. Medical identity theft, such as data breaches, has left patients in a state of destitution as a result of fraudulent data and stolen information.

In their work by J. Kwon et al. [27], market technique can encourage healthcare businesses towards successful enterprising and honorary security initiatives, notwithstanding the ambiguities of healthcare security costs and benefits. The efficiency of market processes, on the other hand, is hampered by the economic dynamics of the defective US healthcare system. As a result, across all sorts of investments, market-driven investments must be complemented with regulatory intervention.

In the work by Z. O. Omogbadegun [28], healthcare informatics indicates that, particularly inside the official health industry, healthcare poses the biggest issues of user control, with disparate, personalized, and sometimes fragile user permission for limited information to assess service quality and little choice. In addition, consulting expertise in a variety of healthcare organization (HCO) IT contexts strongly suggests that technological security foundations are important.

In the study of Y. He and C. W. Johnson [29], it is highlighted that several data breach cases have occurred in the past few years, and patient and clinician confidentiality must continue to be protected. However, the market's multiplicity of privacy goods, methods, and methodologies make it difficult for management to confirm that they've put in place consistent countermeasures to achieve the organization's higher-level goals. This article explores the challenges that health organizations face while developing and maintaining cybersecurity policies. We employ pictorial argumentation strategies to solve these issues. They explain the goal structuring notations (GSN), i.e., how it can be used for more than just adaptation.

In their study, Y. Tao and H. Lee [30], have fostered a multi-layered cloud security system to work with cloud clients' need to coordinate with their security necessities with security arrangements of cloud specialist co-ops (CSPs). Their paper covers research that reviews the holes in spanning MTCS and Singapore's Healthcare IT Security Policy (HITSecP) so CSPs who have been confirmed to MTCS can know how well and best they could meet the security prerequisites of IT frameworks for the medical services industry in Singapore.

In their work, N. Bruce et al. [31], proposed a middleware solution for securing data and networks in an e-healthcare system. Due to the sensor devices' easy deployment area accessibility, e-healthcare systems are a significant concern. Furthermore, they frequently interact intimately with the physical environment and the people around them, increasing security risks in circumstances where they are exposed.

In their work C. H. Ip et al. [32], reported that due of the growing population, the city's rapid growth necessitates the expansion of government healthcare services for the general public. A temporary government healthcare service is set up at a university with a functioning hospital to address the urgent needs of a large number of residents. As a result, resources (medical equipment and IT services) have been reduced.

In their study, J. Kwon and M. E. Johnson [33], reported that, for IT managers, regulatory compliance and data security are critical goals. This study evaluates the impact of IT security resources, functional capabilities, and managerial capabilities on regulatory compliance and data security, based on the resource-based approach. We examine data from 250 healthcare companies using binomial and multinomial log-logistic models. The findings suggest that IT security is important.

In [34], physically, the healthcare system is made up of a variety of sub-networks. It's tough to respond to hazardous traffic like warm viruses that damage entire networks because each sub-network has its own management privileges and policies. In this study, we suggest a high-level policy language for the healthcare system as well as a middle-level data structure. They were given the names Triton and Common.

In their work, Kanghee Lee et al. [35], proposed that the hospital industry is looking at incorporating digital technologies to improve access, lower prices, improve quality, and expand their ability to reach a larger number of people. However, this exposes healthcare organizations' systems to external elements employed within or outside of their facilities, introducing new risks and vulnerabilities in terms of cyber threats and mishaps.

In their work, A. I. Newaz et al. [36], reported that the hospital industry is looking at incorporating digital technologies to improve access, lower prices, improve quality, and expand their ability to reach a larger number of people. However, this exposes healthcare organizations' systems to external elements employed within or outside of their facilities, introducing new risks and vulnerabilities in terms of cyber threats and mishaps.

H. Kupwade Patil and R. Seshadri [37] reported that with the rising expense of healthcare and rising health insurance rates, preventive healthcare and wellness are more important than ever. Furthermore, the healthcare business has undergone a paradigm shift as a result of the current wave of medical record digitization. As a result, the healthcare business is dealing with an increase in data volume, complexity, diversity, and timeliness. Big data emerges as a viable solution with the potential to alter the healthcare industry as healthcare experts hunt for every conceivable way to reduce costs while enhancing the care process, delivery, and management. This shift in focus from reactive to proactive healthcare may result in a reduction in overall health care costs.

In their work, B. C. Kara et al. [38], reported that with innovative innovations, the healthcare sector has progressed from Healthcare 1.0 to Healthcare 4.0. While Healthcare 1.0 is focused on doctors, Healthcare 4.0 employs cutting-edge technologies, such as the Internet of Things (IoT), big data, fog computing, and cloud computing, to share data among several stakeholders. While Healthcare 4.0 has numerous benefits, it has also created significant security and privacy concerns. The security and privacy issues in Healthcare 4.0 are discussed in this paper, as well as the approaches established to address these issues in the literature.

A. Yogeshwar and S. Kamalakkannan [39] reported that the Internet of Things (IoT) has a huge and growing impact all over the world. IoT is a technology that collects data and information from a variety of sensors and other smart devices. Those who benefit from IoT technology can share information and connect with smart devices amongst themselves.

IoT delivers additional convenience to doctors, nurses, and patients in the healthcare sector. It can be more efficient for monitoring and diagnosing people with illnesses while also lowering costs. In the healthcare system, there are several security breaches and malicious assaults that are particularly vulnerable, such as forgery, privacy leakage, and so on.

P. K. Yeng et al. [40] reported that cyber defences have indeed been bolstered by technological countermeasures, and adversaries tend to target easy entry points. Furthermore, healthcare personnel are frequently preoccupied with their primary responsibility of providing healthcare, and have limited experience with information security. Observational measures for successful profiling of healthcare staff were developed using a design science approach (DSA).

In their work, A. K. Alharam and W. Elmedany [41] reported that, a wide range of wearable IoT healthcare applications have been developed and deployed in recent years. The fast proliferation of wearable devices enables the sharing of patients' personal information between devices, while also allowing for the tracking and attack on patients' personal health and wellbeing information. Patient information is protected in medical and wearable devices in a variety of ways. A comparison of the complexity of cybersecurity architecture and its implementation in the IoT healthcare business was conducted in this study. The study's goal is to secure the healthcare business from cyber threats, with a concentration on IoT-based treatment.

In their work, M. Evans et al. [42], tried to gather insights into the underlying problem of health error, that is, the most frequent cause of data security events in a private healthcare business. The IS-CHEC information security human reliability analysis (HRA) technique was proactively applied using a survey questionnaire. The IS-CHEC technique questionnaire determined the most likely core human error causes that could lead to incidents, their likelihood, the most likely tasks that could be affected, suggested remedial and preventive measures, structures or methods that would've been likely to be influenced by human mistakes, as well as vulnerability to health hazards.

In [43], the current security research efforts are mostly motivated by the desire to assure the security and usability of healthcare software. Practitioners are always developing techniques to improve security while maintaining ease of use. Despite the countless efforts made by developers and security professionals in this regard, the degree of usability-security is not what it should be. Furthermore, greater research into the most effective ways for evaluating and improving the usability-security of healthcare technology is required. Quantitative usability and security testing is a key aspect in raising software security requirements in particular.

F. A. Al-Zahrani [44], reported that in industry, public sectors, and in research, electronic health record (EHR) systems have acquired a great amount of attention to neatly enhance the standard of healthcare. However, major issues i.e. security and privacy still require forward investigations. In the acquisition of EHR solutions, the identification of the consequences of different security strands has been done along with a growing research work which has aimed to intercept these issues. In the past few years, monitoring of Security has attracted growing attention, which is one of the issues. A mechanism that detects anomalous behaviour and security violations during an operation is called security monitoring. That type of violation identification can be done at the business layer or at lower technical layers.

In their work, W. Iqbal et al. [45], reported the role of Internet of Things (IoT) in monitoring and controlling of the connected smart objects, is transforming the life of everyone. IoT applications explore a broad scale of services together with smart cities, cars, homes, manufacturing, smart control systems, e-healthcare, transportation, farming, wearables, and many more. The acquisition of these devices is exponentially growing, by offering a considerable amount of data or information for analyzing and processing. These devices are also susceptible to different security challenges and threats, which not only worry the enjoyer for accepting it in a sensitive environment, such as smart home and e-health, but also give rise to hazards for the IoT advancement in upcoming days. The article rigorously reviews the security requirements, threats, pertinent attack vectors, and challenges to the IoT networks. A novel approach that combines a network-based formation of IoT architecture by way of software-defined networking (SDN) is suggested based on the analysis of the gap. The article presents an outline of the software-defined networking along with an all-over discussion on IoT deployment models which are SDN-based, i.e. centralized and decentralized. They further embellished SDN-based security solutions of IoT to present a far-reaching overview of the SDSec (software-defined security) technology. Additionally, based upon the literature, many core issues are underlined that are the main obstacles in unifying all stakeholders of IoT on the same platform and few discoveries that are prominent on network-based security solutions for the IoT standard. Lastly, some future directions of research of SDN-based technologies of IoT security are talked about.

In their work, K. K. Karmakar et al. [46], reported that the smart healthcare zone and the Internet of Medical Things (IoMT) are getting popular. These devices are exposed to attack and are resource-inhibited. IoMT becomes the main target of the adversary because of weak privacy and security measures, as it is associated with the network infrastructure of healthcare. In this concern, they propose a security architecture which is for smart healthcare network infrastructures, in this paper. The proposed architecture uses numerous services and security components that are established as virtual network functions. The security architecture becomes ready because of this concept, for future network frameworks like Open MANO.

4.3 PROPOSED WORK

Proposed work of the current system will be discussed in this section.

4.3.1 Flowchart of the Proposed Work

The development and use of computer systems are able to adapt and learn without following direct instructions, by using statistical models and algorithms to draw and analyse assumptions from data patterns. Or by using a concept that permits the machine to learn from experience and examples, and that without being programmed directly, called machine learning. So rather than writing the code, data is fed to the algorithm or machine, and the algorithm or machine, according to the given data, builds the logic. The application to biological databases has increased day by day of machine learning (Figure 4.6).

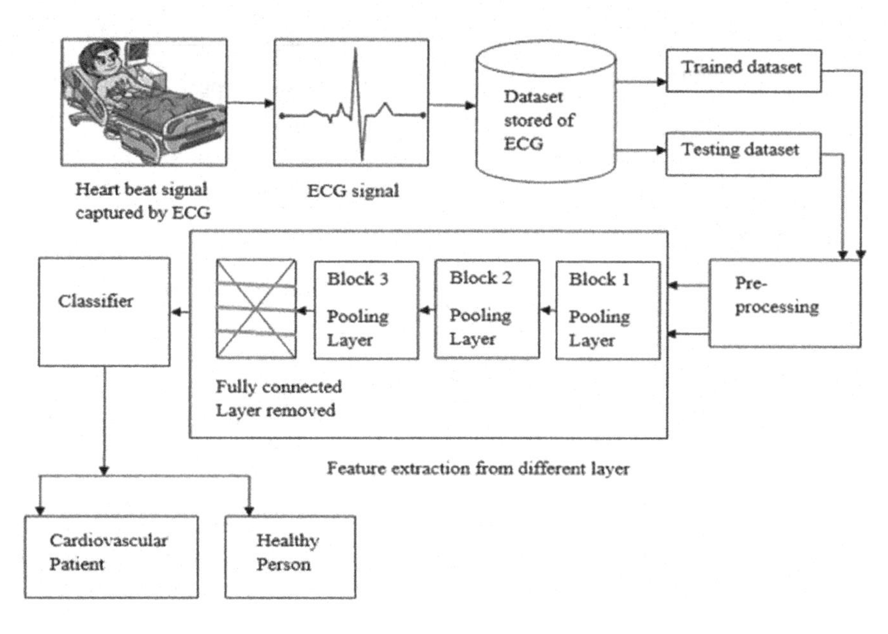

FIGURE 4.6 Proposed model.

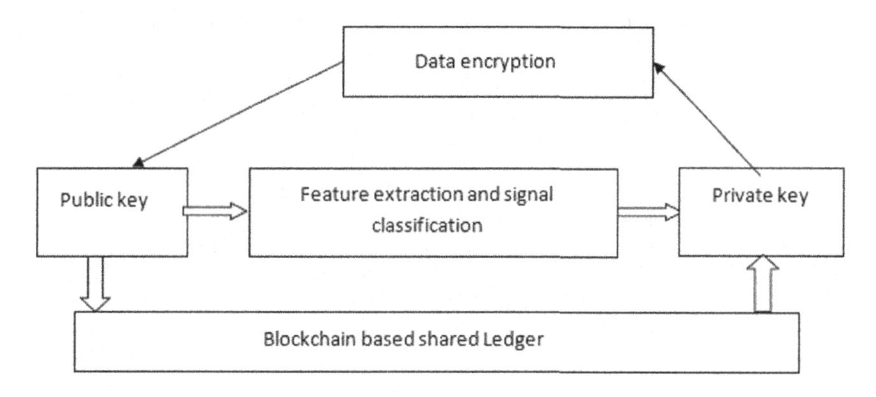

FIGURE 4.7 System overview of data encryption in blockchain-based secured platform.

Data Encryption: In the computing world, the transformation of data from a readable form into an encoded form that can only be processed or read after it's been decrypted is called encryption.

The basic building block of security of data is encryption and is the simplest way to ensure that the information can't be read and stolen by anybody at all who wants to use data for depraved means of a computer system. The motive of data encryption is to protect the confidentiality of digital information as it is residing on a computer system and travelling using computer networks or the internet (Figures 4.7 and 4.8).

4.3.2 Dataset Collection

The dataset was collected from a free website, and ECG was used to collect data. The ECG characteristics of patients with their ages and sex are depicted in Figure (Figure 4.9).

4.3.3 Data Description

Age – age between 29 and 77.

Sex – Gender of patient represented by 1 and 0 for male and female, respectively.

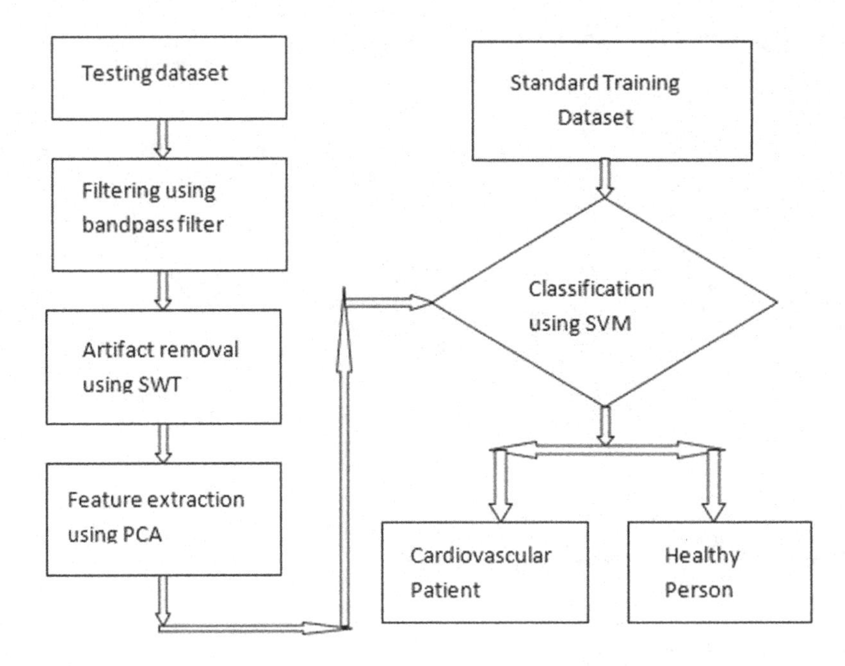

FIGURE 4.8 Flowchart diagram of classification of cardiovascular disease using ML.

	A	B	C	D	E	F	G	H	I	J	K	L	M
1	age	sex	cp	trestbps	chol	fbs	restecg	thalach	exang	oldpeak	slope	thal	target
2	63	1	3	145	233	1	0	150	0	2.3	0	1	1
3	37	1	2	130	250	0	1	187	0	3.5	0	2	1
4	41	0	1	130	204	0	0	172	0	1.4	2	2	1
5	56	1	1	120	236	0	1	178	0	0.8	2	2	1
6	57	0	0	120	354	0	1	163	1	0.6	2	2	1
7	57	1	0	140	192	0	1	148	0	0.4	1	1	1
8	56	0	1	140	294	0	0	153	0	1.3	1	2	1
9	44	1	1	120	263	0	1	173	0	0	2	3	1
10	52	1	2	172	199	1	1	162	0	0.5	2	3	1
11	57	1	2	150	168	0	1	174	0	1.6	2	2	1
12	54	1	0	140	239	0	1	160	0	1.2	2	2	1
13	48	0	2	130	275	0	1	139	0	0.2	2	2	1

FIGURE 4.9 Dataset collection from a free website "https://archive.ics.uci.edu/ml/datasets/Heart+Disease".

Cp – Here Cp stands for chest pain, which has 4 types of values: 0, 1, 2, and 3 for typical angina, atypical angina, non-angina pain, and asymptomatic, respectively.
Trestbps – blood pressure level (in mm/Hg) at resting mode.
Chol – serum cholesterol (in mg/dl).
Fbs – fasting blood sugar greater than 120 mg/dl; here 1 means true and 0 for false.
Rest ECG – result of ECG at resting state, values are 0, 1, and 2.
Thalach – maximum heart rate achieved.
Exang – exercise induced angina (1 means yes and 0 means no).
Oldpeak – ST depression induced by exercise relative to rest.
Slope – the slope of the peak exercise ST segment.
Thal – thal: 0 = normal; 1 = fixed defect; 2 = reversible defect, all are for heart status.
Target – target value is either 0 or 1.

4.3.4 Filtering

A class of signal refinement is called filtering, the filter's defining feature being the partial or complete suppression of signal's in some facet. Commonly, this means removing several frequency bands or frequencies. However, filters do not entirely act in the frequency domain; other numerous targets for filtering are present. Without intervening in the domain of frequency, correlations can be removed for particular frequency components and not for others. Filters are extensively used in radio, audio, television, control systems, recording, image processing, electronics and telecommunication, computer graphics, and radar music synthesis.

Band pass filter within the range between 5 and 50 Hz is used to reduce muscle noise and power line interference.

4.3.5 Artefact Removal

Stationary wavelet transform (SWT) is used to remove motion artefacts from ECG signals. SWT algorithm cleans 0.71 to 0.88 median motion artefacts which are created by the human body with respect to non-contact electrodes.

$$S(k) = f(k) + e(k) \tag{4.1}$$

$S(k)$ denotes signal with noise, $f(k)$ denotes wanted signal, $e(k)$ denotes noise signal.

4.3.6 Feature Extraction and Selection

Feature extraction is a dimensionality reduction process by which more feasible groups of data are formed for processing from an initial fresh data set by reduction. These large types of data sets have greater quantity variables which require much computing resources to process. Feature extraction is a method that selects or merges variables into features, effectively reducing the data amount that must be processed, while still completely and accurately describing the actual data set. The feature extraction process is useful when the number of resources you need to reduce, without losing relevant or important information needed for processing. Feature extraction also can reduce the number of redundant data for a specified analysis. It eases generalization steps and the speed of learning in the process of machine learning.

PCA: Principal component analysis (PCA) is the process of principal components computing, which is used to carry out a change of basis on the data, sometimes taking no notice of the rest and only using the first little principal components.

PCA is used for creating predictive models and in exploratory data analysis. It is often used for the reduction of dimensionality; to obtain lower-dimensional data and preserve as much as possible of the data's variation, it estimates each data point onto only the first little principal components (Table 4.1).

4.3.7 Classification

Classification that needs the use of machine learning algorithms is a task that grasps how to assign a class label from the problem domain to examples. Classification needs a training dataset which has examples of outputs and inputs from which to learn. A model computes how to best map specimens of input data to specific class labels using the training dataset. Thereby, the training dataset essentially has many examples of every class label and must be barely representative of the problem.

Support Vector Machine: In machine learning, supervised learning models are called support vector machines related to learning algorithms which scrutinize data for regression analysis and classification. An SVM maps training examples to spots in space so as to maximize the width of

TABLE 4.1
Feature selection

Attributes	Description	Value	Value Type
Age	Age between 29 and 77 in Integer number	29–77	Numeric
Sex	Male represent as 1, female represent as 0	0,1	Nominal
Cp	Chest paint type: 1 represents the type of typical angina disease, 2 for atypical angina, 3 for non-angina pain, 4 indicates the asymptomatic type of heart disease	1,2,3,4	Nominal
Trestbps	Level of blood pressure when patient is in rest condition (mm/Hg)	94–100	Numeric
Chol	Serum cholesterol (measured by mg/dl)	126–564	Numeric
Fbs	Blood sugar level measured on fasting; fasting blood sugar >120 mg/dl; 1 indicates true, 0 means false	0, 1	Nominal
Rest ECG	Result of ECG at resting state, values are 0, 1, 2	0, 1, 2	Nominal
Thalach	Maximum heart rate achieved	71–202	Numeric
Exang	Exercise-induced angina (1 means yes and 0 means no)	0, 1	Nominal
Old peak	ST depression induced by exercise relative to rest	0, 62	Nominal
Slope	The slope of the peak exercise ST segment. The values are 1 for unsloping, 2 for flat, and 3 for downsloping	1, 2, 3	Nominal
Thal	Heart status illustrated. thal: 0 = normal; 1 = fixed defect; 2 = reversible defect	0, 1, 2	Nominal
Target	Target values are either 0 or 1	0, 1	Nominal

[38]

the aperture between the two categories. New examples are then mapped into that same space for prognosis which category they belong to based on which side they fall of the aperture.

SVMs can efficiently carry out both linear classification and a nonlinear classification, but for nonlinear classification, it uses kernel trick, and absolutely maps their inputs into a high-dimensional feature space.

The result is classified by cardiovascular patients and healthy people.

Training: Learning or determining good values for all the biases and the weights from labelled examples is simply called training a model. Empirical risk minimization is a process in supervised learning, which is a machine learning algorithm that constructs a model and attempts to discover a model with minimal loss by examining many examples.

For a bad prediction, loss is the penalty. That is, loss is a number on an example showing how bad the model's prediction was. If the model's prediction is ideal, the loss is zero; otherwise, the loss is substantial. The aim of training a model that has on average low loss, overall examples by discovering a set of biases and weight.

Testing: In connection to Machine Learning models, the word "testing" is used every time. Mainly it is used for testing the model performance with regard to precision and or accuracy of the model.

In this chapter, we used Equation (4.2) for cardiovascular disease classification.

$$\begin{aligned} H(xi) = +1 if\ w.x + b \geq 0 \quad & \text{"Cardiovascular disease"} \\ -1 if\ w.x + b < 0 \quad & \text{"Healthy person"} \end{aligned} \tag{4.2}$$

```
Algorithm 1: Cardiovascular disease classifier
Start
1.   Collect a dataset using an ECG sensor.
2.   Pre-processing done
```

```
a.  Filtering using a bandpass filter (5-50 Hz).
b.  Artefact removal using stationary wavelet transform (SWT).
```

$$S(k) = f(k) + e(k)$$

```
3.  Feature extraction and selection using principal component analysis
    (PCA).
Age, Sex, Cp, Trestbps, Chol, Fbs, Rest ECG, Thlach, Exang, Old peak,
Slope, Thal, Target.
If(Age>=29 && Age<=77)
"Allow for Test"
If(Sex==0)
"Female"
Else if (Sex==1)
"Male"
If(CP==1)
   "angina disease"
Else if(Cp==2)
   "atypical angina"
Else if(Cp==3)
   "non-angina pain"
Else
   "asymptomatic type of heart disease"
If(Trestbps>=94 &&Trestbps<=100)
   "Normal"
Else
   "Abnormal"
If(Chol>=126 &&Chol<=564)
   "Normal"
Else
   "Abnormal"
If(Fbs>=120)
"Blood sugar"
Else
"Not"
If(Rest_ECG>1)
"Abnormal"
Else
"Normal"
If(Thalach>=71 && Thalach<=202)
"Normal"
Else
"Abnormal"
If(Old_Peak>=0 and Old_Peak<=62)
"ST depression induced by exercise"
If(Slope==1)
"Unslopping"
Else if (slope==2)
"Flat"
Else
"Down sloping"
4.  Classification done by comparing training and testing dataset using
    support vector machine (SVM)
```

$$H(xi) = \begin{cases} +1 \; if \; w.x + b \geq 0 \; "Cardiovascular \; disease" \\ -1 \; if \; w.x + b < 0 \; "HealthyPerson" \end{cases}$$

```
5.  Classification result is not Normal.
6.  Compare with
```

```
a.   Classification result
b.   Retraining Threshold value
7.   Classification result=Normal AND Reconstruction error of
     sample<Retraining threshold
8.   Add sample to sample list.
9.   sample list>=Normal
10.  Add new features to the hidden layer.
11.  Merge similar features
12.  Retrain with new features
13.  Adjust threshold value for anomaly detector.
End
```

4.3.8 Applications and Highlights of the Proposed System

Application of proposed work is in the following areas:

- The proposed work predicts if the user is suffering from cardiovascular disease or not.
- The system can be used in the healthcare system.
- The system is hazardless, so it can help to diagnose heart disease sitting at home.
- The system can help paralyzed and old age people with heartbeat classification.

Highlights of work are as follows:

- It is difficult to store, determine, and predict data manually to overcome this problem. Machine learning techniques are used in our proposed model.
- Above proposed work overcomes challenges from healthcare organizations, the system is diagnosed heart disease at a reasonable price.
- To get accurate results, the proposed model removes noise using a bandpass filter and an acceptable signal range between 5 Hz and 50Hz.
- Stationary wavelet transform is used to remove human motion artefacts so that datasets are cleaner and results more accurately.
- Feature extraction and selection by using principal component analysis that chooses important features for heart disease prediction.
- Support vector machine (SVM) is used to detect heart problems, categorized as suffering from cardiovascular disease or not.

4.4 CONCLUSION AND FUTURE WORK

This chapter is designed to classify heartbeat rate in a simple, efficient, and costless way as the collection of data is done by a widely used method, that is ECG, and then we used machine learning techniques, which itself is a simple and efficient method. In automatic cardiovascular disease detection, the method is secured with a blockchain so the systems are robust to get or predict the result.

In future, this work will be extended to several issues of IoT and ML-based telemedicine systems, and other health care issues will also be taken into account.

REFERENCES

1. V. Harshini, Shreevani Danai, H. Usha and Manjunath R. Kounte, "Health Record Management through Blockchain Technology," in *2019 3rd International Conference on Trends in Electronics and Informatics (ICOEI)*, 2019, pp. 1411–1415. doi: 10.1109/ICOEI.2019.8862594
2. H.Chang, C.Wu, J. Liu and J. R. Jang, "Using Machine Learning Algorithms in Medication for Cardiac Arrest Early Warning System Construction and Forecasting," in *2018 Conference on Technologies and Applications of Artificial Intelligence (TAAI)*, Taichung, 2018, pp. 1–4, doi: 10.1109/TAAI.2018.00010.

3. V. K. Chauhan, V. Chauhan, S. Tiwary and A. Kumar, "Cardiac Arrest Prediction Using Machine Learning Algorithms," in *2019 2nd International Conference on Intelligent Computing, Instrumentation and Control Technologies (ICICICT)*, Kannur, 2019, pp. 886–890, doi: 10.1109/ICICICT46008.2019.8993296.
4. S. Das and A. Bhattacharya, "ECG Assess Heartbeat Rate, Classifying Using BPNN While Watching Movie and Send Movie Rating through Telegram," in Tavares, J. M. R. S., Chakrabarti, S., Bhattacharya, A., and Ghatak, S. (eds), *Emerging Technologies in Data Mining and Information Security. Lecture Notes in Networks and Systems*, vol. 164. Springer, Singapore, 2021, doi: 10.1007/978-981-15-9774-9_43.
5. M. Puppala, T. He, X. Yu, S. Chen, R. Ogunti and S. T. C. Wong, "Data Security and Privacy Management in Healthcare Applications and Clinical Data Warehouse Environment," in *2016 IEEE-EMBS International Conference on Biomedical and Health Informatics (BHI)*, 2016, pp. 5–8, doi: 10.1109/BHI.2016.7455821
6. K. Abouelmehdi, A. Beni-Hssane, H. Khaloufi and M. Saadi, "Big Data Security and Privacy in Healthcare: A Review," *Procedia Computer Science*, vol. 113, 2017, pp. 73–80.
7. S. Das, L. Ghosh and S. Saha "Analyzing Gaming Effects on Cognitive Load Using Artificial Intelligent Tools," 2020 IEEE International Conference on Electronics, Computing and Communication Technologies (CONECCT), 2020, pp. 1–6, doi: 10.1109/CONECCT50063.2020.9198662.
8. A. Prashanth Joshi, M. Han and Y. Wang, "A Survey on Security and Privacy Issues of Blockchain Technology," *Mathematical Foundations of Computing*, vol. 1, no. 2, 2018, pp. 121–147.
9. I.-C. Lin and T.-C. Liao, "A Survey of Blockchain Security Issues and Challenges," *International Journal of Network Security*, vol. 19, pp. 653–659, 2017.
10. L. Sankar, M. Sindhu and M. Sethumadhavan, "Survey of Consensus Protocols on Blockchain Applications," in *2017 4th International Conference on Advanced Computing and Communication Systems (ICACCS)*, 2017, pp. 1–5, doi: 10.1109/ICACCS.2017.8014672
11. S. Modak, K. Majumder and D. De, "Vulnerability of Cloud: Analysis of XML Signature Wrapping Attack and Countermeasures," in Bhattacharjee, D., Kole, D.K., Dey, N., Basu, S., and Plewczynski, D. (eds), *Proceedings of International Conference on Frontiers in Computing and Systems. Advances in Intelligent Systems and Computing*, vol 1255. Springer, Singapore, 2021, doi: 10.1007/978-981-15-7834-2_70.
12. Z. Zheng, S. Xie, H. Dai, X. Chen and H. Wang, "An Overview of Blockchain Technology: Architecture, Consensus, and Future Trends", in *2017 IEEE International Congress on Big Data (BigData Congress)*, 2017. pp. 557–564, doi: 10.1109/BigDataCongress.2017.85
13. M. Alharby and A. van Moorsel, "Blockchain-Based Smart Contracts: A Systematic Mapping Study," *Computer Science & Information Technology (CS & IT)*, 2017, pp. 125–140. https://arxiv.org/abs/1710.06372.
14. N. Rifi, E. Rachkidi, N. Agoulmine and N. Taher, "Towards Using Blockchain Technology for eHealth Data Access Management," in *2017 Fourth International Conference onAdvances in Biomedical Engineering (ICABME)*, Beirut, Lebanon, 2017, doi: 10.1109/ICABME.2017.8167555.
15. A. Azaria, A. Ekblaw, T. Vieira and A. Lippman, "MedRec: Using Blockchain for Medical Data Access and Permission Management," in *2016 2nd International Conference on Open and Big Data (OBD)*, Vienna, 2016, pp. 25–30, doi: 10.1109/OBD.2016.11.
16. S. K. Dwivedi, R. Amin and S. Vollala, "Blockchain Based Secured Information Sharing Protocol in Supply Chain Management System with Key Distribution Mechanism," *Journal of Information Security and Applications*, vol. 54, 2020, p. 102554.
17. Amit Juneja and Michael Marefat, "Leveraging Blockchain for Retraining Deep Learning Architecture in Patient-Specific Arrhythmia Classification," in *2018 IEEE EMBS International Conference on Biomedical & Health Informatics (BHI)*, Las Vegas, NV, 2018, pp. 393–397, doi: 10.1109/BHI.2018.8333451.
18. Venkatasamy Sureshkumar, Ruhul Amin, Mohammad S. Obaidat and Isswarya Karthikeyan, "An Enhanced Mutual Authentication and Key Establishment Protocol for TMIS Using Chaotic Map," *Journal of Information Security and Applications*, vol. 53, 2020, p. 102539.
19. J.-K. Kim, et al., "Adaptive Mining Prediction Model for Content Recommendation to Coronary Heart Disease Patients," *Cluster Computing*, vol. 17, no. 3, 2014, pp. 881–891.
20. M. Gul, S. M. Anwar and M. Majid, "Electrocardiogram Signal Classification to Detect Arrythmia with Improved Features," in *2017 IEEE International Conference on Imaging Systems and Techniques (IST)*, IEEE Press, pp. 1–6, 2017, https://doi.org/10.1109/IST.2017.8261545.
21. A. Mustaqeem, et al., "Wrapper Method for Feature Selection to Classify Cardiac Arrhythmia," in *Engineering in 2017 39th Annual International Conference of the IEEE Medicine and Biology Society (EMBC)*, pp. 3656–3659, 2017, doi: 10.1109/EMBC.2017.8037650. PMID: 29060691.

22. N. Kausar, et al., Systematic Analysis of Applied Data Mining Based Optimization Algorithms in Clinical Attribute Extraction and Classification for Diagnosis of Cardiac Patients," in Noreen Kausar, Sellapan Palaniappan, Samir Brahim Belhaouari, Azween Bin Abdullah and Nilanjan Dey (Eds.), *Applications of Intelligent Optimization in Biology and Medicine*, Springer, 2016, pp. 217–231.
23. M. Zubair, J. Kim and C. Yoon, "An Automated ECG Beat Classification System Using Convolutional Neural Networks," in *2016 6th International Conference on IT Convergence and Security (ICITCS)*, 2016, pp. 1–5, doi: 10.1109/ICITCS.2016.7740310.
24. R. Marshal, K. Gopinath and V. V. Rao, "Proactive Measures to Mitigate Cyber Security Challenges in IoT based Smart Healthcare Networks," in *2021 IEEE International IOT, Electronics and Mechatronics Conference (IEMTRONICS)*, 2021, pp. 1–4, doi: 10.1109/IEMTRONICS52119.2021.9422615.
25. K. Matousek, "Security and Reliability Considerations for Distributed Healthcare Systems," in *2008 42nd Annual IEEE International Carnahan Conference on Security Technology*, 2008, pp. 346–348, doi: 10.1109/CCST.2008.4751326.
26. A. Jayanthilladevi, K. Sangeetha and E. Balamurugan, "Healthcare Biometrics Security and Regulations: Biometrics Data Security and Regulations Governing PHI and HIPAA Act for Patient Privacy," in *2020 International Conference on Emerging Smart Computing and Informatics (ESCI)*, 2020, pp. 244–247, doi: 10.1109/ESCI48226.2020.9167635.
27. J. Kwon and M. E. Johnson, "Protecting Patient Data-The Economic Perspective of Healthcare Security," *IEEE Security & Privacy*, vol. 13, no. 5, pp. 90–95, 2015, doi: 10.1109/MSP.2015.113.
28. Z. O. Omogbadegun, "Security in Healthcare Information Systems," in *2006 ITI 4th International Conference on Information & Communications Technology*, 2006, pp. 1–2, doi: 10.1109/ITICT.2006.358263.
29. Y. He and C. W. Johnson, "Generic Security Cases for Information System Security in Healthcare Systems," in *7th IET International Conference on System Safety, incorporating the Cyber Security Conference 2012*, 2012, pp. 1–6, doi: 10.1049/cp.2012.1507.
30. Y. Tao and H. Lee, "MTCS for Healthcare," in *2017 International Conference on Cloud Computing Research and Innovation (ICCCRI)*, 2017, pp. 14–17, doi: 10.1109/ICCCRI.2017.10.
31. N. Bruce, M. Sain and H. J. Lee, "A Support Middleware Solution for E-Healthcare System Security," in *16th International Conference on Advanced Communication Technology*, 2014, pp. 44–47, doi: 10.1109/ICACT.2014.6778919.
32. C. H. Ip, S. H. Pun, M. I. Vai and P. U. Mak, "The Network Security Regime for the Hybrid Connection of Healthcare Entities," in *2012 International Conference on Biomedical Engineering and Biotechnology*, 2012, pp. 1832–1834, doi: 10.1109/iCBEB.2012.431.
33. J. Kwon and M. E. Johnson, "Healthcare Security Strategies for Regulatory Compliance and Data Security," in *2013 46th Hawaii International Conference on System Sciences*, 2013, pp. 3972–3981, doi: 10.1109/HICSS.2013.246.
34. Kanghee Lee, Zhefan Jiang, Sangok Kim and Sangwook Kim, "Security Policy Management for Healthcare System Network," in *Proceedings of 7th International Workshop on Enterprise Networking and Computing in Healthcare Industry. HEALTHCOM 2005*, 2005, pp. 289–292, doi: 10.1109/HEALTH.2005.1500463.
35. E. Markakis, Y. Nikoloudakis, E. Pallis and M. Manso, "Security Assessment as a Service Cross-Layered System for the Adoption of Digital, Personalised and Trusted Healthcare," in *2019 IEEE 5th World Forum on Internet of Things (WF-IoT)*, 2019, pp. 91–94, doi: 10.1109/WF-IoT.2019.8767249.
36. A. I. Newaz, A. K. Sikder, M. A. Rahman and A. S. Uluagac, "HealthGuard: A Machine Learning-Based Security Framework for Smart Healthcare Systems," in *2019 Sixth International Conference on Social Networks Analysis, Management and Security (SNAMS)*, 2019, pp. 389–396, doi: 10.1109/SNAMS.2019.8931716.
37. H. Kupwade Patil and R. Seshadri, "Big Data Security and Privacy Issues in Healthcare," in *2014 IEEE International Congress on Big Data*, 2014, pp. 762–765, doi: 10.1109/BigData.Congress.2014.112.
38. B. C. Kara and C. Eyüpoğlu, "*Sağlık 4.0*'da Mahremiyet ve Güvenlik Sorunları Privacy and Security Problems in Healthcare 4.0," in *2020 4th International Symposium on Multidisciplinary Studies and Innovative Technologies (ISMSIT)*, 2020, pp. 1–12, doi: 10.1109/ISMSIT50672.2020.9255155.
39. A. Yogeshwar and S. Kamalakkannan, "Healthcare Domain in IoT with Blockchain Based Security- A Researcher's Perspectives," in *2021 5th International Conference on Intelligent Computing and Control Systems (ICICCS)*, 2021, pp. 1–9, doi: 10.1109/ICICCS51141.2021.9432198.
40. P. K. Yeng, B. Yang and E. A. Snekkenes, "Framework for Healthcare Security Practice Analysis, Modeling and Incentivization," in *2019 IEEE International Conference on Big Data (Big Data)*, 2019, pp. 3242–3251, doi: 10.1109/BigData47090.2019.9006529.

41. A. K. Alharam and W. Elmedany, "Complexity of Cyber Security Architecture for IoT Healthcare Industry: A Comparative Study," in *2017 5th International Conference on Future Internet of Things and Cloud Workshops (FiCloudW)*, 2017, pp. 246–250, doi: 10.1109/FiCloudW.2017.100.
42. M. Evans, Y. He, C. Luo, I. Yevseyeva, H. Janicke and L. A. Maglaras, "Employee Perspective on Information Security Related Human Error in Healthcare: Proactive Use of IS-CHEC in Questionnaire Form," *IEEE Access*, vol. 7, pp. 102087–102101, 2019, doi: 10.1109/ACCESS.2019.2927195.
43. F. A. Al-Zahrani, "Evaluating the Usable-Security of Healthcare Software Through Unified Technique of Fuzzy Logic, ANP and TOPSIS," *IEEE Access*, vol. 8, pp. 109905–109916, 2020, doi: 10.1109/ACCESS.2020.3001996.
44. B. Katt, "A Comprehensive Overview of Security Monitoring Solutions for E-Health Systems," in *2014 IEEE International Conference on Healthcare Informatics*, 2014, pp. 364–364, doi: 10.1109/ICHI.2014.59.
45. W. Iqbal, H. Abbas, M. Daneshmand, B. Rauf and Y. A. Bangash, "An In-Depth Analysis of IoT Security Requirements, Challenges, and Their Countermeasures via Software-Defined Security," *IEEE Internet of Things Journal*, vol. 7, no. 10, pp. 10250–10276, 2020, doi: 10.1109/JIOT.2020.2997651.
46. K. K. Karmakar, V. Varadharajan, U. Tupakula, S. Nepal and C. Thapa, "Towards a Security Enhanced Virtualised Network Infrastructure for Internet of Medical Things (IoMT)," in *2020 6th IEEE Conference on Network Softwarization (NetSoft)*, 2020, pp. 257–261, doi: 10.1109/NetSoft48620.2020.9165387.

5 IoT-Centered Household Security and Person's Healthcare System Predominantly Aimed at Epidemic Circumstances

S. Kavitha, K.R. Gokul Anand, T. Poornima, and H. Sathiya Girija

CONTENTS

DOI: 10.1201/9781003217398-5

5.1 INTRODUCTION: BACKGROUND AND DRIVING FORCES

The COVID-19 pandemic, as we all know, wreaked havoc on the world and altered our way of life. Today, Internet of Things (IoT) is active in a variety of fields, including security, monitoring, control, and healthcare. There's nothing quite like a sweet home, but we can make our homes smart and healthy enough to endure current endemic and panic situations! IoT allows us to make our homes smarter by connecting computing equipment via a network utilizing unique identifiers (UIDs) and transferring data without the need for human-to-human (H2H) or human-to-computer (H2M) interactions. These IoT gadgets can potentially be utilized to automate our homes.

The role of IoT in healthcare is also predominantly increasing and aids in saving lives in peril by speedy responsiveness via medics. IoT in fitness bands will be the future of patient health monitoring service provision. An IoT-based healthcare system can provide service quickly, potentially saving millions of lives.

Pandemic extortions, housetrains, delinquencies, fire misfortunes, and LPG gas leaks are all too common these days. What is remarkable is the general public's awareness of various sensors, security cameras, and, above all, IoT, artificial intelligence (AI) embedded in controllers [1]. It's also challenging to integrate all of these distinct detectors into a single unit. Contemporary research and advances head towards home security and automation and health safety in two distinct trails. Since the working environment for any person is inevitable and switchable [Both Home + Office], even in a situation like a pandemic, for sure, one has to substantiate one's own well-being before stepping in and out. This chapter, however, deliberates on bringing the two major rudiments into a conjoint.

Since the late 1970s, the concept of home safety automation has been around. The first home automation technology was created in 1975 with the help of a network technology called X10. It utilized electric power transmission wiring for signaling and controlling various electrical equipment. To control any digital electronic gadget put in a residence, the signals use radio frequency as digital data. However, because of the high cost of data storage and the lag in high-speed data transmission, researchers and technicians are working on advanced technologies such as the IoT and AI. Home automation, with the help of sophisticated hardware and Free Open Source Software (FOSS), can now turn a dream house into a reality.

5.2 PROPOSED SYSTEM SETUP FOR HOME AUTOMATION AND HEALTH SECURITY SYSTEM

The main advantage of this proposed system is the integrated work done for assuring people's safety, home safety, security and control, which has not been discussed so far. Figure 5.1 affords rudimentary knowledge about the system considered for study further down this chapter.

5.3 TECHNICAL DETAILS OF DEVICES AND CONNECTIONS

The architecture mentioned in Figure 5.2 allows users to control and automate several IoT devices from a remote location using a smartphone and the Internet via a controller. IoT devices are able to send data to a smartphone app such as room temperature, visitor details, gas leakage, or fire event, enabling remote monitoring and control of homes.

5.4 IoT GADGETS FOR HOME SECURITY

A number of IoT devices and sensors can be used for home automation and security. Wall switches, voltage sensors, energy monitors, thermostats, smart door locks, air conditioners, and surveillance cameras are the most basic [2]. Aside from the IoT devices described above, a home may have a range of other gadgets to increase convenience and automation. Our system uses the devices as shown in Figure 5.3.

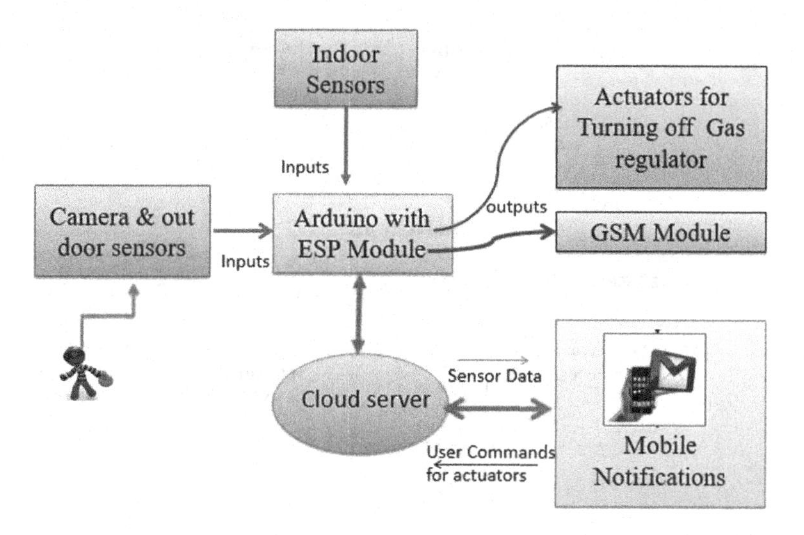

FIGURE 5.1 Overall block diagram of IoT-based household person's health safety and security system.

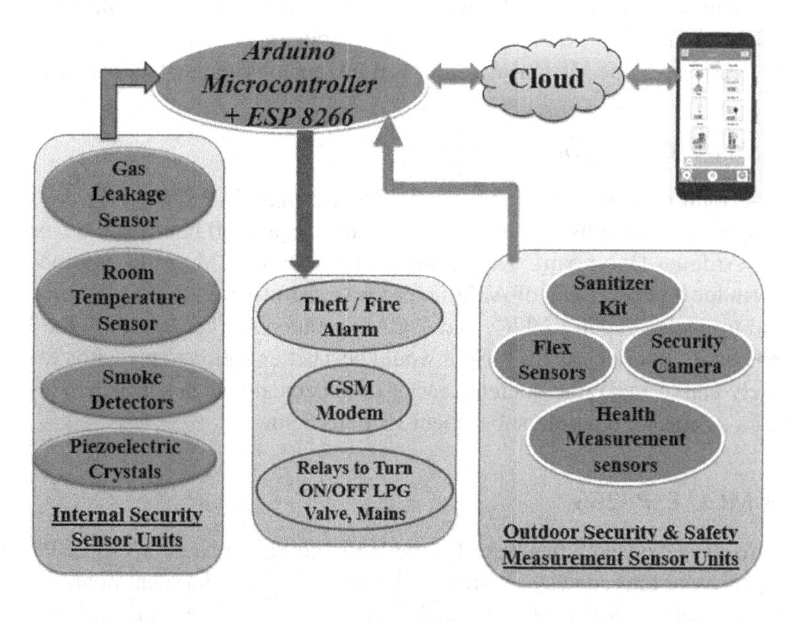

FIGURE 5.2 Home automation and health security setup.

5.5 BRAIN OF THE SETUP

Basically, a router linked to the Internet and a controller/hub connected to the IoT devices or sensors are required for home automation. IoT devices can connect to a cloud network through the Internet using a controller/hub and router. Hence, the controller/hub is the most significant part of the system since it controls all the IoT devices/sensors put in a home. Both wired and wireless connections are available, with wireless being the recommended choice [3]. The four most common operational protocols for home automation technologies are Wi-Fi, Z-Wave, Zigbee, and Bluetooth Low Energy (BLE). The most extensively used one is Wi-Fi. Hundreds of IoT devices/sensors in a home can be connected and operated automatically via a smartphone app using such a controller/hub. Your home automation hubs, for example, can turn out the lights, lock the doors, and arm the security system when it's time for you to go to bed. If you have an Amazon Echo, all you have to do is issue a voice

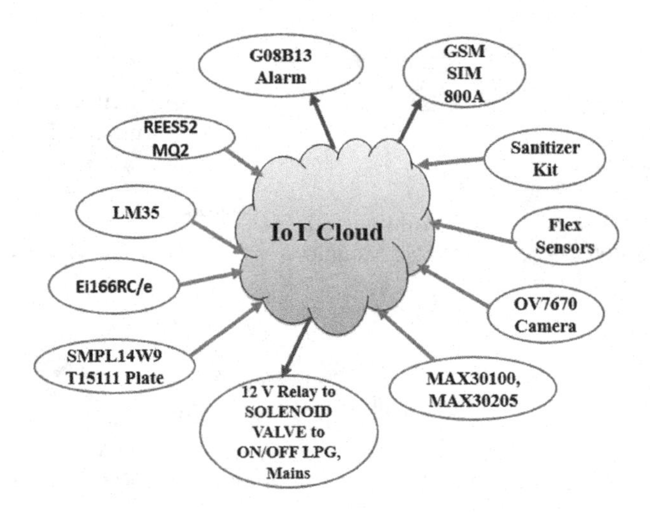

FIGURE 5.3 IoT devices.

command. Wink and SmartThings are the most popular IoT controllers for home automation, which are commercially available [4]. The Arduino microcontroller acts as a controller/hub in this study. In our case, the ESP8266 Node MCU web server is used, and it is connected to a wireless router [5].

5.5.1 Arduino Microcontroller

In this project, a total of nine analogue sensors and five digital output pins were used for both internal and external connections. We used the Arduino Mega 2560 board while working. We can also employ the Arduino Duo board. The 32-bit Arduino Duo ARM cortex microcontroller is an excellent platform for robust scaling of Arduino projects, featuring 54 digital I/O pins, 12 analogue inputs, 2 digital-to-analog inputs, 2 I2C, and 2 CAN protocols. The Arduino Duo board, unlike earlier Arduino boards, operates at 3.3 V. So it would be a better option to try with. To deliberate the matter exclusively and to make the contents easier to understand, each subsystem is demonstrated with the help of a basic Uno board in subsequent sections below.

5.5.2 Node MCU ESP8266

Espressif systems have devised a firmware for the Wi-Fi so-called Node MCU ESP8266, which is a 32-bit RISC processor and comes as a single silicon on chip development board. This processor runs at a clock frequency of 80 to 160 MHz and has provisions for operating with real-time operating systems (RTOS). It has got 128 KB of RAM and 4 MB of flash memory for the purpose of data storage. In-built features like high computing power, built-in Wi-Fi, Bluetooth, and deep sleep operating modes make it perfect for IoT applications. An external supply or a USB jack can be used for powering up the Node MCU. Simply, when you configure the ESP8266 as an access point, it creates its own Wi-Fi network to which adjacent Wi-Fi devices can connect.

Over the cloud network, they may be controlled using a FOSS or a mobile app. There are several FOSS choices for home automation. The most prominent are OpenHAB, Jeedom, and Calaos. Some other examples include Home Assistant, Domoticz, OpenMotics, LinuxMCE, PiDome, MisterHouse, and Smarthomatic. From a "lovely home" to a "smart home," there's a lot to consider. By opting for the right choice of hardware and software, it is possible to make home automation more secure and intelligent. Home automation can also help you save money on your electric bill by lowering your total power consumption. Now, for ease of understanding, we will discuss outdoor and indoor security and safety aspects separately [6].

5.6 OUTDOOR HEALTH SAFETY ASPECTS AND SECURITY MONITORING

Our prototype aims at measuring the person's health conditions while entering the home in this pandemic era. We propose the measurement of human temperature, pulse rate, and oxygen level using the sensors MAX30205 and MAX30100. These two sensors are packed and placed at the door entrance as a module. Whenever the person wants to enter the house, he/she has to place his finger on the smart health sensor module fixed at the door and find his/her health parameters to be normal on the LCD display fixed to the door, and then unlock the door through a face recognition system using a camera module for authenticating the house members or relatives for digital unlocking. We have also fixed the automatic sanitizer dispenser kit at the main door entrance to ensure the safety of children and the aged at home. The door will remain unlocked until we complete a health examination, sanitization, and face recognition. A flex sensor is attached to the door lever/handle, which will measure the rate of opening of the door to ensure safekeeping. If an intruder attempts to open the door vastly with severe force on the door handle, the sensor will read an abnormal change in resistance and intimate it to the owner through an IOT server update (Figure 5.4).

5.6.1 Health Parameter Measurement Sensors

In the present Covid-19 situation, it's critical to step inside our home after work without knowing the viral suspects. Hence, the health vigilant kit at the main door entrance includes two main sensors:

5.6.1.1 Body Temperature Sensor [MAX30205]

Body temperature variation is the first-level indication for a clinician to confirm the reaction of the human immune system to foreign substances like bacteria/viruses. The most straightforward technique for determining a person's body temperature is to take it directly from their skin. In medical

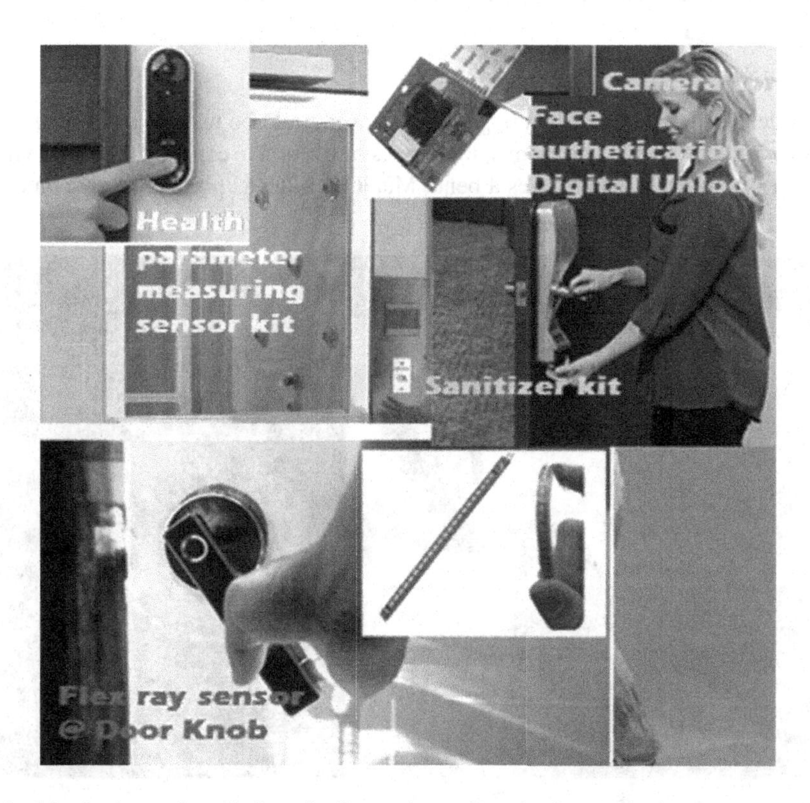

FIGURE 5.4 Monitoring and regulation of safety and security criteria at main door entrance outside.

applications, infrared (IR) temperature sensors are used to measure temperature without touching anything. Ear, forehead, and skin measurements are the most common. The MAX30205 is a popular thermometer that monitors a person's body temperature. The MAX30205 digital thermometer temperature sensor uses an in-built ADC unit with a high resolution of 16 bits (0.00390625 °C) to convert temperature readings to digital form and is accurate to 0.1°C across a measuring range of 37°C to 39°C. A hysteresis thermal alarm, often known as a thermostat, is included in the MAX30205. Energy is saved by using the one-shot and shutdown modes. This particular sensor requires a low input supply and current, which makes it ideal for wearable fitness and medical applications.

5.6.1.2 MAX30100 Sensor

The oxygen level of the blood is also a very important parameter being studied in this pandemic. Hence, we use MAX30100 that monitors pulse rate and blood oxygen levels and communicates data to the Internet through a Wi-Fi network. It has 14 pins and it's a better option for medical portables. It transmits the SPO2 and pulse details through I2C communication to the controller. It consists of two LEDs (red and green IR LEDs), a photo detector, improved optics, and low-noise electronics. The MAX30100 breakout board runs between 1.8V and 5.5V. The LED current can be set anywhere between 0 and 50 mA. The I2C pins' pull-up resistors are provided in the module. It has a typical ultra-low shutdown current of 0.7A. The MAX30100's primary job is to read the absorption levels of both light sources (Normal Red and Infrared) and store them in a buffer. Since the pulse rate is obtained by calculating the time difference between the rise and fall of oxygenated and deoxygenated blood, we can check the entering person's oxygen level and guarantee that he/she is in good health in this manner. These health values can be displayed on the door if needed using an LCD. Since it's updated on the mobile app through notification and its connection details are well known, the LCD part is not discussed here (Figure 5.5).

5.6.2 Flex Sensor

A flex sensor detects deflection or bending. A flex sensor could be used to determine the opening status of doors/windows by placing them at lock edges or livers. We can read the change in the resistance of this sensor when it experiences a bend. Materials such as plastic and carbon can be used

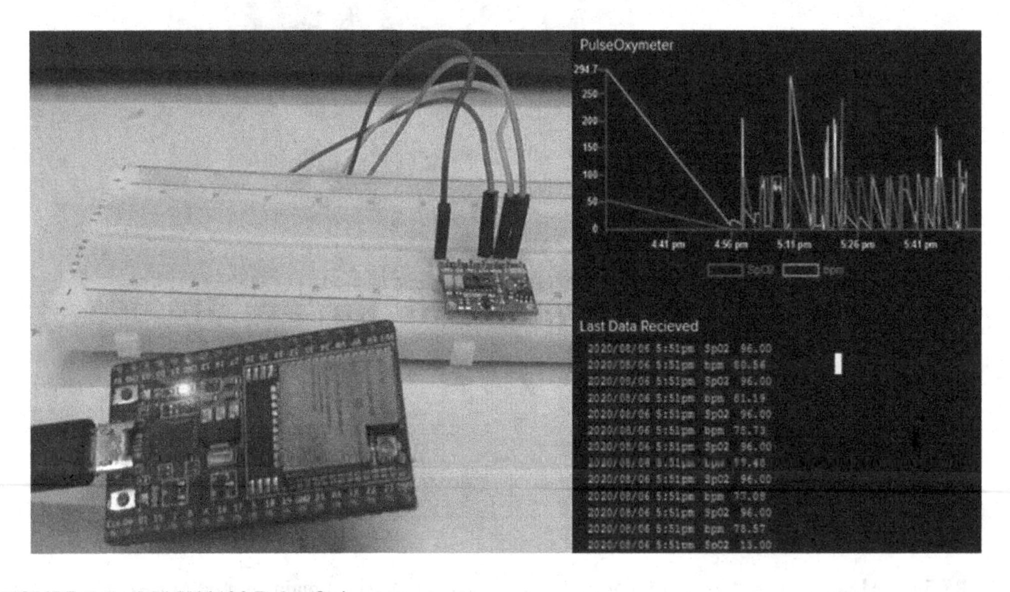

FIGURE 5.5 MAX30100 Pulse Oximeter outputs.

in the design of this sensor. The carbon surface is set on a plastic strip, which can be turned away to modify the sensor's resistance. With the use of any controller, this change in value can be read.

This sort of sensor is utilized in a variety of applications, including computer peripheral interface, rehabilitation, servo motor control, security systems, intensity control, and medical instruments, robotics, physical therapy, virtual motion (gaming), musical instruments, and robotics. The flex sensor has two pins which are connected to positive and negative terminals. The sensor requires a voltage between 3.3 and 5 volts DC to operate. The peak power rating is 1 Watt, and the constant power level is 0.5 Watt. The operating temperature varies from −45 to +80°C where 25K is the flat resistance. Bend resistance will be in the region of 45K to 125K Ohms. The resistance tolerance will be 30 percent. In this work, we have set the tolerance to 50K, and above 80K, it is observed to be an intruder's door opening for security purposes.

5.6.3 OV7670 Camera Module for Face Authentication

Cameras have traditionally dominated the electronics sector because they offer a wide range of applications, including visitor monitoring systems, surveillance systems, and attendance systems. Today's cameras are intelligent, with several functions that were not available in previous models. Artificial intelligence and machine learning are utilized to process the captured frames, which are subsequently employed in motion detection and facial recognition. The most extensively used camera module, the OV7670, has been interfaced with Arduino in this project (Figure 5.6).

Serial camera control bus (SCCB), an I2C interface (SIOC, SIOD) with a maximum clock frequency of 400 KHz, is used to control the OV7670 image sensor. The programming begins with the inclusion of OV7670's required library along with util/twi.h for I2C. After that, the registers must be configured to accommodate OV7670. The camera must be configured once the Arduino has been configured. The default register values must be adjusted to custom values. In addition, depending on the microcontroller frequency, add the needed delay. We'll be capturing images with a resolution of 320 × 240 pixels for this project.

This project was intended to provide an overview of how to use an Arduino with a camera module. Because the Arduino has less memory, you can utilize other processors/controllers with higher processing memory such as Raspberry Pi (Figure 5.7).

5.6.4 Intuitive Hand Disinfectant Machine

COVID-19 disease has not yet ended, and our government and doctors are reminding us that the only way to prevent it is to wash our hands frequently. Alcohol and hand sanitizers are essential

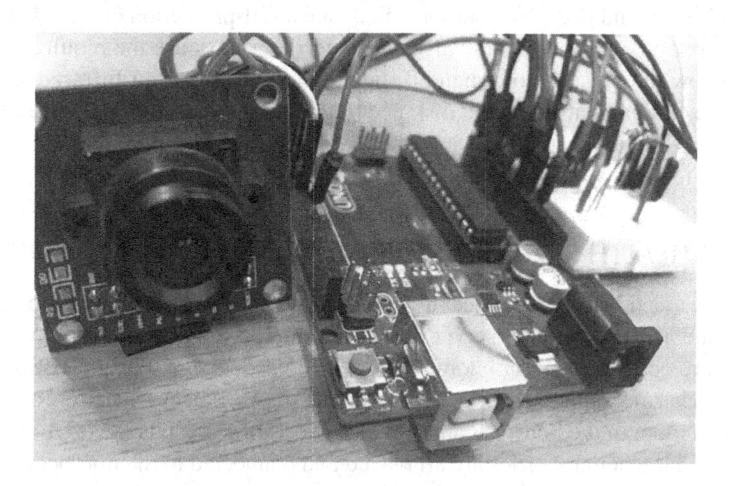

FIGURE 5.6 OV7670 Camera interface with Arduino microcontoller.

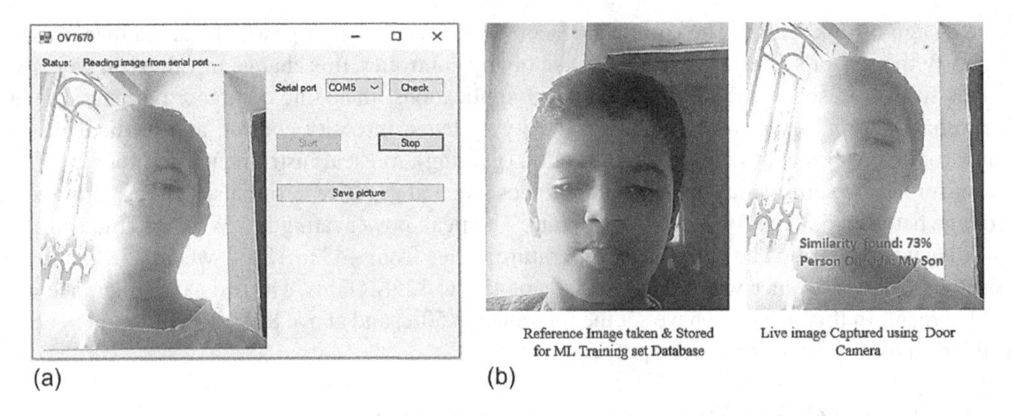

FIGURE 5.7 (a) Sample images taken from the OV7670; (b) output after ML comparison.

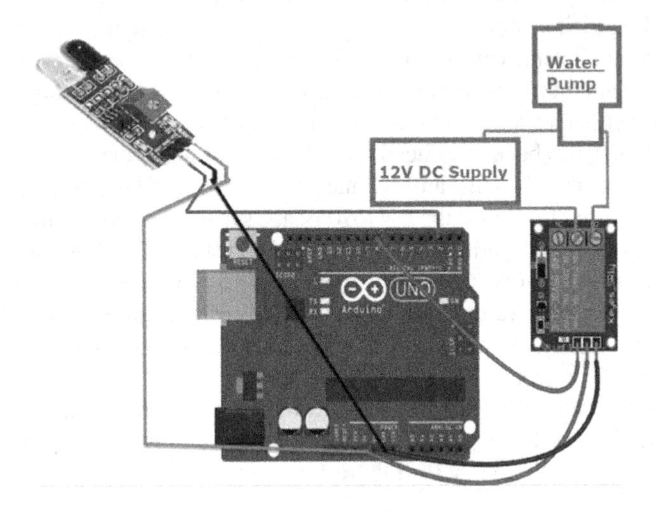

FIGURE 5.8 Automatic hand sanitizer dispenser circuit.

fluids in this situation, but they must be used correctly. When contaminated hands touch alcohol containers or hand sanitizers, the virus can be transferred to the next person. Hence, the goal was to discover the simplest and cheapest solution and create a self-protection circuit. The ultrasonic/IR sensor, Arduino, relay, water pump and valves, and sterilizer flask are the required hardware. The controller will know the presence of a hand through an ultrasonic or an Infrared sensor that indicates the presence of a hand at a specific distance (ultrasonic was used in our case). If the distance between the sensor and the relay module is less than 10 cm, the relay module will immediately turn on the 12V DC water pump and spray the liquid [7] (Figure 5.8).

5.7 INDOOR HEALTH SAFETY ASPECTS AND HOUSEHOLD MONITORING

The internal safety assembly in this project uses four different sensors from which data are collected and updated to the ThingSpeak webserver through a microcontroller. The following sensors are employed to ensure complete internal home safety: The gas leakage sensor (REES52 MQ2), temperature sensor (Thermocouple sensor/LM35), optical smoke detectors (Ei166RC/e) mounted on the ceiling of each room in the house, and piezoelectric ceramic crystals (SMPL14W9T15111) fixed to the bathroom and kitchen floor tiles are all placed and connected to the microcontroller unit. The controller will continuously read all these sensor values, and the controller will update them to the cloud using the IoT module (Figure 5.9).

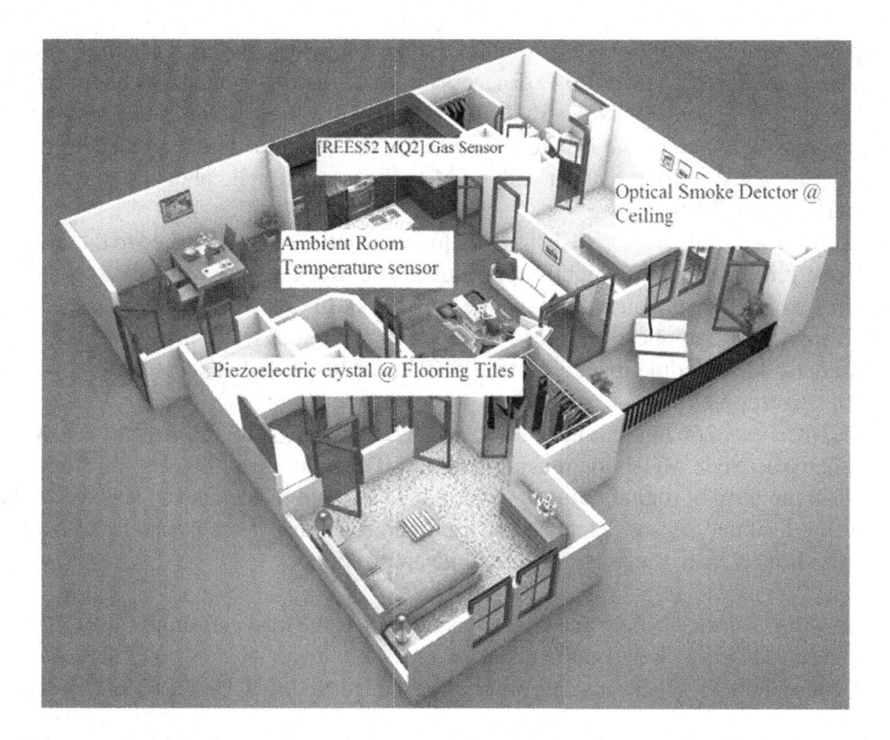

FIGURE 5.9 Monitoring and mechanization of safety and security inside the house.

5.7.1 Gas Sensor (MQ-X)

Gas sensors are used to track air quality. The rising toxic gases and emissions can affect human health. It has the potential to affect people's comfort, well-being, and productivity. Oxygen, carbon monoxide, and carbon dioxide are the three most popular types of air quality sensors. All MQ-X sensors produce analogue signals that may be read with Arduino-compatible controllers.

5.7.2 MQ2 Sensor

In the MQ2 type, concentrated gases can be detected via a meek power divider network. It can notice gases such as LPG, smoke, alcohol, propane, hydrogen, methane, and carbon monoxide ranging between 200 and 10,000 PPM. Since we are observing flammable gases, it guarantees that the furnace component inside does not trigger an explosion unless detected. Oxygen gets coated on it when the tin gets heated up to a high temperature. In the presence of clean air, donors of tin elements get attracted toward O_2 on the surface of the sensor element. Hence, the flow of electric current is restricted. However, in the presence of toxic gases, the surface intensity of O_2 decreases. Tin dioxide is subsequently bombarded with electrons, permitting the flow of electric current easily through the sensor. Thus, the controller reads changes in incoming electrical parameters [8].

This section provides a unique solution for preventing leaks and indicating when the cylinder needs to be refilled using an IoT application. The gas sensor MQ2 detects cylinder leakage and transmits the information to the Node MCU with a Wi-Fi module. The sensor values are processed using an open-source IoT platform. Additionally, data is provided to the user using a Google Firebase cloud mobile app. The major goal of this subsystem is to warn users about the risk of a fire in their home due to LPG leakage, even if they are far away from home or in another area [9].

The cylinder's weight is measured by a load cell weighing sensor, which communicates the information to Node MCU. In Node MCU, the data collected from the sensors is processed. It verifies the data using the code installed. When the data from the gas sensor equals one, the data is transferred to the cloud, from where a display warning "There is an emergency & Kindly shut down the power" will be sent to the user's mobile, following which the relay for the LPG system's solenoid valve is triggered to turn it off. If necessary, the exhaust fan can also be turned on. The load cell data is then received by Node MCU and processed by the system. If the weight is greater than the upper threshold, no action is taken. However, if the weight is less than the lower set value, for example, 5 kg, a text will be sent through GSM to the user's mobile phone, saying "Refill your LPG cylinder" (Figure 5.10).

The data processed by the Node MCU IOT platform is continuously delivered to the cloud, where it is stored, and it is also sent to a mobile application. The user can access the data on the cloud at any time using a mobile application, making the house, industry, or any commercial location more secure. This smartphone application is also designed to make it easy for users to check the status of their cylinders. This module includes: Node MCU esp8266, Gas Sensor – MQ2, load cell, and Arduino [10] (Figures 5.11 and 5.12).

The Node MCU esp8266 board is attached to an MQ2 sensor. To process the function, MQ2 code is deployed onto the Node MCU board using Arduino IDE. The sensor detects gas from LPG and delivers data in the form of digital output to Node MCU as input if there is any leakage. If the LPG level is low, the load cell sensor detects it and communicates the data continually to Node MCU, which then sends an alert to the user via the mobile application.

1. Join the MQ2 sensor's supply and GND pins, as well as the load cell supply and GND pins, to the Node MCU's +5V and GND pins.
2. Next, connect the MQ2 sensor's data pin and load cell to Node MCU's GPIO, or Physical Pin.

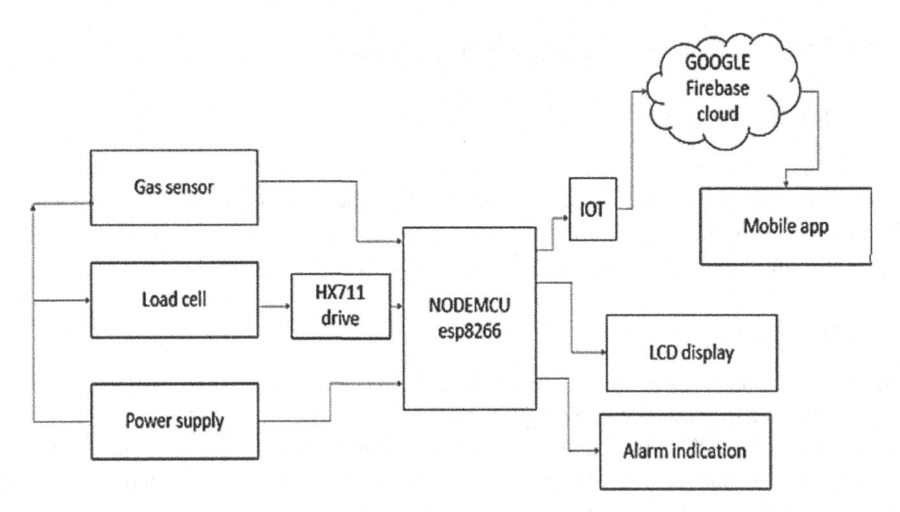

FIGURE 5.10 Block diagram of automatic alert system for LPG based on IOT.

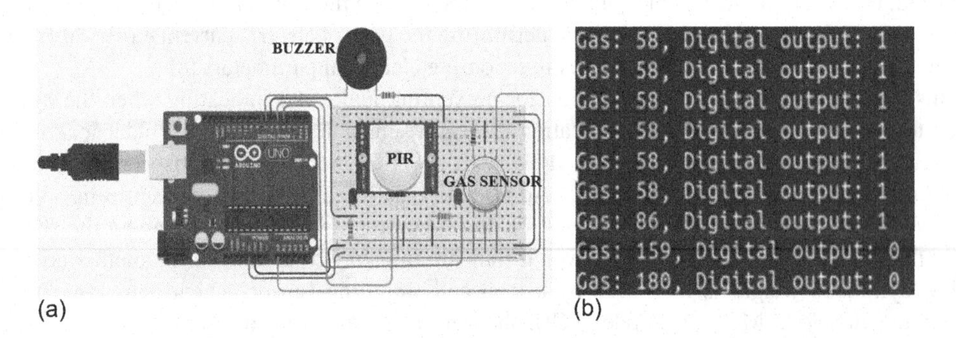

FIGURE 5.11 (a) Connection diagram; (b) simulation result for gas sensor interfacing.

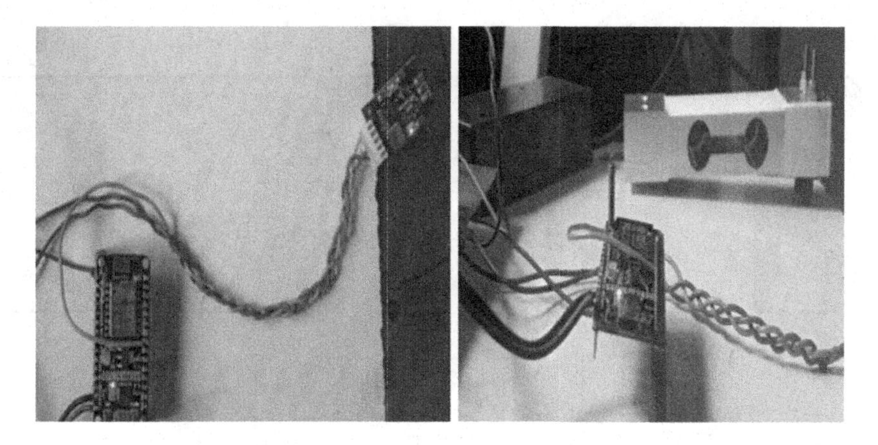

FIGURE 5.12 Hardware connections gas sensor MQ2 and load cell with Node MCU.

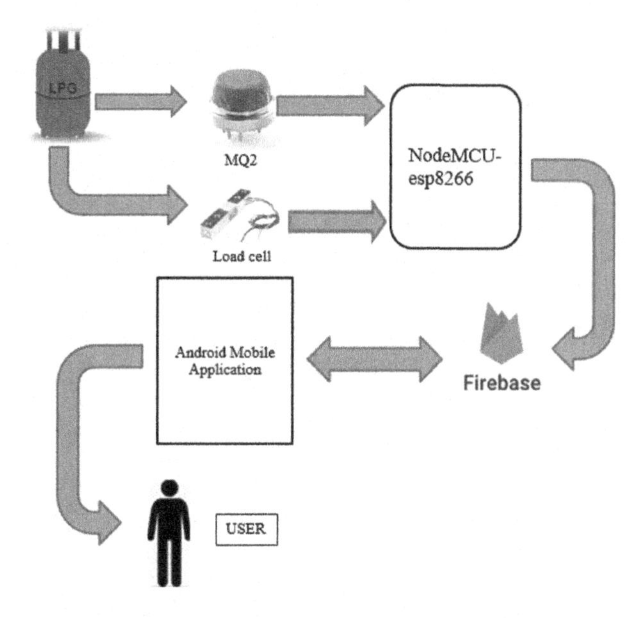

FIGURE 5.13 Flow diagram indicating the application of Firebase for mobile app development.

5.7.2.1 Google Firebase and Flutter

We have finished the mobile app development and verified the working of the same using gas sensors using Google Firebase and its outputs are shown below. Firebase cloud messaging (FCM) supports message sending and receiving through a mobile app. It uses a NoSQL database, which synchronizes users in real-time applications. It has a modest and very time-consuming sign-in process via Google/Facebook/Twitter/GitHub account [11]. Flutter is mainly used for developing user interfaces in our work [12] (Figures 5.13, 5.14, and 5.15).

5.7.2.2 Application Setup

The mobile application for this project comes with a login and signup page. The customer has to sign up, to register his/her username, password, and phone number. Getting a phone number on the sign-up page is used for the automatic booking of the gas cylinder. After signing up, the customer can log in to this app (Figures 5.16, 5.17, and 5.18).

When a customer logs in, a new page appears with three menu bars: gas leakage, gas level (indication), and gas booking. The leakage status detail page displays the leakage's current state in terms

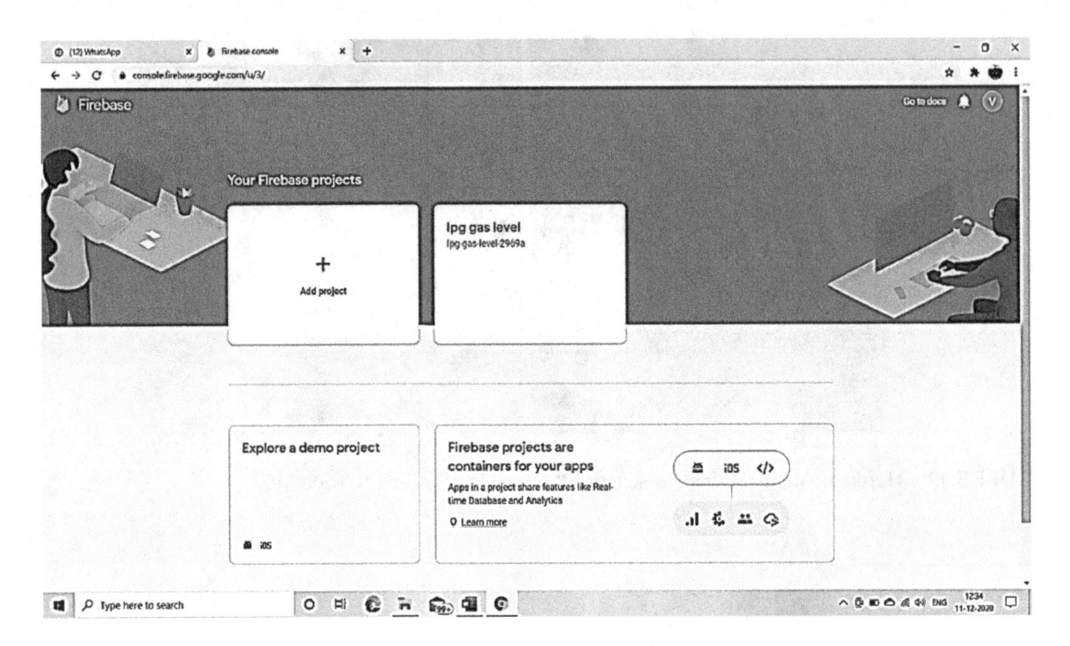

FIGURE 5.14 Firebase project created.

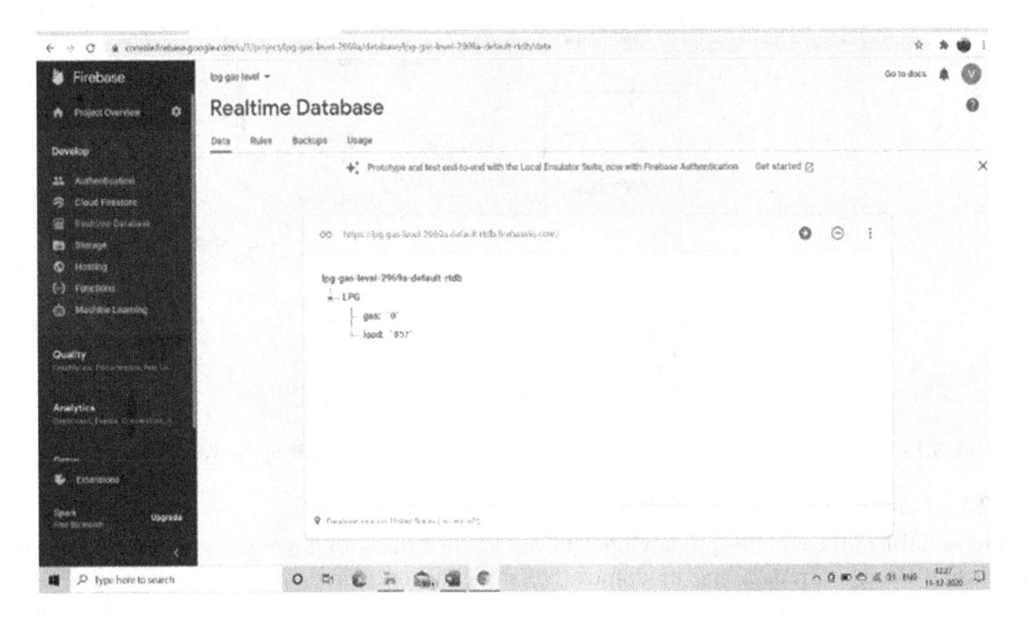

FIGURE 5.15 Real-time data storage.

of running time, with color coding (Red as ON and Green as OFF). When the status of the leak is ON, a notification with the words "Emergency alert!" will appear at the top of the screen. There is a leak in your LPG gas. Check your LPG and get in touch with your supplier. The state of the gas level will be tracked on the gas level page, as well as an estimate of the date for future reference. If the customer decides to book manually, a message ("Alert! Your LPG gas level is very low") will show when the level reaches its limit (5 kg). If the customer chooses to book automatically, the page will be displayed with the details and the only step they should take is to click "send". The other option is to use the automatic booking type, which sends an SMS to the dealer when the level reaches its lower limit (e.g., 5 kg). Before beginning any process, users should be aware of their mobile number,

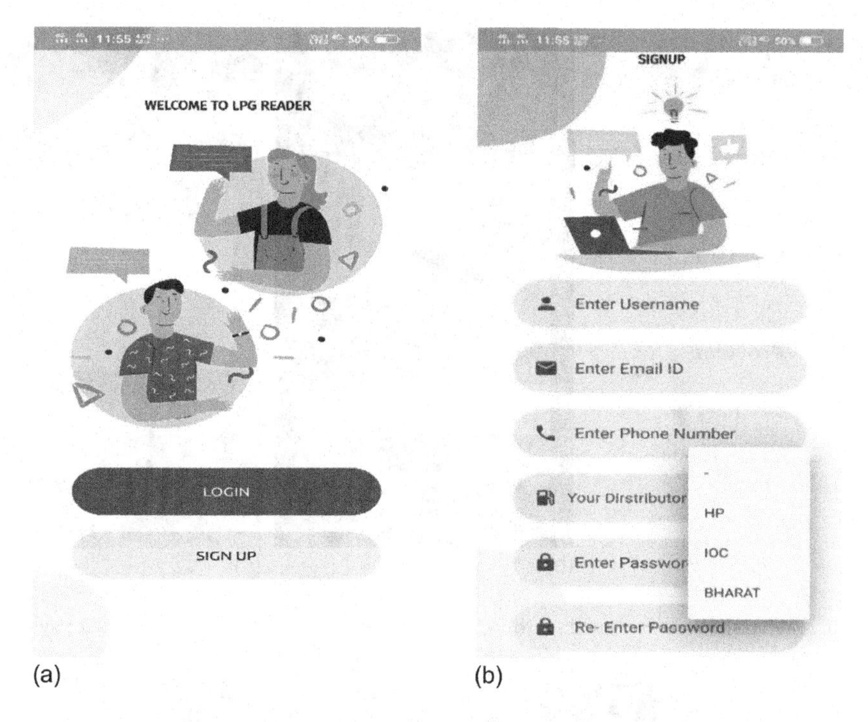

FIGURE 5.16 (a) Application logo page, login or signup page; (b) menu bar page, distributor fixation.

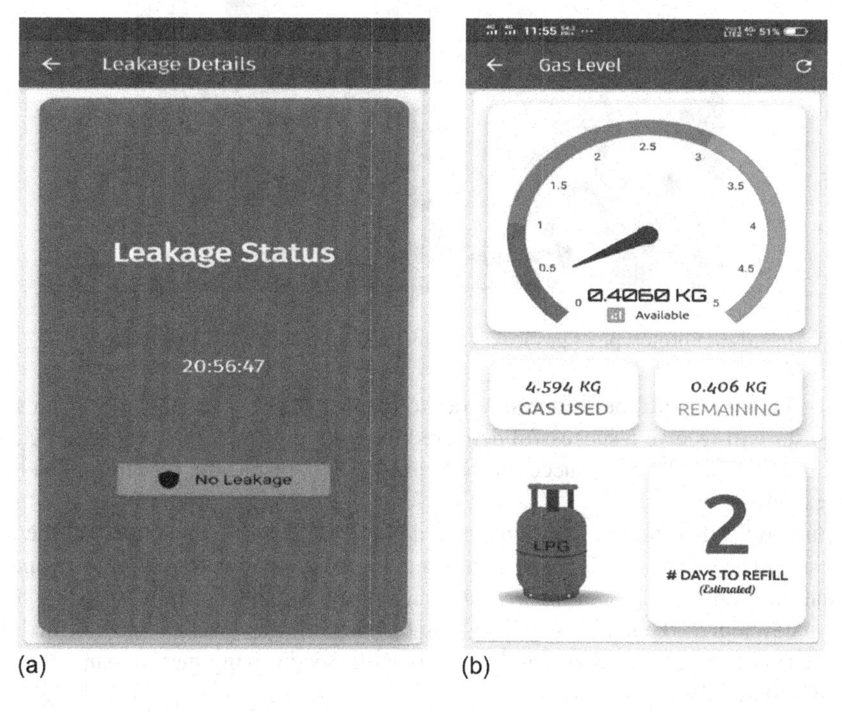

FIGURE 5.17 (a) Leakage status (b) gas-level indication page.

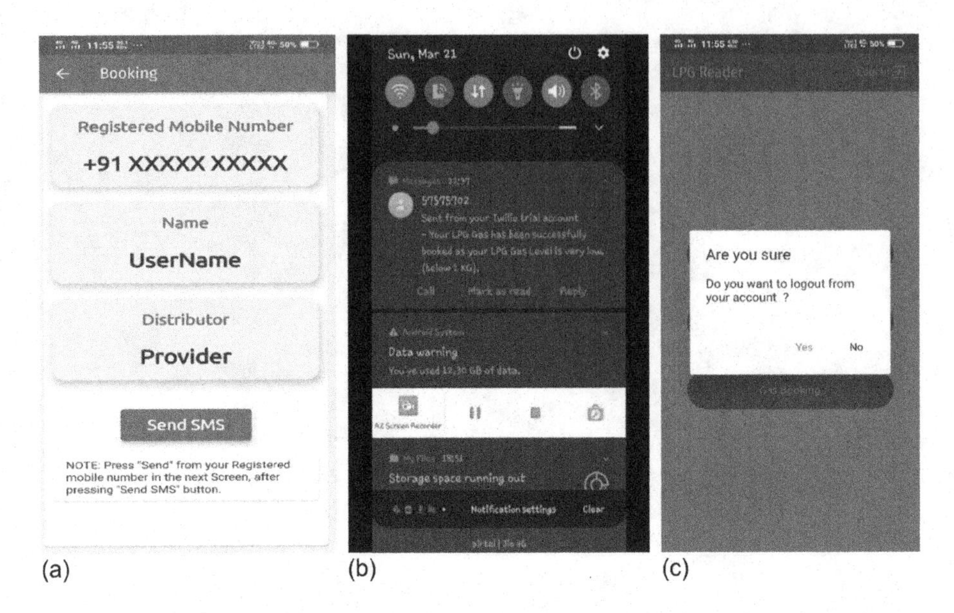

FIGURE 5.18 (a) Notification for booking, (b) acknowledge message for booking, (c) logout page.

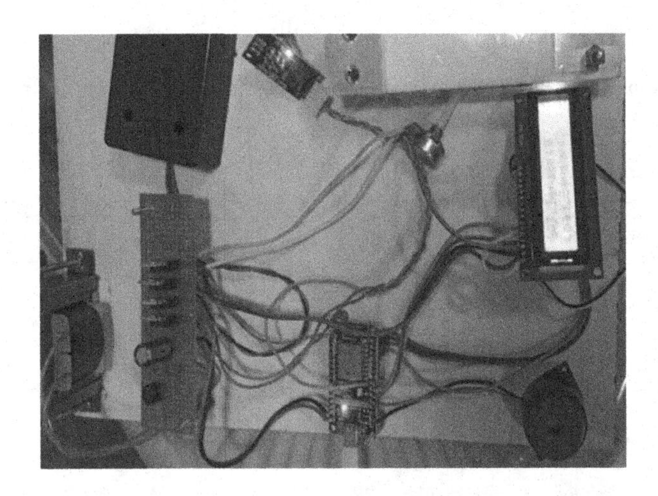

FIGURE 5.19 Hardware prototype of gas leakage detector, automatic booking subsystem.

which they have linked with the dealer, in order to confirm whether an SMS has been sent to the dealer. The user will receive a successful delivered message in their inbox, followed by a message stating, "Your LPG gas has been successfully booked." As a result, the procedure has been completed successfully.

The prototype for this project with sensors and Node MCU was completed, and the automatic alarm system for LPG based on IOT was completed. Firebase cloud was used to store and view the data. The data was obtained from Firebase and entered into an application setup using flutter, a UI interface app developer. The user can use this app to check the gas level and get notified if there is a leak. Furthermore, when the level is reduced, an automatic booking mechanism is built to book the cylinder (Figure 5.19).

5.7.3 Optical Smoke Detectors

Smoke, heat, and flame are the three basic indicators of fire. Optical smoke detectors, ionized smoke detectors, and beam-type smoke detectors are the three types of smoke detectors. The most common smoke detectors are optical smoke detectors. They're found in homes, hospitals, hotels, and retail centers, among other places. They are unsung heroes who save us from the devastation of a fire. The working of optical smoke detectors is based on the idea of light scattering. IR LEDs emit infrared light beams in their natural state. The optical chamber has a barrier that stops IR light from reaching the photodiode. Smoke particles enter the optical chamber of a smoke detector in the event of a fire. IR light from an IR LED scatters and bends onto the Light detector. It conveys to a fire alarm control panel, when scattered IR light beams reach the photo detector. Smoke sensors measure the amount of particles and gases in the air. They've been around for a while, but with the advancement of IoT, they can now alert consumers to problems quickly.

The Ei166RC/e model was used in our study. This is an optical smoke alarm that operates on 230V AC mains power and includes tamper-proof Lithium cells that serve as a battery backup in the event of a power outage. They are manufactured by AICO and have an alarm sound output of 85 decibels at 3 meters [13] (Figure 5.20).

5.7.4 Piezoelectric Sensor

Vibration detection and measurement are critical for a variety of applications, including decision-making and warning circuits. The piezoelectric approach is the most effective way to detect vibration. It converts mechanical strain into an electrical parameter. Piezoelectric materials come in a variety of shapes and sizes. Natural single crystal quartz, bone, and artificially made materials such as PZT ceramic are only a few examples of piezoelectric materials.

A picoactuator piezoelectric crystal moves in an extremely linear and hysteresis-free manner. As a result, picoactuator is perfect for extremely dynamic scanning while consuming minimal electrical power.

A difference in potential is generated whenever a person falls on the floor, since the piezoelectric substance converts this physical change into a measurable electrical quantity. Piezoelectric plates have been placed along with bathroom floor tiles, and the readings were observed for people in fallen condition and non-fallen condition. The Arduino board connection for the same has been shown in Figure 5.21.

5.7.5 Temperature Sensors for Room Temperature Monitoring

Temperature sensors detect temperature changes by measuring heat. They've been used to control room temperature by automatic turning on/off of heaters and air conditioners for years, but with the

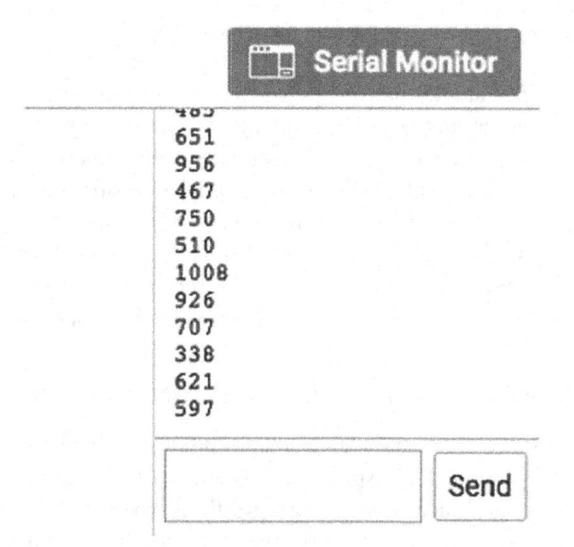

FIGURE 5.20 Optical smoke detector output seen in Arduino IDE Serial Monitor.

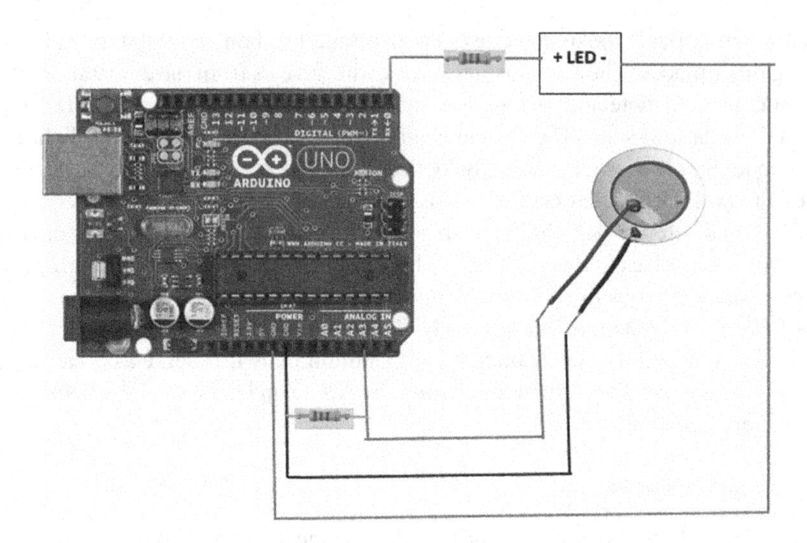

FIGURE 5.21 Piezoelectric sensor interfacing with Arduino.

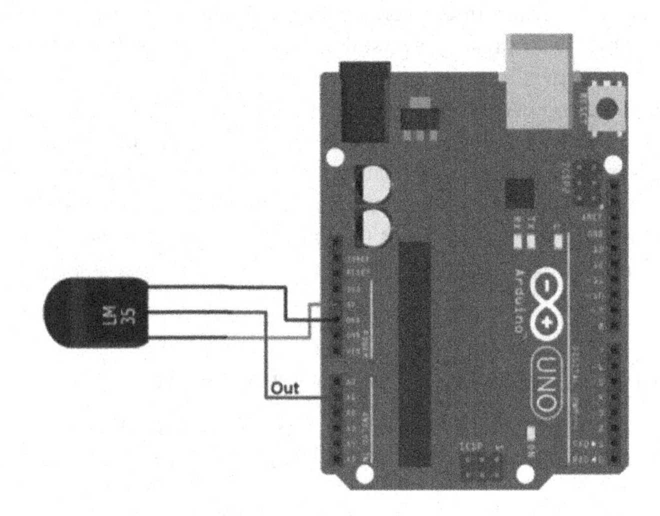

FIGURE 5.22 Temperature sensor connection with microcontroller.

advent of the IoT, they've found a lot more uses too. Semiconductor-based sensors, thermocouple, resistance temperature detector, and negative temperature coefficient thermistor are the four types of temperature sensors. Very abnormal room temperatures mean uneven fire or heat occurrences. In this prototype, we used a standard LM35 room temperature sensor element for detecting any fire suspicious when the temperature exceeds a certain threshold. It can also be used to save electricity by turning off the AC automatically by measuring room temperature. We will limit our discussion to this because most of us have enough experience with interfacing and reading temperature sensors. The circuit below shows the LM35 connection with our microcontroller [14] (Figure 5.22).

5.8 FEATURING ROLE OF IOT AND AI – MACHINE LEARNING

The IoT server will continuously monitor and update the cloud about the person's arrival at the house and internal security and safety aspects. The owner of the house is given a mobile app to personally monitor everything. Machine learning algorithms have been employed to make the controller take effective control actions on actuators for first responding to emergencies.

In our case, the following parameters are monitored and controlled.

1. If the gas sensor witnesses a leakage event, the LPG cylinder is turned off using a solenoid valve.
2. If any abnormalities like personal falls are sensed by piezoelectric crystals attached to the kitchen and bath space (since the probability of falling is high in these two areas, it is alone considered here), then the controller will make a call to 108 or nearby hospitals' emergency number + care taker/relatives' personal number through GSM modem.
3. When optical smoke detectors in every room give high output, the controller will make a call to the nearby fire service emergency number and also to neighboring + house owners' mobile numbers.

Thus, at the time of security collapse or during any health sickness, IoT-based devices can be used to take control of remedies and this prototype acts exactly like a first responder network. This project idea is getting robust by providing all the sensory data to machine learning algorithms and making the controller take perfect decisions without human interaction. Because humans cannot always keep on monitoring cloud updation due to non-availability of the Internet in certain localities, due to substantial assignments at work, and during unavoidable situations like driving, conferences, function/event halls, etc. own situations where the proprietor cannot always have his mobile with him to monitor the parameters when he is out of home. Under those circumstances, the machine learning algorithm developed aids the embedded controller in taking up the decision. The following section elucidates in detail each of the functional sensor subsystems, discretely for better understanding by the readers.

Since sensor devices in IoT have limited power and battery life, establishing a balance between security and resource efficiency while demanding IoTs is particularly important. For this reason, we're looking for machine intelligence to make decisions that are as efficient as human decision-making. For this purpose, we rely on artificial intelligence (AI) and hence use machine learning (ML) techniques, which is a subset of AI.

Machine learning is "the study of giving computers the ability to learn without being explicitly taught." When it comes to making decisions, such a system should be equivalent to a human. "A computer Programme is said to learn from experience 'E' with respect to a class of tasks 'T' and achieve a performance measure of 'P'. Note: 'P' increases with experience, 'E'" [15].

The major types of machine learning algorithms are supervised learning, unsupervised learning, and reinforcement learning.

1. Supervised learning: Here, the computer gets exposed to examples as well as labels or data sets/values. The data labels assist the algorithm in correlating the features. Classification and regression are two major classifications of supervised learning strategies.
2. Unsupervised Learning: Here the system tries to find patterns in the data through unclassified and unlabeled data. The instances aren't given a label or a goal. Clustering is a typical task that involves grouping related items together.
3. Reinforcement Learning: This method refers to goal-oriented algorithms that learn over many steps how to achieve a difficult target (goal) or maximize along a specific dimension. In order to increase their productivity, this technology allows machines and software agents to automatically select the appropriate behavior in a given situation. Simple reward feedback is required for the agent to learn which action is better; this is known as the reinforcement signal. [16].

In our case, decision making is required in three phases:

1. First, when employing a surveillance camera, the ML algorithm should recognize the face correctly, using the data set already recorded on a comparison basis using a classifier algorithm.

2. The second phase is to activate the theft alarm when an intruder attempts to break down the door. When the camera detects an unknown face output, Flex sensor reads a sudden variation, and the health parameter kit and automatic sanitizer outputs are idle/unused during that time, this is bound to happen. Because house guests, family members, friends, and delivery guys will undoubtedly use the health kit and sanitizer and gently open the door.
3. The third stage of deception involves indoor security issues, such as when a person falls or a fire event is recorded, or when LPG leakage is detected. In those situations, the microcontroller must be programmed to activate the emergency alert and instruct the GSM modem to contact an emergency number like a fire station without waiting for user commands, which is where the ML algorithm comes in handy (Figures 5.23 and 5.24).

On observing the above cases, it is observed that based on the four independent sensor events, one dependent output device has to be either turned on or off, i.e., provided with either Logic 1/ Logic 0 at its port value. Hence, the logistic regression algorithm will best suit this consideration.

5.8.1 Logistic Regression Algorithm

Logistic regression is the most frequently employed supervised learning technique. It's a technique for forecasting a firm's dependent variable from a set of independent variables. It is a binary classification method. The output of logistic training may be 1/0 or High/Low or Yes/No. As a result, we can consider logistic regression to be a single-layer neural network. The most often used neural network model for image categorization is convolutional neural networks (CNNs).

Three types of Logistic regression are as follows [17]:

- Binomial: Here, the dependent output variables can be 0/1, Pass/Fail, etc.
- Multimodal: In this type, the dependent variable can be one of three or more unordered kinds, like "cat," "dogs," or "sheep."

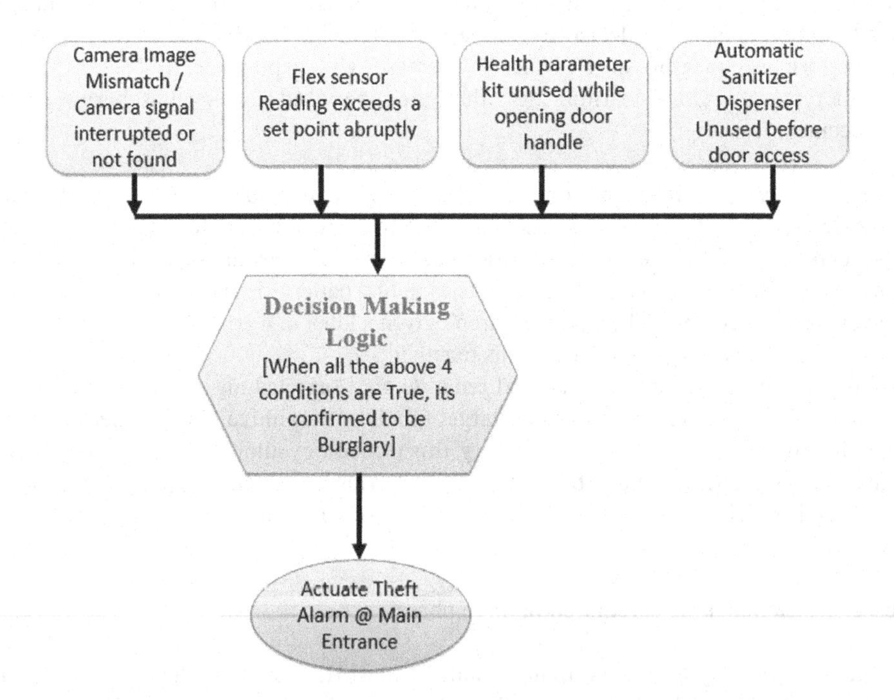

FIGURE 5.23 Decision-making logic used in ML Algorithm for Outdoor drives.

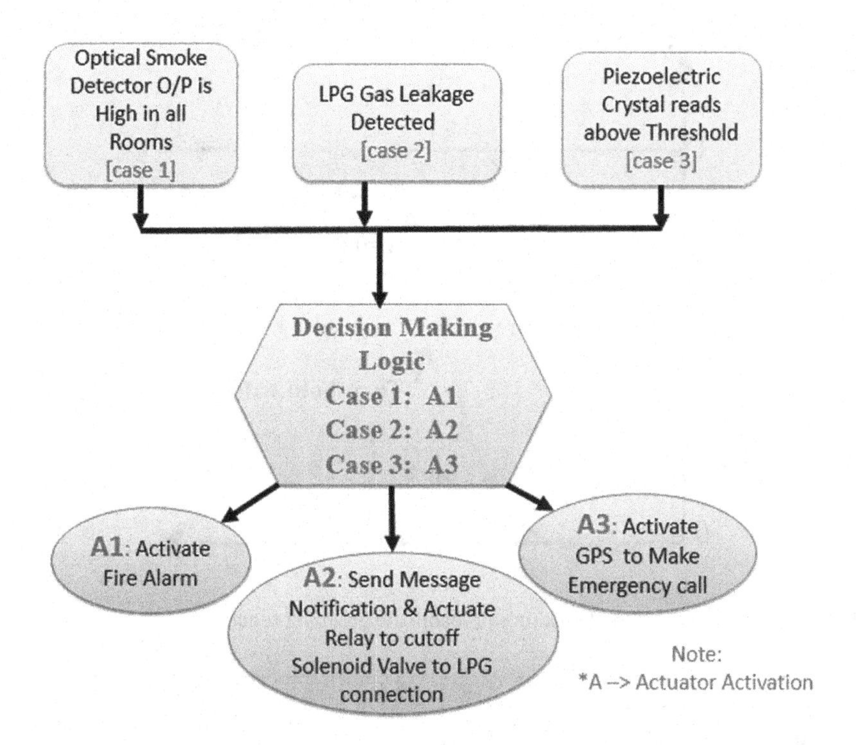

FIGURE 5.24 Decision making logic in ML algorithm for indoor drives.

- Ordinal: Here output can be three or more types of well-organized reliant variables, such as "low," "medium," or "high."

The mathematical model used to represent this particular algorithm is given below:

[Equation Credits: 17]

$$\log\left[\frac{y}{1-y}\right] = b_0 + b_1x_1 + b_2x_2 + b_3x_3 + \ldots b_nx_n \tag{5.1}$$

The mathematical model uses a sigmoidal function. This function transforms predicted values into the likelihood of decisive outputs (0/1, T/F, etc.). In logistic regression, rather than fitting into a regression line, we fit into an "S"-shaped curve. Here, the threshold value is used to describe the chance of falling into either 0 or 1. Values more than or equal to the threshold value are likely to be 1, while those less than or equal to the threshold value tend to be 0. [17]. Figure 5.25 [R17] shows the function used.

5.8.2 Steps Followed in Logistic Regression Algorithm

The steps for implementing Logistic Regression design are as follows:

1. Data acquisition and processing: As far as the initial stage is concerned, we'll collect and process the input data to make it flawless to train the network. The dataset is acquired as the result of running the function/code using Python or MATLAB tools. From the obtained sensor dataset, dependent and independent variables are separated and segregated into two parts: a training vector and a test vector. We will utilize feature scaling in

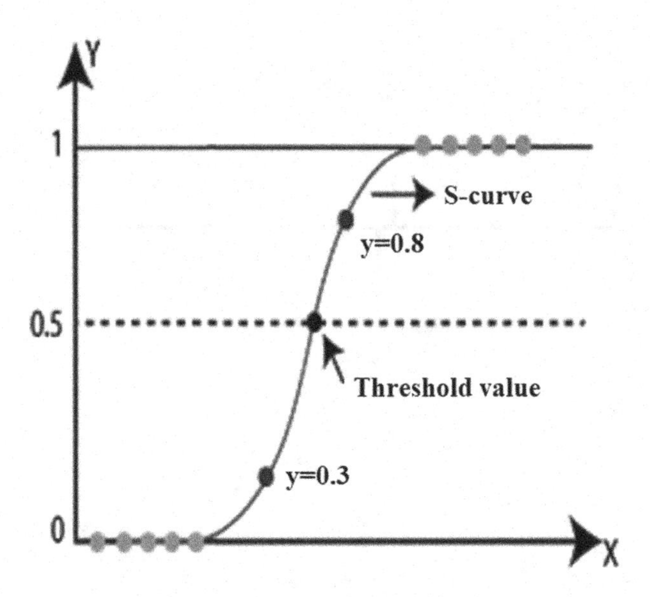

FIGURE 5.25 Logistic regression algorithm's probabilistic grouping function.

TABLE 5.1
Dataset Dispensation

Index	Parameters Measured/Action Taken	Independent/Dependent Variable [IV/DV]	Training Set/Test Set
1	Camera output comparison result	IV	Training data
2	Flex sensor value	IV	Training data
3	Health parameter values	IV	Training data
4	Automatic sanitizer dispenser used/not	IV	Training data
5	Theft alarm	DV	Test data
6	MQ2 gas sensor – leakage detection	IV	Training data
7	Optical smoke detectors	IV	Training data
8	Piezoelectric crystal output	IV	Training data
9	GSM call to fire station on smoke detector output	DV	Test data
10	GSM call to emergency care taker /hospital on piezoelectric output	DV	Test data
11	Activation of fire alarm	DV	Test data

logistic regression since we want precise predictions. Because the dependent variable only has 0 and 1 values, we shall only scale the independent variable (Table 5.1).

2. Training the dataset: We've prudently organized our dataset, and in this step, we'll use the logistic regressive function to train the refined dataset. We can use library functions in the build process. We'll create a classifier object after importing the class and use it to fit the model to the logistic regression. As a result, our model fits the training set perfectly.
3. Forecasting the test outcome: Since this model has got proficient training from a logistic function using the input and target vectors, we will now use test data to predict the outcome. When you run the code, it will generate a new vector (y_pred). Results are shown as (Figure 5.26):

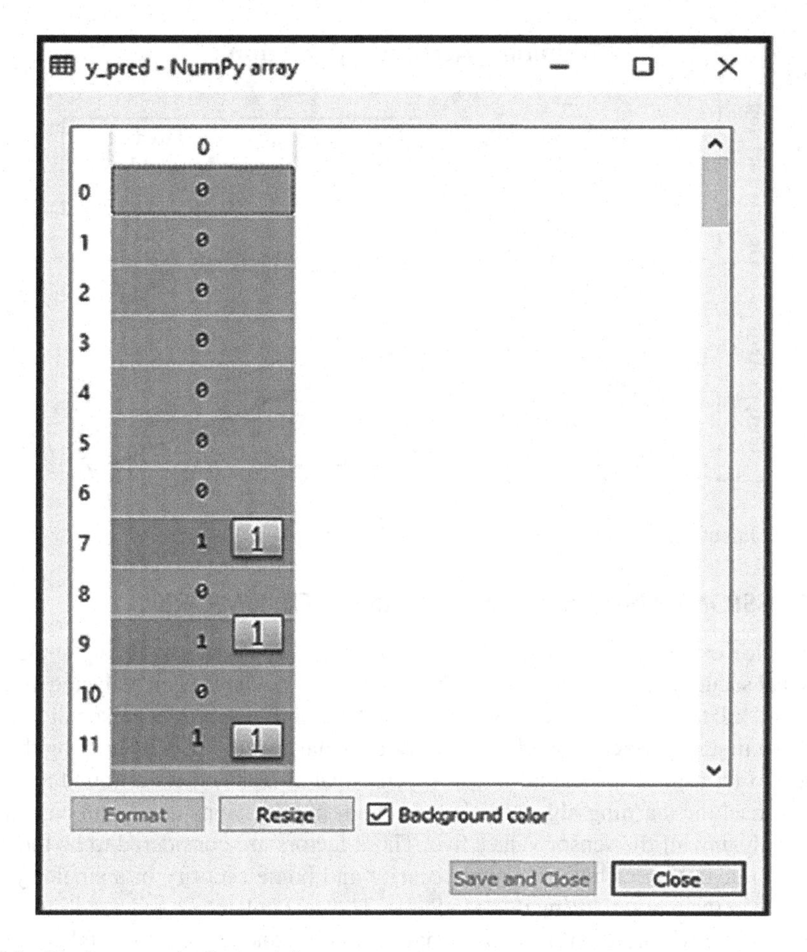

FIGURE 5.26 Final test result after training.

The corresponding values for actuating the outputs, based on sensor data, are shown in the output image above. Here, index "7" is high as optical sensors read high, index "9" goes high, indicating a fire service emergency call from GSM, and index "11," indicating fire alarm output goes high.

4. Testing the result accuracy: The confusion matrix can be used to determine the accuracy of the projected result.
5. Visualizing the test set result: Using the training dataset, we have a well-trained model. Now we'll see how the results look for the fresh test vectors. The graph in Figure 5.27 shows the test vectors attained. Thus, our model is fairly accurate and capable of making new predictions for this categorization challenge (Figure 5.27).

The above plot proves the efficiency of a trained network. It casts off sensor values along horizontal axes and actuator on/off along vertical axes. We can also estimate from the graph that most of the time, sensor values are normal and hence output remains normal. For verification purposes, the prototype was purposefully made to raise sensor values above a threshold and output actuators were getting Logic 1.

The classifier's purpose: We've successfully visualized the logistic regression training set results, and our goal for this classification is to make the best use of the sensor data to manage output alarms with the same efficiency as a human.

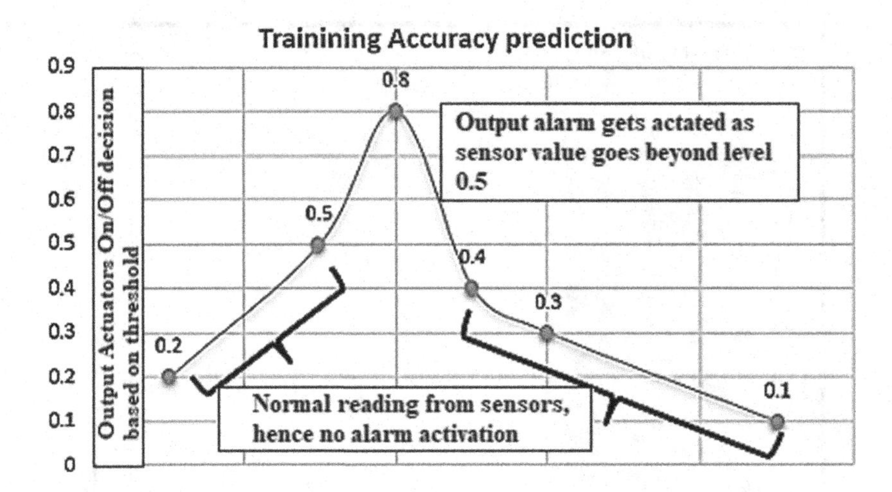

FIGURE 5.27 Output Test vector set results.

5.9 DISCUSSIONS AND PROS AND CONS OF OUR WORK

The accessible IoT expertise has been best utilized for the purpose of preserving home security as well as personal security in this work. The numerous sensor data have been collected and processed with the help of IoT technologies and cloud updation helped in rescuing a person at critical condition similar to a first responder network. This work also alarmed the person entering the home that he/she is safe to intersperse or should keep oneself isolated from others if found abnormal. The integration of machine learning algorithm helped in taking decisions during an emergency crisis alone, after analyzing all the sensor values live. These factors are considered to be the pros of our work since the integration of both personal security and home security in a single system is not mostly available in the market during this pandemic. The data collection and handling from all sensor nodes using a single controller unit was a challenging hit, and this could be taken care of in the future by reemploying smart sensors.

5.10 CONCLUSION

Healthcare and security of one's own are the two biggest challenges humans have been facing since a long time. These expectations have even grown in this pandemic situation to the peak and are demanding good solutions. Although technologies excel in their own way to provide solutions for these two big problems, some loop hovels still take back the issues. The problems encountered while developing an integrated system were handling of massive sensor data in real time, energy feeding to devices in an uninterrupted fashion, difficulty in maintaining one controller source for data collection from sensors, algorithm development, and testing of hardware. Developments in big data handling and energy harvesting will surely answer the above-mentioned issues. This chapter deliberated successfully about an integrated approach for maintaining both human and home security and safety aspects by making use of IoT and logistic regressive decision-making techniques. In future work, readers may try energy harvesting methods to produce energy needed by circuitry and use big data methods to handle and process enormous sensor data.

REFERENCES

1. Amani Aldahiri, Bashair Alrashed, Walayat Hussain, "Trends in Using IoT with Machine Learning in Health Prediction Systems", *Forecasting*, vol. 3, pp. 181–206, 2021, https://doi.org/10.3390/forecast3010012.

2. A. Anitha, "Home Security System Using Internet of Things", *Conference Series: Materials Science and Engineering*, vol. 263, 042026, 2017, doi: 10.1088/1757-899x/263/4/042026
3. P. Gupta, D. Agrawal, J. Chhabra and P. K. Dhir, "IoT Based Smart Healthcare Kit", 2016 International Conference on Computational Techniques in Information and Communication Technologies (ICCTICT), pp. 237–242, 2016, doi: 10.1109/ICCTICT.2016.7514585.
4. Ravi Kishore Kodali, V. Jain, S. Bose and L. Boppana, "IoT Based Smart Security and Home Automation System", 2016 International Conference on Computing, Communication and Automation (ICCCA), pp. 1286–1289, 2016, doi: 10.1109/CCAA.2016.7813916
5. D. M. Jeya Priyadharsan, K. Sanjay, S. Kathiresan, K. Karthik, and K. Prasath, "Patient Health Monitoring Using IoT with Machine Learning", *International Research Journal of Engineering and Technology*, vol. 6, no. 03, pp. 7514–7518, March 2019.
6. Chnar Mustafa, Shavan Askar, "Machine Learning for IoT Healthcare Applications: A Review", *Journal of Science and Business*, vol. 5, no. 3, pp. 42–51. https://doi.org/10.5281/zenodo.4496904.
7. https://robu.in/automatic-hand-sanitizer-dispenser-using-arduino/
8. Priyanka Raut, Surabhi Bondre, Ankita Girde, "LPG Leakage Detection and Alarming System", *International Journal of Scientific Research & Engineering Trends*, vol. 6, no. 2, pp. 496–498, March–April 2020.
9. S. Shyamaladevi, V. G. Rajaramya, P. Rajasekar, P. Sebastin Ashok, "ARM7 Based Automated High-Performance System for LPG Refill Booking & Leakage Detection", *International Journal of Engineering Research and Science and Technology*, vol. 3, no. 2, pp. 1–7, May, 2014.
10. B. B. Didpaye, S. K. Nanda, "Automated Unified System for LPG Using Microcontroller and GSM Module", *International Journal of Advanced Research in Computer and Communication Engineering*, vol. 4, no. 1, pp. 209–212, January 2015.
11. L. Fraiwan, K. Lweesy, A. Bani-Salma, N. Mani, "A Wireless Home Safety Gas Leakage Detection System", 2011 1st Middle East Conference on Biomedical Engineering, pp. 11–14, 2011, doi: 10.1109/MECBME.2011.5752053.
12. Hussain A. Attia Halah Y. Ali, "Electronic Design of Liquefied Petroleum Gas Leakage Monitoring, Alarm, and Protection System Based on Discrete Components", *International Journal of Applied Engineering Research*, vol. 11, no. 19, pp. 9721–9726, 2016.
13. https://www.pressac.com/insights/types-of-smart-building-sensor-and-how-they-work/
14. https://www.researchgate.net/publication/323622487_Smart_temperature_sensors_and_temperature_sensor_systems
15. https://towardsdatascience.com/machine-learning-basics-part-1-a36d38c7916
16. https://machinelearningmastery.com/a-tour-of-machine-learning-algorithms/
17. https://www.javatpoint.com/logistic-regression-in-machine-learning

6 Artificial Intelligence-Based Categorization of Healthcare Text

Omer Koksal

CONTENTS

DOI: 10.1201/9781003217398-6

6.1 INTRODUCTION

The process of classifying text data in healthcare systems is of particular importance. It is vital to collect, classify, disseminate, and manage information for applications and decision support systems used in healthcare. The number of text classification applications is increasing in parallel with the rise of AI applications in the healthcare domain. Categorizing healthcare text data (e.g., patients' symptom description) according to diseases using a text classifier is a critical process that determines the healthcare procedures to be followed, such as online healthcare counseling and information advice. At this stage, the most significant factor determining the accuracy of the provided services is the high accuracy obtained in text classification. Thus, decisions in healthcare are crucial, and attempts to make up for them later are also very costly. This chapter presents the common techniques and classifiers used in healthcare text classification to develop robust healthcare applications with high accuracy. Text classification is the automated process of categorizing text data depending on its content. In earlier applications, text classification was used in information retrieval systems. Nowadays, text classification is a vital natural language processing (NLP) task widely employed in various domains such as medicine, biology, social sciences, and engineering. Diverse text classification tasks are used in these areas, such as document categorization, document summarization, information filtering, sentiment analysis, spam e-mail detection, topic tagging, and intent detection.

Text classification processes use fundamental text mining techniques. However, with the rise of artificial intelligence (AI), learning-based algorithms have become the most important part of the text classification process. This chapter describes the main steps of the text classification process and techniques and explains the fundamentals of learning-based classifiers. Please refer to cited references for more details on the mathematical formulations of the algorithms.

6.2 TEXT CLASSIFICATION

As defined above, text classification can be described as classifying text data depending on its content. Text classification can be conducted utilizing learning-based or rule-based techniques, as shown in Figure 6.1. Further, hybrid methods are used in particular applications. In this chapter, we focus on learning-based text classification algorithms.

A text classification process has one or more datasets and uses rule-based or learning-based methods to extract valuable information from datasets. Some applications use hybrid methods that consist of both rule-based and learning-based methods. Various metrics might be used to evaluate the performance of text classification processes.

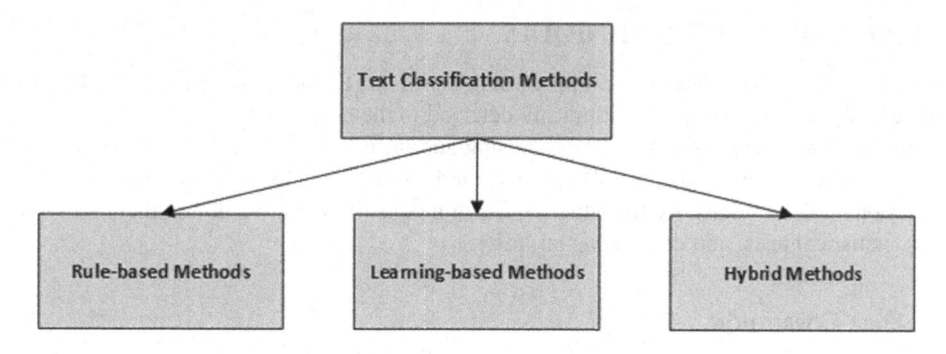

FIGURE 6.1 Text classification methods.

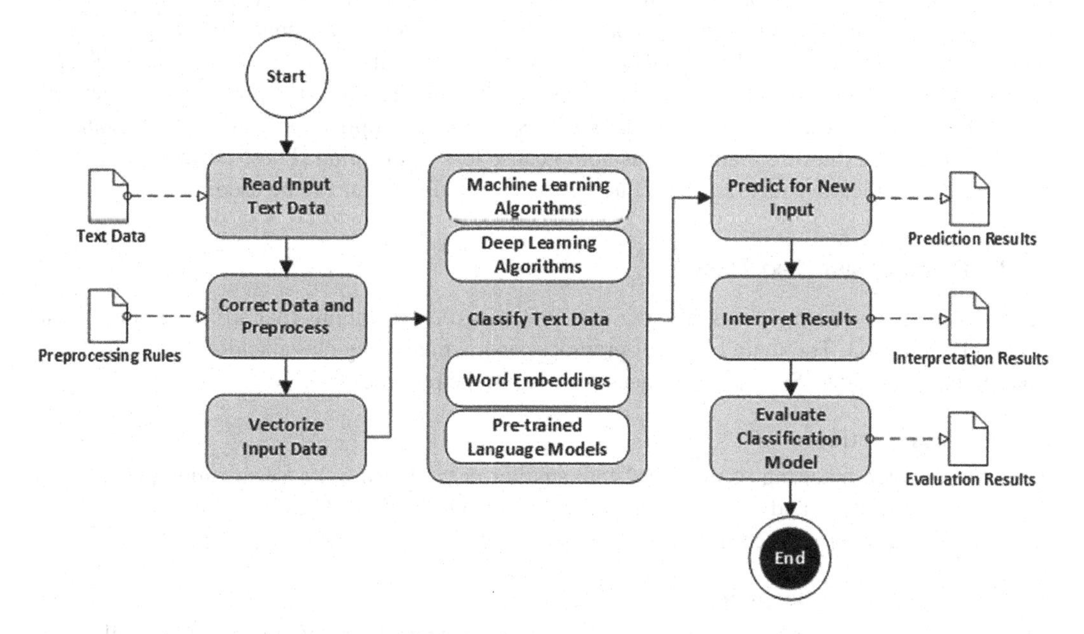

FIGURE 6.2 Text classification framework.

6.2.1 Text Classification Framework

This section defines a typical framework for text classification that is given in Figure 6.2. This framework covers all the main steps of text classification. However, some steps might be skipped depending on the data used and application type, such as preprocessing and correction.

The classification process starts with reading input text data that might be in a structured or unstructured format. It can be accessed via a database or crawled from the internet. Generally, this input text shall be corrected and preprocessed using the provided rules.

Several techniques are used in this step, such as removing punctuations and correcting misspelled words with a spell checker. At this point, the input text data shall be converted into numbers by vectorization techniques for further processing for classifying. Since the dimension of the vectors is very big to process, the dimension reduction takes place, and the features which mostly affect the classification accuracy are extracted.

The test data used in the prediction step is classified using the classification model. In this step, obtaining interpretable results is crucial. The final step is the evaluation of the whole process using appropriate metrics.

6.3 TEXT PROCESSING TECHNIQUES

In this section, we introduced major text processing topics and techniques used in the text classification process. The classification algorithms are deferred to the next chapter.

We start with an overview of text preprocessing and introduce two fundamental feature extraction methods: the bag-of-words (BOW) approach and word embeddings. Then we investigate feature selection methods. Later we introduce N-Gram models. Finally, we briefly mention sampling methods, statistical tests, and document similarity.

6.3.1 Data Correction

In many text classification applications, the input text data has errors. Apart from misspelled words, there might be several forms of intentional or unintentional errors in the text. For example, in sentiment analysis of a product, customer feedbacks are in an unstructured format. They might include comments with several misspelled words and intentional errors like "baddd" instead of "bad" and "cmputr" instead of "computer". Several techniques (e.g., similarity metrics) are used to detect and correct these errors. Although spell checkers are used in some applications, these errors shall be corrected in a context-aware manner so as not to cause loss of meaning. These corrections help to increase the classification accuracy by reducing the feature dimensions to be used.

6.3.2 Preprocessing Text Data

Preprocessing is converting raw input text data into new representations that are more convenient for text classification. The main object of preprocessing is improving classification accuracy while reducing input data size. Several techniques are used in the preprocessing step.

6.3.2.1 Tokenization

Tokenization is the breaking of input text into smaller parts. During the tokenization process, all punctuation, delimiters, and extra spaces are removed from the data. Thus, the assessed token is a valued part of the unstructured input data.

6.3.2.2 Lowercase Conversion

Lowercase conversion converts all input text to a lowercase format, one of the most commonly used techniques in the preprocessing phase. This conversion reduces feature dimension and improves the classification accuracy almost in all cases. However, this technique shall not be applied where the uppercase and lowercase of words have different meanings. For instance, "Opera" is a browser and "opera" is a kind of music. In such cases, the lowercase conversion process causes the loss of meaning [1].

6.3.2.3 Stop Word Removal

Stop word removal is another commonly used technique in text preprocessing. The most commonly used words in a particular language are called stop words. Stop words are assumed to be irrelevant within the working domain and have no effect on classification. The stop word removal process filters out these words before the classification process. Hence, the stop word removal process provides dimensionality reduction.

6.3.2.4 Stemming

Stemming can be defined as acquiring the stem or root form of an inflected word by removing the suffix. Stemming is a language-specific process providing a common form for the variants of words. Hence, word frequencies are typically counted after the stemming process in the vectorization process.

6.3.2.5 Lemmatizing

The lemmatizing process results in the lemma of an inflected word based on the intended meaning. Moreover, the lemmatizing takes morphological information into account, whereas stemming only crops the beginning of the end of the word to obtain the root of a word.

6.3.3 Feature Extraction

Text classification requires converting text data into numerical forms to perform further processing. Transforming text data into vector space models is called feature extraction.

6.3.3.1 Bag-of-Words Approach

The bag-of-words (BOW) approach is the characteristic technique used in traditional text classification applications to vectorize the text input. In this model, input text data is represented as vectors, and all terms correspond to features. Put it differently, distinct words in documents figure out the dimension of the feature space used. The BOW model does not retain word order in the text; it just distinguishes the existence of a word in the document.

The weights of the extracted features are determined utilizing diverse methods with the BOW approach [2]. We present three main vector weighting techniques.

Binary Assignment

Binary assignment is the elementary vector weighting method that just checks the existence of terms in each document.

The Term Frequency

The term frequency (TF) method takes the terms frequencies that appear in each text into account. Thus, the TF can be expressed as given as follows in Equation (6.1):

$$\mathrm{TF}(t,d) = \log\left(1 + \mathrm{freq}(t,d)\right) \tag{6.1}$$

Term Frequency–Inverse Document Frequency (TF-IDF)

TF-IDF is an advanced weighting method that takes the frequencies in a whole collection into account. In TF-IDF, the importance of terms is related to their frequencies in the particular document while being inversely proportional to the term's frequency in the batch. The TF-IDF can be expressed as given in Equations (6.2 and 6.3):

$$\mathrm{TF-IDF}(t,d,D) = \mathrm{TF}(t,d) \times \mathrm{IDF}(t,D) \tag{6.2}$$

where

$$\mathrm{IDF}(t,D) = \log\left(N/\mathrm{count}\left(\mathrm{d}\varepsilon D : t\varepsilon d\right)\right) \tag{6.3}$$

6.3.3.2 Word Embeddings

A more recent approach in feature extraction is using word embeddings. Word embeddings acquire the meaning of words or phrases mapped to vector representations, enabling similar text grouping in a new vector space. Word embeddings might be more efficient than the BOW models. In the BOW models, the broadness of document collection and tagging at the index position causes data sparsity problems. However, word embeddings take the token's surrounding words into account to solve the data sparsity problem. The given text's information is transferred to the model to end up with dense vectors. In this continuous vector space representation, semantically alike words are close to each other. This deduction can either be ensured by utilizing neural networks for language modeling, predicting a word in a sentence, given the nearby words as input, or capturing the training corpus's statistical properties. When predicting words in similar context inputs, neural networks generate similar predicted word outputs, resulting in a semantic representation space with the desired property. The following subsections present some well-known word embedding techniques briefly.

Word2Vec

Word2Vec is a statistical predictive method [3]. It utilizes two neural networks to learn a particular word embedding from a given text collection. The continuous BOW (CBOW) model is the first neural network used by Word2Vec. CBOW foresees the word in the middle of a sequence. However, the second neural network named the skip-gram model predicts the context.

Doc2Vec

Doc2Vec is supposed to be an extension of the Word2Vec model, also called a paragraph vector [4]. Doc2Vec generates vectors for sentences, paragraphs, and documents; however, Word2Vec generates vectors just for words.

Global Vectors for Word Representation

Global Vectors for Word Representation (GLOVE) is essentially an unsupervised algorithm. To construct word embeddings from a corpus, GLOVE assembles a comprehensive word co-occurrence matrix [5]. GLOVE carries out dimensionality reduction on the co-occurrence information to learn vectors. GLOVE is a count-based model and easier to parallelize compared to the Word2Vec method.

FastText

FastText treats each word as composed of character n-grams instead of Word2Vec [6]. Thus, for rare words, FastText results in better word embeddings. Further, it can generate a vector for an out of vocabulary word that does not exist in the training corpus. This feature is not possible with either Word2Vec or Glove.

6.3.4 Feature Selection Methods

Feature selection reduces the number of input variables manually or automatically to figure out the most important features for the prediction. By eliminating less redundant and misleading data, feature selection methods help reduce training time and overfitting and improve classification accuracy [7,8]. We provide several feature selection methods typically used in text classification in the following subsections.

6.3.4.1 Chi-Square

Chi-Square (CHI) is used to check the correlation between two variables statistically. This method measures the independence between features and categories by comparing them with a CHI distribution. High dependence means more influence of a feature on selecting the compared category and vice versa.

6.3.4.2 Correlation Coefficient

The correlation coefficient (CC) method measures the strength of the statistical relationship between a feature and a category.

6.3.4.3 Information Gain

Information gain (IG) measures the reduction of the class variable's entropy having the feature's values observed. IG determines how common a feature is in a particular class when compared to the other classes.

6.3.5 N-Gram-Based Language Models

Several NLP applications utilize N-Gram-based models, especially in language identification and machine translation tasks [9]. In these models, data is parsed to have "N" words in each token. For example, the single-word language model is called unigram, size two is bigram, and size three is trigram. Despite their vast usage, these models lack long-range dependency representation in the text classification tasks.

6.3.6 Sampling Methods

In the text classification process, selecting the training and test datasets might dramatically affect the classification accuracy and cause misleading results. So, selecting these datasets to reflect the characteristics of the whole dataset is important. Sampling is the process of selecting suitable samples from a dataset. In classification tasks, to have reliable predictions, several resampling methods such as N-Fold cross-validation (N-Fold CV), holdout, and bootstrap can be used. In this subsection, we briefly mention the N-Fold cross-validation sampling method.

6.3.6.1 N-Fold Cross-Validation

N-Fold CV is the most commonly used sampling method in text classification. It randomly partitions the data into "N" subsets where "N" experiments are performed. In each experiment, "N–1" subsets are used for training, and the remaining one is used for testing. The CV method is named depending on the number "N", such as 3-fold CV or 10-fold CV.

6.3.7 Statistical Tests

In many text classification applications, the machine learning application's performance might be different on specific datasets. In these cases, the results (or dataset) shall be checked if a significant difference exists statistically. In this part, we present two commonly used statistical tests to provide a solution in these situations.

6.3.7.1 *T*-Test

T-test is a statistical hypothesis test. It is applied to check whether the difference between the means of the two sets is significantly different.

6.3.7.2 Kappa Coefficient

To measure agreement between two raters, the Kappa coefficient is used. These coefficients are evaluated using the guidelines of Landis and Koch [10].

6.3.8 Document Similarity

In the text classification applications, semantically similar documents are considered similar. The similarity between documents is measured by converting input documents to real-valued vectors. In this part, we present two document similarity methods.

6.3.8.1 Cosine Similarity

The cosine similarity CS method indicates the semantic similarity of documents by utilizing the cosine of the angle between vectors.

6.3.8.2 Okapi BM25

Okapi BM25 (and its variants such as BM25F and BM25Ext) is a ranking function that uses a probabilistic retrieval framework to estimate the relevance between documents.

6.4 CLASSIFICATION ALGORITHMS

As mentioned earlier, text classification is the automated process of categorizing text data depending on its content. Diverse learning-based algorithms are used to classify text data. In this section, we introduce several algorithms used in text classification. We use the terms algorithm and classifier interchangeably throughout the text. Although in all of these classification algorithms, features are the input variables, and the output attribute is the predicted class or category, they use different techniques and models to improve the accuracy of the classification. Hence, we group these algorithms into three main categories: machine learning-based classifiers, deep learning-based classifiers, and pre-trained language models. In the following subsections, we present several details of these algorithms.

6.4.1 Machine Learning-Based Classifiers

This section presents common machine learning-based text classification techniques and algorithms. We mainly group these classifiers into two fundamental types: supervised and unsupervised classifiers. Further, we present semi-supervised learning. It shall be noted that, since we focus on classification algorithms, the terms algorithm and classifier are used interchangeably throughout the paper.

6.4.1.1 Supervised Machine Learning-Based Classifiers

Supervised machine learning algorithms use training data to build a mathematical model. This model predicts the label (classification) or value (regression) of the test data. In contrast, unsupervised algorithms try to detect previously undetected patterns in the previously unlabeled dataset. This subsection briefly describes the traditional supervised machine learning algorithms.

Naïve Bayes

Naïve Bayes (NB) is widely used in classification tasks as a probabilistic classifier. NB requires low computation time and is interpretable. However, NB is grounded on the Bayes Theorem, assuming a specific feature's value does not depend on other features [11]. This assumption is not always valid in real life. Several versions of NB classifiers are developed to overcome the limitations of NB's independence assumption. Multinomial NB, Complement NB, and Bernoulli NB are the well-known variants of the NB classifier.

Logistic Regression

Logistic regression (LR) is another classification algorithm as opposed to what its name implies. Although the mathematical formulation of LR is similar to linear regression, LR performs classification by comparing the logistic function's output with a determined threshold value depending on the problem domain [12].

Support Vector Machine

Since support vector machine (SVM) outperforms other traditional machine learning algorithms in many applications, it is a popular classifier used in text classification applications. SVM constructs optimal hyperplanes to classify data, called the decision surfaces. SVM uses these hyperplanes iteratively to minimize the error. A hyperplane is drawn between the support vectors that belong to the different categories. The closest data points to the hyperplanes are named support vectors. To construct hyperplanes, SVM utilizes particular kernels. Linear, polynomial, radial basis function, and sigmoid kernel are the most commonly used SVM kernels. The kernel might provide higher classification accuracy depending on data type and particular size [12] Therefore, SVM can be used instead of deep learning-based classifiers for small data since it provides similar performance with fewer training times. Further, neural network-based classifiers might suffer from interpretability problems.

K-Nearest Neighbors

K-nearest neighbors (KNN) algorithm is based on feature similarity and has no assumption for data distribution. KNN predicts based on the neighbor data points. "K" is the only input parameter of the algorithm. The training phase of KNN is fast. KNN is especially important when processing data with no prior knowledge.

Decision Tree

Decision tree (DT) is a predictive modeling approach that uses a tree structure to break down complex data into more manageable parts. In this structure, internal nodes correspond to tests on attributes, branches represent the outcomes of the tests, and leaf nodes denote class labels. In DT, classification is performed iteratively by initializing at the root node, testing the node's attributes, and reaching down according to the test's outcome.

Maximum Entropy

Maximum entropy (ME) classifier assesses the conditional distribution of the category tags in the document based on probabilistic distribution. In addition, the ME classifier uses the training data to assess the expected value of the word counts based on classes [13].

Latent Dirichlet Allocation

Latent dirichlet allocation (LDA) is categorized as a generative probabilistic model and is especially used in topic modeling [14]. LDA's primary objective is to find the topics that a document belongs to, using the words in that document.

6.4.1.2 Unsupervised Machine Learning Classifiers

Unsupervised machine learning classifiers try to find previously undetected patterns in the unlabeled dataset. Unsupervised learning allows the modeling of probability densities over inputs. Unsupervised learning aims to learn new feature space capturing the original space's characteristics by maximizing objective function and minimizing the loss. In this part, we briefly present the principal unsupervised machine learning classifiers.

K-Means

K-Means uses vector quantization to separate data into groups with equal variances minimizing inertia or the sum of squares within a cluster. Kadena's Mining Algorithm (KDA) takes the number of cluster values as the single input. This clustering algorithm stores the centroids to describe the clusters. Based on the current centroids and data points' assignments, K-means aims to determine the most proper centroid for the given data [15].

Latent Semantic Analysis

Latent semantic analysis (LSA) is an unsupervised classifier commonly used in topic modeling [16]. LSA assumes that the words that are closer in their meaning occur in a similar fragment of the text. LSA classifies topics using the matrix generated by existing words in the paragraphs. Singular value decomposition (SVD) is utilized to deduct the number of rows retaining the similar structure among columns. LSA employs cosine similarity to compare documents. Similar documents have values close to 1, whereas dissimilar documents are close to zero.

6.4.1.3 Semi-supervised Learning

Semi-supervised learning classifiers might be more suitable for classification tasks when a dataset has many unlabeled instances and a few labeled instances. The labeled instances are used for training a supervised learning model. Most semi-supervised learning classifiers utilize clustering techniques to check the existence of multiple tagged or unlabeled data points in a unique cluster [17].

6.4.1.4 Ensemble Learning-Based Classifiers

Several learning techniques such as active learning, transfer learning, and ensemble learning are used in machine learning applications. In this section, we provide several ensemble learning techniques that are widely used in classification tasks.

Bagging

The bagging (or bootstrap aggregating) algorithm [18] is generated by utilizing different bootstrap samples. It improves the machine learning algorithms' stability and accuracy in classification and prevents overfitting. Bagging is typically implemented in DTs.

Boosting

Boosting is another popular ensemble-learning algorithm. One of the most popular versions of boosting algorithms is adaptive boosting (AdaBoost), proposed in 1999 [19]. In this algorithm, the weak learners' outputs' weighted sum determines the boosted classifier's output. The AdaBoost classifier is sensitive to outliers and noisy data. However, even if the individual learners are weak, as long as each weak learner's performance is better than random predictions, the boosting model can converge to a strong learner.

Majority Voting

Majority voting is a combined model that consists of two or more classifiers. For each data instance, all classifiers make their own prediction. Then, the majority of the votes acquired from the involved classifiers determine the label of the data instance [20].

Random Forest

Random Forest (RF) consists of assemblies of DTs. RF can be presented as ensembles of DTs and generally outperforms them. The predictions are determined by voting after training all trees in the forest. RFs are very fast to train text data. However, they are slower in predictions compared to deep learning-based classifiers.

6.4.2 Deep Learning-Based Classifiers

The functional aspects of human thinking inspire the deep learning concept. Deep learning-based classifiers and architectures are widely used in text classification applications with remarkable performances. There are several assets of using Deep Learning classifiers in text classification. Firstly, in natural language processing, deep learning replaces existing linear models with better-performing models that are capable of learning and exploiting nonlinear relationships. Also, deep learning methods simplify the development of new models. Another dominance of deep learning methods is learning feature representations rather than requiring experts to specify and extract features manually. Besides, deep learning enables rapid improvement on compelling problems. Further, deep learning techniques can develop and train end-to-end models, resulting in faster and simpler solutions in NLP tasks. This section presents common deep learning architectures used for text classification in the following subsections.

6.4.2.1 Deep Neural Networks

Deep neural networks (DNNs) are artificial neural networks (ANNs) that are devised for learning by multi-connection layers. The architecture of DNNs includes one input layer, one output layer, and one or more hidden layers between them, as shown in Figure 6.3.

The input feature space of the text data constitutes the input layer of the DNN. The input can be constructed with feature extraction methods like TF, TF-IDF, or word embeddings in the text classification process. The output layer has one node in binary classification and has nodes as much

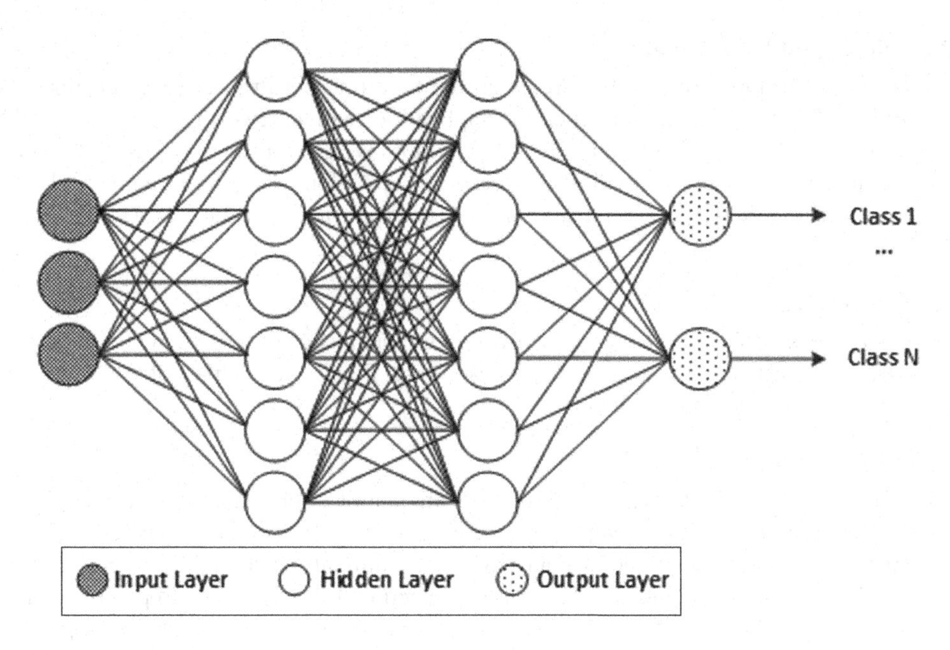

FIGURE 6.3 The architectural design of the deep neural network for text classification.

as the number of classes in multi-class classification. DNN uses a standard back-propagation algorithm with an activation function. The activation function is sigmoid or RELU functions in many applications. The sigmoid and RELU functions can be defined as shown in the Equations (6.4 and 6.5), respectively:

$$\text{SIGMOID}(x) = 1/\left(1+\exp(-x)\right) \tag{6.4}$$

$$\text{RELU}(x) = \max(0, x) \tag{6.5}$$

With the help of the presented architecture, DNN's extract features from the input text data. Then, the model is trained to optimize weight and bias values in the neural network structure. Finally, the trained model is used to predict the class of the new text input. In DNNs, the output of the multi-class classification shall be the Softmax function. The definition of the Softmax function [17] is given in Equation (6.6).

$$\sigma(Z)_j = \exp(Z_j)/\Sigma_k\left(\exp(Z_k)\right) \quad \text{where } k = 1\ldots K \tag{6.6}$$

6.4.2.2 Convolutional Neural Network

Convolutional neural network (CNN) was initially designed for image processing using the deep learning architecture, but it is also used in text classification and hierarchical document classification [21]. CNN's hidden layers comprise several convolutional layers, also called feature maps, convolved with multiplication or other dot product. In CNN, typically, RELU is used as the activation function followed by pooling layers that enable additional convolutions. Then comes fully connected layers, normalization layers, and the output layer. While using CNN in text classification, the feature space's size might cause a problem. In image classification applications, few channels (e.g., three channels in RGB) are needed. But, for text classification applications, this feature space might be massive.

6.4.2.3 Recurrent Neural Network

Since recurrent neural network (RNN) architecture fits well to perform sequence or time-based analysis, it is widely used for text classification applications with noteworthy performance. RNN evaluates the previous nodes' information and puts more weight on the previous data points in the input sequence. RNN is used within bidirectional RNN, long short-term memory (LSTM), or gated recurrent unit (GRU) architectures to overcome vanishing and exploding gradient problems.

Bidirectional RNN

Bidirectional RNNs perform predictions by merging the outputs of two RNNs. One of the RNNs processes data forward, and the other processes backward. Finally, the outputs of these two RNNs are combined to make the final prediction.

Long Short-Term Memory

LSTM utilizes various gates to arrange each node's amount of information [22]. A typical LSTM gate comprises three gates (input, output, and forget) and a cell. With its feedback connections, LSTM processes an entire data sequence, and hence it is commonly used in applications like speech recognition, handwriting recognition, and intrusion detection. It is well suited to process and classifying time series data. In addition, LSTM is successful in overcoming the vanishing gradient problem of RNN.

Gated Recurrent Unit

GRUs are RNNs with gating mechanisms and perform better than the traditional tanh function in RNNs [23]. Hence, GRUs can be evaluated as simplified versions of LSTM architectures. Although GRU's performance is similar to that of LSTMs on certain tasks (like speech processing and NLP), they might have higher performance in particular smaller and less frequent datasets. However, LSTM performs unbounded counting and outperforms GRU to learn simple languages [24] and perform machine translation [25].

6.4.3 Pre-trained Language Models

The use of pre-trained language models is emerging due to their valuable performance in the NLP domain. With the introduction of encoder–decoder models in the transformer architecture [26], pre-trained language models have seen increasing research interest. Encoder models take input text and generate high-dimensional latent embeddings that do not necessarily belong to a semantic space. Decoder models convert these embeddings back into the natural language to accomplish a language modeling task. Pre-trained language models utilize dynamic representations of words, also referred to as contextual embeddings. The pre-training procedure is carried on using domain-independent large corpora. Deploying such models for downstream applications requires a fine-tuning step that optimizes the model for the task using smaller, domain-specific data. This section presents some of the widely used pre-trained language models briefly.

6.4.3.1 Embeddings from Language Models

Based on the LSTM model, embeddings from language models (ELMO) generate word representations as functions of the entire input sentence [27]. Further, ELMO has a prediction task to guess the next word in a sentence. Prediction is performed based on the information captured from the previous words in the hidden state vectors of LSTM. By combining forward and backward language modeling, ELMO associates context information with the word representations. Thus, ELMO deviates from the other word embedding algorithms that generate static word vectors with its dynamically computed word vectors.

6.4.3.2 Efficiently Learning an Encoder that Classifies Token Replacements Accurately

Efficiently learning an encoder that classifies token replacements accurately (ELECTRA) [28] utilizes a similar architecture to generative adversarial networks (GAN), training the generator in the architecture with a masked language modeling task. The masked language modeling task replaces a randomly chosen token in the input with a "[MASK]" token and expects the model to predict the original token. ELECTRA's main advantage is using smaller generator networks to decrease the computational complexity while achieving competitive accuracy.

6.4.3.3 Bidirectional Encoder Representations from Transformers

Bidirectional encoder representations from transformers (BERT) is a multilayer transformer encoder model. BERT is trained over a large corpus with a masked language modeling task and a next sentence prediction task simultaneously [29] It uses an attention mechanism to model long-range dependencies in the input text. The language modeling in BERT is bidirectional, as its name implies. This bidirectional model aims to capture the prediction process's contextual information. The next sentence prediction task samples the next sentence in the input with another sentence at random. It expects the model to predict whether the chosen sentence naturally follows the first sentence. This task enables BERT to develop a broader understanding of natural language by working at the sentence level. BERT brings a compelling basis for a variety of downstream tasks through its fine-tuning feature. The BERT fine-tuning enables the use of additional domain-specific data to adapt pre-trained BERT. For the classification task, the BERT embedding vector for the special "(CLS)" token placed at the beginning of the input sequence is used to encode the entire sequence. An additional fully connected layer maps the sequence embedding to the classification probabilities. BERT has several parameters for improving performance, such as the epoch size, maximum input sequence length, and pre-trained model choice. The literature shows that BERT outperformed other pre-trained language models in diverse NLP tasks [30]. BERT can incorporate smaller, task-specific data in the more lightweight fine-tuning process. So, it becomes widely adopted for high-accuracy gains in a range of downstream tasks [31].

6.5 EVALUATION METRICS

This section presents several vital metrics used for assessing the classification's performance. Most of the evaluation metrics of classification tasks are built on the confusion matrix (also called as error matrix) concept that reveals the prediction results of the classification model for the test set. The confusion matrix allows visualization of a classifier's performance in supervised learning.

The confusion matrix is a two-by-two matrix in a binary classification where the columns present the instances of the predicted classes. In contrast, the rows represent values for the actual classes. The confusion matrix is not limited to binary classification and can be used for multi-class classification tasks similarly. This representation reports true positives, true negatives, false positives, and false negatives, as shown in Table 6.1.

TABLE 6.1
Representation of True Positives, True Negatives, False Positives, and False Negatives

	Predicted Positive	Predicted Negative
Actual Positive	True positive (TP)	False negative (FN)
Actual Negative	False positive (FP)	True negative (TN)

The confusion matrix indicates the ways our model is confused in predicting classes where TP presents the predicted positive instances whose actual classes are positive (i.e., no confusion). Similarly, TN shows the instances that are predicted as negative, which are also true. On the other hand, FP and FN show instances predicted as positive and negative, respectively, which are false. The next subsections present evaluation measures based on the confusion matrix.

6.5.1 Accuracy

Accuracy can be defined as dividing the sum of correct predictions (TP and TN) to all instances, as given in Equation (6.7).

$$\text{Accuracy}(\text{A}) = (\text{TP}+\text{TN})/(\text{TP}+\text{TN}+\text{FP}+\text{FN}) \tag{6.7}$$

Accuracy is a practical score to evaluate classifiers' performance and can be misleading for imbalanced data. For imbalanced data, separately indicating precision and recall measures would be more interpretive for evaluating the classification results. The definitions of the precision and recall measures are introduced below.

6.5.2 Precision

Precision shows the accuracy of the positive class. Precision is the division of TP to the total positive predictions (TP and FP) as shown in Equation (6.8):

$$\text{Precision}(\text{P}) = \text{TP}/(\text{TP}+\text{FP}) \tag{6.8}$$

A perfect precision measure of 1 shows that every sample the model identified as belonging to a specific class, the actual class of each sample. However, this value does not show the model misclassified how many other samples belong to that class.

6.5.3 Recall

Recall (or sensitivity) shows the ratio of correctly detected positive classes, and it is defined as TP divided by the sum of positive classes (TP and FN) as shown in Equation (6.9):

$$\text{Recall}(\text{R}) = \text{TP}/(\text{TP}+\text{FN}) \tag{6.9}$$

A perfect recall measure of 1 shows that the model correctly classifies all the samples belonging to that class; however, this measure does not show how many are incorrectly classified as belonging to that class.

The usefulness of precision and recall measures are broadly context-dependent. For example, high precision would be more important in some classification tasks, and in some other tasks, the recall measure may be more critical. Hence, the classification models can be tuned for either metric, trading-off the other, depending on the context.

6.5.4 F-Measure

F-Measure compares models having different precision and recall values with a single evaluation measure. F-Measure can be defined as the harmonic mean of precision and recall as shown in Equation (6.10):

$$F_{\alpha} = (1+\alpha^2)*(\text{P}\times\text{R})/(\text{P}+\text{R}) \tag{6.10}$$

There are several variations of F-measure based on Equation (6.10), with varying α values. A higher α value indicates that recall measure is more emphasized in evaluation. Among several F measures, the F1 measure is widely used, keeping the α value as 1. Then the F1 measure can be interpreted as below in Equation (6.11).

$$F1 = 2*(P \times R)/(P + R) \tag{6.11}$$

6.5.4.1 Receiving Operational Characteristics

Receiving operating characteristics (ROC) is a graphical plot that shows the performance of a classification model at all classification thresholds by plotting the true positive rate (TPR) vs. false positive rate (FPR) at various threshold settings. The TPR is also known as sensitivity or recall. The FPR is called the probability of false alarm.

6.5.4.2 Area Under ROC Curve

Area under ROC curve (AUC) is an accumulated measure showing the performance across all possible classification thresholds between 0 and 1. Hence, AUC can be obtained using ROC. An AUC value closer to 0 is considered worse, whereas an AUC value closer to 1 is evaluated as better. AUC is one of the most robust measures used in the literature since it summarizes the classification model's indicative ability in a single number.

6.6 CONCLUSION

Classification of healthcare text is a crucial process. In the healthcare domain, the text categorization process might determine the healthcare procedures to be followed. Hence, obtained results and classification accuracy are of extreme importance. So, in this section, we presented the details of the algorithms and techniques used in the artificial intelligence-based categorization of healthcare text to develop robust healthcare applications with high accuracy. The classification process of healthcare text requires a well-established understanding of text mining and information retrieval techniques used in the text classification process. Hence, firstly, we presented a framework that shows all the main steps of the text classification process. Then, we explained fundamental text processing techniques, including data correction, preprocessing, vectorization, N-Gram language models, document similarity models, and sampling techniques. Further, we presented several machine learning-based classifiers widely used in healthcare text classification applications. Apart from traditional machine learning-based classifiers, we also present word embeddings and deep learning-based classifiers. Finally, we presented the pre-trained language models that are evaluated as state-of-the-art in several NLP tasks. Further, we mentioned metrics used to evaluate the performance of the classification algorithms. We believe that this chapter would be beneficial for further research in the healthcare text classification. We have presented diverse techniques and learning-based classifiers used in healthcare text classification. Therefore, this chapter will be gainful for both researchers and practitioners. Researchers might quickly outline the reported techniques and classifiers. In this respect, the outcomes of this study can be a short reference for the research activities of future studies related to the healthcare text classification. On the other hand, practitioners might utilize the presented techniques to analyze the relevant approaches and decide their applicability to develop reliable healthcare applications.

REFERENCE LIST

1. Işık, Muhittin, and Hasan Dağ. 2020. "The Impact of Text Preprocessing on the Prediction of Review Ratings." *Turkish Journal of Electrical Engineering and Computer Sciences* 28 (3): 1405–21.
2. Gomes, Luiz Alberto Ferreira, Ricardo da Silva Torres, and Mario Lúcio Côrtes. 2019. "Bug Report Severity Level Prediction in Open Source Software: A Survey and Research Opportunities." *Information and Software Technology*, vol. 115, C (Nov 2019), pp. 58–78. https://doi.org/10.1016/j.infsof.2019.07.009.

3. Mikolov, Tomas, Kai Chen, Greg Corrado, and Jeffrey Dean. 2013. “Efficient Estimation of Word Representations in Vector Space.” In *1st International Conference on Learning Representations, ICLR 2013 - Workshop Track Proceedings*. arXiv. https://doi.org/10.48550/arxiv.1301.3781
4. Le, Quoc V., and Tomas Mikolov. 2014. “Distributed Representations of Sentences and Documents.” *31st International Conference on Machine Learning, ICML 2014*, 4 (May): 2931–39.
5. Pennington, Jeffrey, Richard Socher, and Christopher Manning. 2014. “GloVe: Global Vectors for Word Representation.” In *Proceedings of the 2014 Conference on Empirical Methods in Natural Language Processing (EMNLP)*, 1532–43. Doha, Qatar. Association for Computational Linguistics.
6. Bojanowski, Piotr, Edouard Grave, Armand Joulin, and Tomas Mikolov. 2017. “Enriching Word Vectors with Subword Information.” *Transactions of the Association for Computational Linguistics* 5 (December): 135–46.
7. Asim, Muhammad Nabeel, Muhammad Wasim, Muhammad Sajid Ali, and Abdur Rehman. 2017. “Comparison of Feature Selection Methods in Text Classification on Highly Skewed Datasets.” In *2017 1st International Conference on Latest Trends in Electrical Engineering and Computing Technologies, INTELLECT 2017*, pp. 1–8, doi: 10.1109/INTELLECT.2017.8277634.
8. Deng, Xuelian, Yuqing Li, Jian Weng, and Jilian Zhang. 2019. “Feature Selection for Text Classification: A Review.” *Multimedia Tools and Applications* 78 (3): 3797–816.
9. Peng, Fuchun, and Dale Schuurmans. 2003. “Combining Naive Bayes and N-Gram Language Models for Text Classification.” *Lecture Notes in Computer Science (Including Subseries Lecture Notes in Artificial Intelligence and Lecture Notes in Bioinformatics)* 2633: 335–50.
10. Landis, J. Richard, and Gary G. Koch. 1977. “The Measurement of Observer Agreement for Categorical Data.” *Biometrics* 33 (1): 159.
11. Alpaydin, Ethem. 2016. *Machine Learning: The New AI*. The MIT Press, Camabridge.
12. Koksal, Omer, and Ömer Köksal. 2020. “Tuning the Turkish Text Classification Process Using Supervised Machine Learning-Based Algorithms.” In *2020 International Conference on INnovations in Intelligent SysTems and Applications (INISTA)*. Novi Sad, Serbia. IEEE.
13. Nigam, Kamal, John Lafferty, and Andrew McCallum. 1999. “Using Maximum Entropy for Text Classification.” In *IJCAI-99 Workshop on Machine Learning for Information Filtering*, 61–67. Stockholm, Sweden.
14. Blei, David M., Andrew Y. Ng, and Jordan@cs Berkeley Edu. 2003. “Latent Dirichlet Allocation Michael I. Jordan.” *Journal of Machine Learning Research* 3: 993–1022.
15. Dogan, Turgut, and Alper Kursat Uysal. 2020. “A Novel Term Weighting Scheme for Text Classification: TF-MONO.” *Journal of Informetrics* 14 (4): 101076.
16. Suleman, Raja Muhammad, and Ioannis Korkontzelos. 2021. “Extending Latent Semantic Analysis to Manage Its Syntactic Blindness.” *Expert Systems with Applications* 165 (March): 114130.
17. Kowsari, Kamran, Kiana Jafari Meimandi, Mojtaba Heidarysafa, Sanjana Mendu, Laura E. Barnes, and Donald E. Brown. 2019. “Text Classification Algorithms: A Survey.” *Information (Switzerland)* 10 (4),: 150.
18. Breiman, Leo. 1996. “Bagging Predictors.” *Machine Learning* 24 (2): 123–40.
19. Schapire, Robert E. 1999. “A Brief Introduction to Boosting.” In *Proceedings of the 16th International Joint Conference on Artificial Intelligence - Volume 2*, 1401–6. IJCAI’99. San Francisco, CA: Morgan Kaufmann Publishers Inc.
20. Randhawa, Kuldeep, Chu Kiong Loo, Manjeevan Seera, Chee Peng Lim, and Asoke K. Nandi. 2018. “Credit Card Fraud Detection Using AdaBoost and Majority Voting.” *IEEE Access* 6 (February): 14277–84.
21. Akhter, Muhammad Pervez, Zheng Jiangbin, Irfan Raza Naqvi, Mohammed Abdelmajeed, Atif Mehmood, and Muhammad Tariq Sadiq. 2020. “Document-Level Text Classification Using Single-Layer Multisize Filters Convolutional Neural Network.” *IEEE Access* 8: 42689–707.
22. Hochreiter, Sepp, and Jürgen Schmidhuber. 1997. “Long Short-Term Memory.” *Neural Computation* 9 (8): 1735–80.
23. Chung, Junyoung, Caglar Gulcehre, KyungHyun Cho, and Yoshua Bengio. 2014. “Empirical Evaluation of Gated Recurrent Neural Networks on Sequence Modeling,” December. doi: 10.48550/ARXIV.1412.3555
24. Weiss, Gail, Yoav Goldberg, and Eran Yahav. 2018. “On the Practical Computational Power of Finite Precision RNNs for Language Recognition.” In Proceedings of the 56th Annual Meeting of the Association for Computational Linguistics *(Long Papers)*, vol. 2 (May): 740–45, Melbourne, Australia, Association for Computational Linguistics.

25. Britz, Denny, Anna Goldie, Minh Thang Luong, and Quoc V. Le. 2017. "Massive Exploration of Neural Machine Translation Architectures." In *EMNLP 2017 - Conference on Empirical Methods in Natural Language Processing, Proceedings*, 1442–51, Copenhagen, Denmark, Association for Computational Linguistics (ACL).
26. Vaswani, Ashish, Noam Shazeer, Niki Parmar, Jakob Uszkoreit, Llion Jones, Aidan N. Gomez, Łukasz Kaiser, Illia Polosukhin, Lukasz Kaiser, and Illia Polosukhin. 2017. "Attention Is All You Need." In I. Guyon, U. Von Luxburg, S. Bengio, H. Wallach, R. Fergus, S. Vishwanathan and R. Garnett (Eds.), *Advances in Neural Information Processing Systems*, 2017 December, 5999–6009. Neural Information Processing Systems Foundation.
27. Peters, Matthew E., Mark Neumann, Mohit Iyyer, Matt Gardner, Christopher Clark, Kenton Lee, and Luke Zettlemoyer. 2018. "Deep Contextualized Word Representations." In *Proceedings of the 2018 Conference of the North American Chapter of the Association for Computational Linguistics: Human Language Technologies, Volume 1 (Long Papers)*, 1:2227–37. New Orleans, LA: Association for Computational Linguistics.
28. Clark, Kevin, Minh-Thang Luong, Quoc V. Le, and Christopher D. Manning. 2020. "ELECTRA: Pre-Training Text Encoders as Discriminators Rather than Generators." doi: 10.48550/ARXIV.2003.10555
29. Devlin, Jacob, Ming-Wei Chang, Kenton Lee, and Kristina Toutanova. 2019. "BERT: Pre-Training of Deep Bidirectional Transformers for Language Understanding." In *Proceedings of the 2019 Conference of the North American Chapter of the Association for Computational Linguistics: Human Language Technologies, Volume 1 (Long and Short Papers)*, 4171–86. Minneapolis, MN: Association for Computational Linguistics.
30. Koksal, Omer. 2021. "Enhancing Turkish Sentiment Analysis Using Pre-Trained Language Models." In *2021 29th Signal Processing and Communications Applications Conference (SIU)*, pp. 1–4, doi: 10.1109/SIU53274.2021.9477908
31. Ambalavanan, Ashwin Karthik, and Murthy V. Devarakonda. 2020. "Using the Contextual Language Model BERT for Multi-Criteria Classification of Scientific Articles." *Journal of Biomedical Informatics* 112 (December), https://doi.org/10.1016/j.jbi.2020.103578.

7 Multilayer Perceptron Mode and IoT to Assess the Economic Impact and Human Health in Rural Areas – Alcoholism

Ann Roseela Jayaprakash, T. Nalini, L.R. Sassykova, N. Kanimozhi, S. Geetha, K. Bhaskar, K. Gomathi, and S. Sendilvelan

CONTENTS

7.1 INTRODUCTION

IoT systems are varied and amenable with regard to the range, strength, and extent of services and the situations in which IoT services are provided. Therefore, they are well suited to fulfilling the diverse requirements of individuals with substance-use-related disorders. Theoretically, IoT forms a transitional stage of ambulant care, providing services wherein the IoT systems assess a person's level of intoxication and help develop a treatment plan and subsequent services.

The extent of intoxication can be assessed using sensor data from gadgets like smartwatches integrated with IoT software. The accumulated data can be stored and then be transmitted to cloud storage for analysis. The accessibility of local data storage is vital to avoiding the erratic latencies arising from wireless data transmission to the cloud. The data should be secured both at rest – local or cloud storage – and during transmission. This requires the end-to-end security of the cloud data center from sensors or edge.

The IoT systems enable patients with alcohol dependence to assess their health, through provider-support IoT applications. For instance, IoT systems can potentially connect several sensors for assessing vitals in the intensive-care units or emergency units wirelessly. These systems improve the health assessment, with data analytics uncovering cryptic correlations amid vital health signs. Novel health assessment frameworks assess the health implications of individuals' alcohol consumption

DOI: 10.1201/9781003217398-7

in their working environment by making use of the data acquirement capability of smart sensors as well as the data processing capability of cloud and fog computing.

After data collection, data processing is performed in the cloud to ascertain if there is an association between every kind of sensor's value and the logged blood alcohol content values obtained from the smartwatches. For this purpose, the gathered data should be pre-processed and also visualized. Subsequently, varied machine learning algorithms are exercised to the gathered sensor information to acquire the most precise predictor of blood alcohol values. Figure 7.1 illustrates the major framework employed for a standard data collection as well as an analysis routine. The data acquisition software executing on the smartphone, also referred to as a gateway, utilizes a set of software modules to handle the low-level particulars of the data gathering process.

The data collection module also accomplishes certain aggregation on the gathered data before directing them for storage in the cloud. This is followed by the exercise of data analytics exclusively within the cloud with high-performance computational engines and diverse big data analytics as well as visualization tools. After deriving a model from data analysis, the particulars are stored and integrated to form an Alcohol Prediction software. After a patient has commenced alcohol consumption, constant health assessment becomes more vital than prevention and well-being. The main objective of IoT systems is to handle this trial through the integration of the related data streams for precise assessment of the alcohol user's health. IoT devices such as implantable, wearables, and gadgets, enable monitoring clinical information such as alcohol content in blood as described above, adherence information to assess the intake of prescribed medications, and user health data.

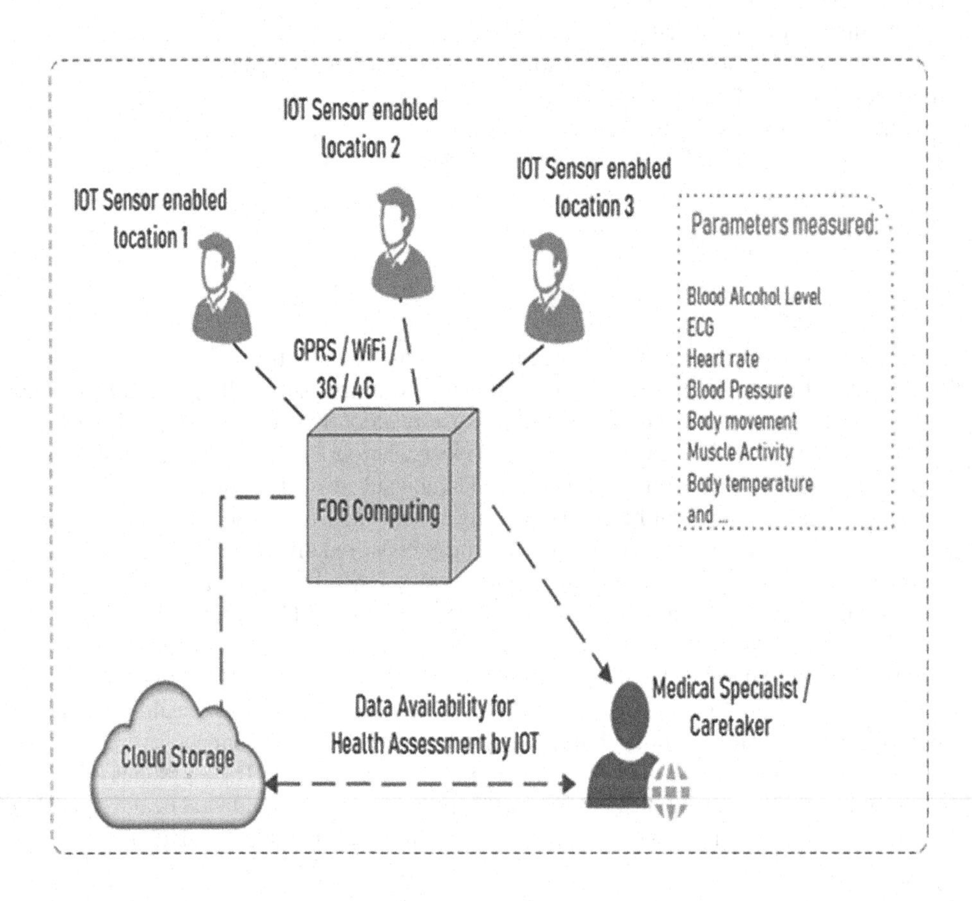

FIGURE 7.1 IoT-based health assessment of alcohol dependence.

7.2 DATA ANALYSIS OF HEALTH IMPACT

This encompasses analysis of health impact, behavioral, environmental, and physical, or postural circumstances of an individual's alcohol dependence by utilizing IoT-oriented interconnected smart sensors technologies. The health dataset holds values of several health-related parameters. The health parameters are assessed and monitored using the bio-sensors and wearables embedded in the surroundings of an individual. The dataset about the environment comprises information relating to air quality, noise, temperature, and cleanliness. This is required for individuals with low health immunity to be very sensitive to their environment. The behavioral datasets assess information relevant to stress and anxiety levels of individuals with alcohol substance usage.

Most of the sensor information is heterogeneous with both numerical and non-numerical data owing to the differences in the architecture of the various sensors. Hence, it gets obligatory to modify the data to a generic format ahead of transmission to the various modules of the health assessment IoT software. To attain synchronization amongst the acquired data, a gateway (programmed) is included between the IoT as well as the fog layer providing transient time-related synchronization in various datasets. The assessed and pre-processed data is additionally relocated to its linked cloud for determining the severity level of health. For data security from the unconstitutional neighborhoods in the course transmission, the network channel is secured with a secure socket layer (SSL) protocol working on transmission control protocol (TCP) as shown in Figure 7.1.

7.3 DETERMINATION OF IRREGULARITIES

The irregularities can be ascertained by integrating distributed data handling techniques of fog technology to retain the sensitiveness of the human health assessment. The gathered data determine the health condition of alcohol-consuming individuals. This data is classified into two groups – normal and abnormal. The abnormal group holds the events influencing the health of the individuals and may stimulate a severe medical problem. On the contrary, a normal group handles situations coherent with physical immunity and does not impact individual well-being. The emergency or warning alerts generated by a fog layer make the framework more efficient for instant decision-making related to the individual's health.

Determination of Severity of Health Condition ascertains the severity of health by using the efficacy of machine learning-aided data handling solutions within the cloud layer. The method of predicting the severity of health enables measurement of the individual's throughput by taking into account the susceptibility of the health and is reliant on the various assessments about health, environmental, behavioral, and postural datasets.

Warning generation mechanism by IOT related to heath severity, initiation is exercised to optimize usage of medical resources by informing the health caretakers as well as medical authorities to enable active and prompt decision-making relevant to the extent of an individual's health gravity. A warning-centered mobile alert notification has an important role in the assessment of individuals' health impact under alcohol dependence and helps to update the present health condition of the individual under substance consumption to their caretakers. The warning and crisis-based notifications are created. This two-stage warning generation mechanism enables the optimized use of medical-related services at a substantial level. The method is completely dependent on the competence to predict the health severity of an individual. Warnings signify the less critical and irregular health status that can be controlled at the custodian level. But an emergency warning outlines the health status of the individual causing the serious state of well-being mandating medical assistance. As compared to manual assessment of health conditions of individuals under alcohol usage, IoT systems have higher accuracy especially with regard to irregular health situations during the time of assessment and accurate prediction of health-related abnormalities concluding that IoT systems efficiently predict irregular conditions in health, posture-related, and environmental and behavioral events with health criticality level determination in comparison with classical manual health assessment methods.

In case of emergencies or critical health conditions, the IoT system can direct the proximate hospitals to pull over for medical assistance. In situations where real-time health-relevant data analysis is needed and conventional interruptions associated with cloud computing cannot be endured, fog computing provides needed assistance. Fog forms an intermediary stage between the cloud and the user, reducing possible latencies by carrying out data analysis rather than transmitting such enormous amounts of user data to cloud for further processing.

7.4 VITAL ROLE OF IOT SYSTEMS IN IDENTIFICATION OF ALCOHOL RELEVANT HEALTH IRREGULARITIES AND MANAGEMENT

The interrelatedness nurtured by IoT along with the learning capabilities of artificial intelligence presents possibilities for handling a broader spectrum of issues. Though not the last thing on everyone's thoughts, addiction to alcohol substances is one such issue against which AI and IoT have the potential to function together. This will entirely transform rehabilitation and enable remote treatments of alcohol dependence amidst pandemics, where in-person-based treatment becomes less viable.

With the ability to tactfully monitor and assess alcohol addictive habits, IoT, as well as AI-centered devices, can furnish users with comprehensive analytics about how often individuals engage in substance addiction and dependence. Through extensive usage of sensor networks, an individual's alcohol dependence can be continually monitored. For instance, usage of applications with AI learning algorithms helps to track alcohol usages and respond by dynamically attempting to treat alcohol addiction with distractions and incentive systems like points-oriented systems. This appealing tactic motivates to knock out obsessive habits.

When an individual has the readiness to hold themselves responsible, IoT devices like Pavlok transmit an electric shock when he/she is about to engage in alcohol usage. Here, the individual with his/her willingness is required to deliver shock on his own when about to consume. Nevertheless, AI recognition provides the device with a greater extent of automation thereby shocking individuals irrespective of whether they press the device button or not.

As part of health assessment and combating alcohol dependence, sensors embedded within fitness bands, virtual glasses as well as smartwatches are capable of detecting an individual's extent of intoxication based on their walking mannerisms, recording the variation in one's pace involving walking towards the bar and later moving out from the bar. If the vehicle is connected to the IoT system, the car or any vehicle can be rendered to not start until a defined period, or until the individual establishes himself to be clearheaded.

There exist IoT models wherein vehicles are fortified with sensors detecting an individual's extent of intoxication. As a response, the vehicle could switch off its ignition and send direct warning messages to family or friends. Sensors can also identify how repeatedly an individual's eyes close to deducing drowsiness. The vehicle is inbuilt with the potential of responding with vibrations or sounds to wake up the person driving. Despite not being directly relevant to alcohol dependence, advancements in technologies related to recognition of eye patterns enable inferring whether the individual is under the usage of alcohol impacting eye movements and postural differences.

The IoT-led developments hold higher potentials to prevent alcohol-dependent individuals from receiving harm. IoT analyzers can thus detect one's blood alcohol levels assessed from the individual's breath and track alcohol consumption, such as the frequency and timings of consumption. The count of drinks an individual consumes is difficult to assess and would be difficult to track, but with alcohol levels interpreted, the IoT systems can provide unvarying measurements, thereby IoT systems eventually help in the assessment of impact of alcohol consumption and subsequent treatment on health.

IoT-centered smart alcohol rehabilitation facilities lessen the issue of limited medical resources owing to the increased number of individuals with alcohol dependence. It can be regarded as an IoT healthcare system interconnecting all the accessible resources within a network to accomplish healthcare activities like diagnosis, specialist care, as well as surgeries performed from remote via the internet. Such an IoT-based framework provides healthcare-related services from communities and hospitals directly to homes. Wireless technologies are broadly employed in integrating the various health conditions assessment devices, with the front-end considered as a network manager. The IoT system interconnects the obtainable medical resources such as hospitals, doctors, rehabilitation units, nurses, assistance devices, and ambulances, with alcohol-dependent patients. The server is operational with a centralized form of the database system. A transitional data processing proxy is accountable to perform data analysis, merger, the discovery of critical incidents, and formation of rehabilitation schemes. An automated allocator for the resources is devised to identify solutions for rehabilitation straightaway to accomplish requirements from the individual alcohol dependents.

Medical relevant decision-making has a vital task in the analysis and assessment of an individual's health condition because of alcohol consumption. Traditional assessment approaches need frequent human involvement to determine the severity of the alcohol's health impact. But defects in medical assessment can develop unfavorable effects on the individual's health. The IoT fortified intensive-care units enable efficient analysis of the severity of the impacted individual's health consequence since it is founded on personalized health-relevant threshold parameter values and health conditions.

It is not practical for medical specialists to read through the extensive data or analyses obtained from IoT sensors. For practical clinical usage, the outcomes from the data analytics engine should be provided to specialists in a perceptive format that can be easily understood. Visualization is acknowledged as a self-regulating and crucial research arena with a broad range of applications in science as well as real-world scenarios. Though health data signifies a fortune trove to perform machine learning and deduction, it is challenging for the medical specialist to easily visualize and interrelate with the data without the usage of tools. The time-fluctuating and multidimensional characteristics of the data about health impacts of alcohol dependence present challenges since they have traditionally not been utilized in healthcare practice despite temporal disparities and progression of health data, as well as analyses outcomes, are of specific concern for diagnosis. The interactivity accessible via touch interfaces provided in prevailing mobile devices proffers a specifically desirable opportunity to visualize temporal relations. By maximizing interactivity, such interfaces enable visualization of changes over some time. Latest IoT systems enable interactive usage intuitively permitting the medical caregivers to review health conditions and levels of substance dependence of the individuals using tablet and smartphone devices previously deployed in the offices.

In this IoT-based alcohol detection system, an MQ135 sensor and an ESP8266 Node MCU development board are interfaced and programmed using Arduino IDE and its parameters are monitored on the Blynk application. I2C and SPI communication protocols can be used to connect with the MQ135 sensor.

An alcohol sensor detects the presence of alcohol gas in the air, and the output measurement is an analogue voltage. With a power supply of less than 150 Ma to 5V, the sensor can activate at temperatures ranging from −10°C to 50°C. The sensing range is 0.04 to 4 mg/L, which is appropriate for breath analyzers. The MQ series of gas sensors have an electrochemical sensor and a small heater within. They are sensitive to a wide range of gases and can be utilized at ambient temperature. MQ135 alcohol sensor consists of SnO_2 with reduced clean air conductivity. When the required explosive gas is present, the sensor's conductivity rises in tandem with the growing levels of the gas concentration. It transforms the charge of conductivity to the corresponding output signal of gas concentration utilizing basic electrical circuits. Alcohol detection through tin dioxide (SnO2), a perspective layer inside aluminum oxide microtubes, and a heating element inside a tubular case make up the MQ-135 alcohol sensor. A stainless-steel net surrounds the sensor's end face, and the connecting terminals are located on the backside. Passing over the heating element, ethyl alcohol in the breath is converted to acetic acid with the ethyl alcohol cascade on the tin dioxide sensing layer, the resistance decreases as shown in Figure 7.2.

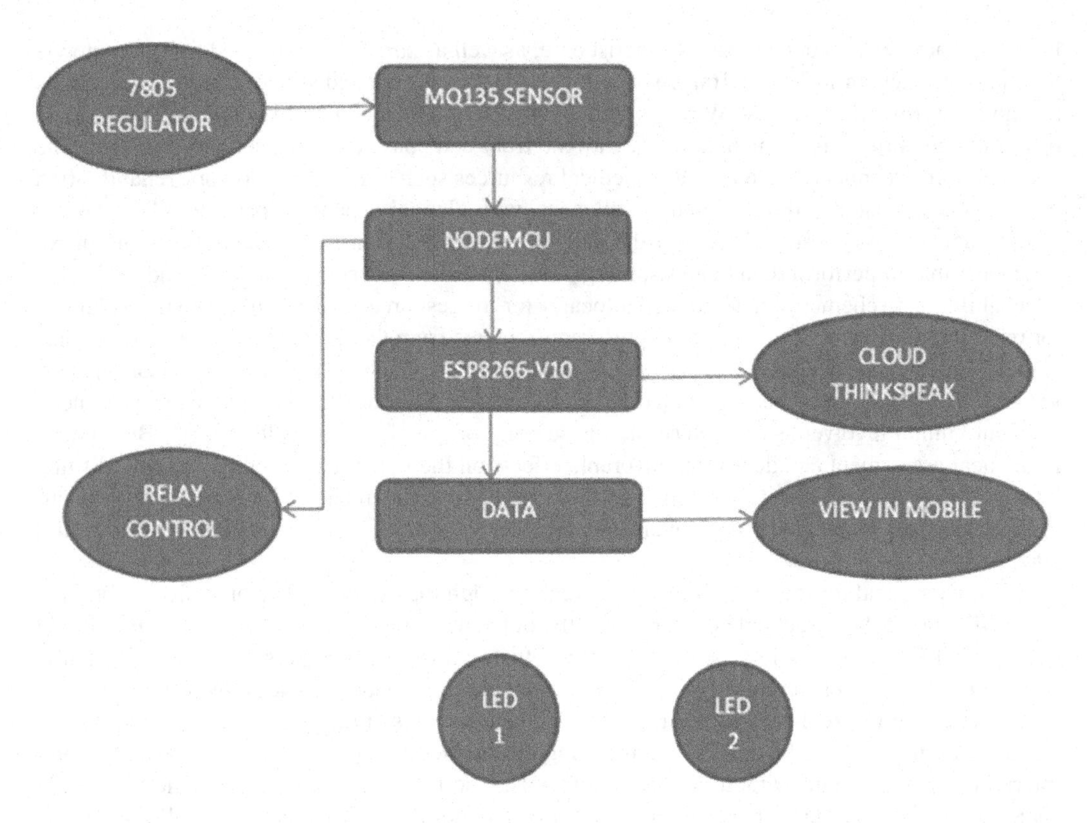

FIGURE 7.2 Process flow diagram.

The resistance goes down. The resistance fluctuation is transformed into a suitable voltage variation by employing the external load resistance. An MQ135 alcohol circuit diagram and connection setup are illustrated below as shown in Figures 7.3 and 7.4.

The alcohol sensor is an MQ3 sensor that detects ethanol and is configured with the Blynk app dashboard. The MQ135 sensor and the ESP8266 Node MCU development board are connected and programmed using the Arduino IDE, and the parameters are monitored using the Blynk app, which has access to the cloud server with the most recent MQ135 sensor reading. Data can be accessed on your smartphone from any network, anywhere in the globe.

This application facilitates the integration of some specific special devices and a special type of sensor. They also allow integration and access of a few instruments related to the field of engineering. This scheme will increase the productivity and accuracy of data collection. IoT systems in health care are becoming the state of the art. They magnify the stretch out and cover a wide range of specialists. This scheme increases the accuracy, precision, and dimension of medical data related to alcohol addicts on a large scale from diversified real cases worldwide.

It uses well-ordered environs and helpers to monitor the leftover examinations in the field of alcohol de-addiction. IoT-based de-addiction paves way for a piece of wealthy real-time information for the data from de-addiction centers followed by analysis and testing. IoT can distribute related data of good quality with typical analytics through various sensors that are integrated to perform research on alcoholism. IoT-based integration provides a lot of important information relating to alcoholism and de-addiction. This technology supports de-addiction in the healthcare domain by offering highly consistent and real-world data thereby providing the solution to unforeseen issues that may arise in the future. It also permits researchers and physicians to avoid risks by gathering data without appropriate testing on the human-race. It then discloses the pattern and lost data in de-addiction-related healthcare applications.

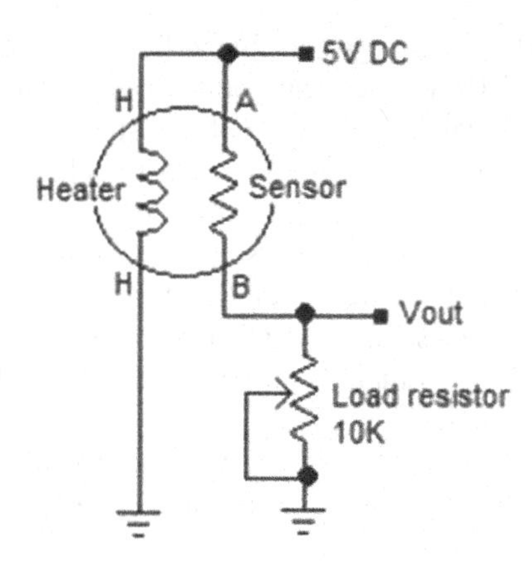

FIGURE 7.3 MQ-135 circuit diagram.

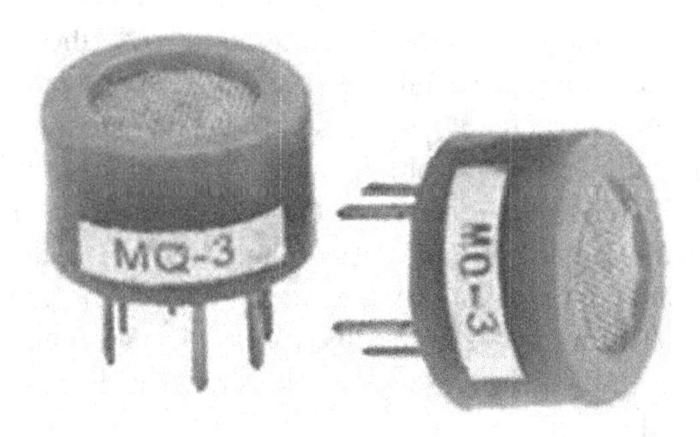

FIGURE 7.4 Alcohol sensor.

Conceivably the utmost development IoT brings to de-addiction in the field of healthcare is in the real practice of medicine since it permits the better usage of the knowledge by healthcare professionals to recover a patient who is addicted to alcohol. They utilize good quality sensors which provide the relevant data in a more precise manner. The decision-making is not affected by the noisy or irrelevant data that is to affect the quality of the entire scheme.

One of the challenges in de-addiction is the circulation of correct and recent information to the addicts. De-addiction care also tackles the complex nature involved in the guidance. IoT devices stretch a straight, 24×7 admission to the alcohol addicts in a noninvasive method as compared with the existing methods. They take de-addiction facilities to home, office, or social space. They motivate the addicts to take care of their health and get relieved from the influence of alcohol. This kind of motivation reduces road accidents resulting from rash driving under the influence of alcohol, deaths due to liver cirrhosis, and healthier precautionary care.

The innovative computerization and analytics of IoT permit more dominant emergency support services to d-addiction centers, which classically suffer from disconnection due to limited resources and fundamental facilities. It offers a method to examine an emergency more comprehensively from a long distance. It also gives more access to alcohol addicts. IoT gives critical facts for providing indispensable care for alcohol addicts. It also increases the care given to alcohol addicts when there is an emergency taking place. This decreases the related losses and recovers emergency healthcare to de-addiction centers.

7.5 ALCOHOL ADDICTION AND USE OF IoT

Humans mostly have used alcohol as an intoxicating chemical substance from time immemorial. Originally, alcohol was not a liquid, but a powder [2]. In Arabian literature, a powder is named as 'al-kuhul', which means 'the kohl' for the eyes or 'finely-divided spirit' [7, 23]. Alcohol has its own distinct properties with many different chemical compounds. Methanol and Isopropanol are the varieties of alcohol used in chemical laboratories and industries. [3, 28]. For cleaning the household equipment, this isopropanol is generally used in industries [27, 39]. It is commonly known as 'rubbing alcohol' [22, 34]. Cleaning solvents and paint removers also contain alcohol [8, 20]. In photocopiers, developer and anti-freeze solutions also have a considerable amount of alcohol. In the manufacturing of alcohol, the ethanol is extracted and the formaldehyde obtained as the end product is poisonous [37, 47]. Consuming even small amounts of methanol, which is another type of alcohol, leads to blindness and death [32, 33]. Ethanol is a type of alcohol [19]. Alcohol, unless otherwise specified, refers to ethanol or ethyl alcohol.

In most states, the important source of revenue generation is alcohol and also it has been an important international trade [46, 18]. It is the responsibility of researchers to provide necessary information to policy providers or program planners to make necessary decisions about the allocation of resources. A health care problem and comparison of the problem with others could be studied using this indicator of the magnitude. There exists economics in alcohol addiction reported nationally and internationally. It is a multidimensional technique to study the economics behind alcohol consumption [31]. Without assessing the social and psychological problems, it is not an easy task to predict the alcohol addicts in a particular area. If the prediction rate is not up to the mark, then it affects the economy of the nation starting from the individual and his family [41]. This study could be an eye-opener for people, make them aware of the consequences of alcoholism, and facilitate the statutory bodies and health organizations to orient their focus on eradication of alcoholism [42].

There exists a perception about alcohol products that the alcohol content may vary and certain products like beer serve as a hydrating agent. In some cases, it has become a social norm to consume alcohol in public gatherings. In this way, there are various reasons discussed by the alcohol addicts to justify their addiction, rather than admitting the fact that they have turned in to alcohol addicts over years of consumption. A symbolism and drinking occasion structure may be more interesting than how much is being drunk in actuality [5]. The health perspective comes in front of the public. Morbidity and mortalities are the agents of alcoholic beverages [4, 43].

In modern times, major community health issues are created because of alcohol addicts, financial crises may occur worldwide because drinking alcohol is emerging as a strong worrisome factor now and also in the future. The economic cost of alcohol is the need of the hour and it is also almost self-evident. For policymakers in public, researchers in academic, and public health doctors, the estimation of alcohol consumption and economic burden and also health care is a major concern; this study is potentially a valuable source of information. This study not just concludes the economic impact of alcoholism and the cost of the drink, the entire spectrum of problems it creates upon the related community and produces impact worldwide. The direct cost includes hospital charges, purchase of alcohol, doctor charges, visits to the hospitals and other expenditures. The indirect costs include gambling charges, loans and mortgages etc. and criminal justice costs like driving the car after drinking, and property damage etc. Apart from this family burden of neglected children, parents' drinking problems could spoil the family relationship [15, 38].

Through blood circulation, alcohol is absorbed and gets distributed with the help of organs, tissues, and cells from the stomach and the small intestines [48]. The liver absorbs the alcohol rapidly from blood circulation. Alcohol is converted into carbon dioxide, water, and energy [16, 26]. Kidney excretes the chemicals by 94–99% of the alcohol consumed, while the remaining 1–5% comes out through sweat, breath, and urine [29].

Dependence on alcoholism is characterized as a chronic disabling addictive disorder due to the use and repeated use of excessive alcoholic beverages, withdrawal identity leads to morbidity, including decreased ability or cirrhosis to function vocationally and socially (Bajaj, 2018). Two billion people take alcoholic beverages worldwide as per the World Health Organization, with 80 million patients with alcohol-use disorder (World Health Organization, 2001). 87% of males addicted in Europe ranked first followed by Americans with 85% [25]. The prevalence of alcoholism is varied for numerous reasons like occupation, civilization, educational qualification, caste, community, financial, and living standards of the people.

Widespread attitudinal shift to more normalization of the use of alcohol, and the impact of globalization, is greater in India being a 'dry' or 'abstaining' country. Due to this, there is a significant age-lowering initiation of drinking. The report revealed the prevalence of alcoholism among males 15 years and above in Punjab is 50%, similarly 42% prevalence of alcoholism in north India [45], with 48% of alcoholics doing unskilled or semi-skilled work. Some more reports show that the male's prevalence of alcoholism admitted to a psychiatric hospital was 42% [21]. The rural male prevalence of alcoholism is 37% at the age of above 15. Some reports categorized illiterate married men as a vulnerable group for alcoholism. The age groups of males are 20–35 and doing unskilled or semi-skilled occupations also residing with the nuclear family.

A study has reported that in the state of Goa, 49% of rural males are addicts to alcohol, with 14.3% of binge drinking [13]. In the remote hills of Arunachal Pradesh, 45% of males use alcohol with 65.2% of the population being current drinkers [9]. 25.7% of male inpatients in a rural hospital are from the prevalence of alcoholism [6]. Dutta et al. discussed the existence of alcohol consumption in Tamilnadu among male members in the villages as 33.8% [12]. According to the report mentioned, the existence of alcohol addicts accounts to 46.6%. Radhakrishnan et al. stated that among the 19–48 age group of men, 35.9% reported alcohol-related problems [36]. In that study, daily 21.1% of the alcohol consumed, and weekly 28.3% alcohol. Kavi et al. reported that in Karnataka, the men and women folk were diagnosed to be under the influence of alcohol and it accounts for 44% of the people in that village [41, 24]. In that report, 29.7% of the males used alcohol four times a week, while every week 23.8% of males consumed alcohol. Dasgupta et al. reported the prevalence of alcoholism as 65.8% in the urban slums of Kolkata [11]. Fathima et al. inferred around 33% existence of alcohol among the male members in villages [14]

The consumption of alcohol continuously makes us alcohol dependent and has been creating issues of great concern and this effect stays for a longer time; harmful effects of alcohol create health issues for the consumer body. Alcohol-related problems are divided as follows:

- Day-to-day effects of alcohol
- Alcohol use and the consequences

Background variables were calculated using descriptive statistics together with the data related to structured population and their social and economic attributes, alcohol consumption information, its usage, and dependence on alcoholism. Dependence of alcoholism was calculated with the 95% confidence interval and also drinking methods, problematic drinkers, and social problem creators. The outcome of alcoholism creates dispersion of data viability and economics. Statistical significance investigation with Chi-square was used. For comparison purposes, *t*-test was conducted to identify the expenses related to alcohol addicts and occasional drinkers.

This study was done at a primary health center in Poonamallee near Chennai, Tamilnadu. Questionnaires were used to study alcohol prevalence; alcohol-use disorder identification tests were done by using a questionnaire. Michigan alcohol screening tests were used to assess psychosocial problems. Males of 19 years or more living in that area were considered for the study, for a minimum period of one year. Voter lists were used to draw sampling frames randomly. The population was identified using simple random methods. The size of the sample selected was 545. All gave consent forms signed and were incorporated in the process study. Demographic characteristics are reported in Table 7.1.

In the study reported in Table 7.1, 23.9 % of men have been found in the age group of 34–45 years, 19.1% of men in the 25–34 age group, 18.7% of men in the 45–54 age group, 15.8% of men in the 18–24 age group, 10.8% of men in the 55–64 age group, and 11.7% of men in the 64+ age group. As per the study, the majority of men were Hindus with 80.7%, then the Christian men with

TABLE 7.1
Statistical data of alcohol addiction in Men

Statistics	No. of Men (Total = 545)	Men (%)
	Age (in Years)	
18–24	86	15.8
25–34	104	19.1
35–44	130	23.9
45–54	102	18.7
55–64	59	10.8
65 and above	64	11.7
	Religion of Men	
Hindu	440	80.7
Muslim	20	3.7
Christian	85	15.6
Others	0	0
	Marital Status of Men	
Unmarried	148	27.2
Married	370	67.9
Widower	25	4.6
Separated/Divorcee	2	0.3
	Family Type	
Nuclear	305	56
Extended nuclear	155	28.4
Joint	85	15.6

15.6%, and Muslims with 3.7%. In the statistics, 27.2% of men were unmarried, 67.9% of men were married, 4.6% of them were widowers, and 0.3% of them were separated/divorced.

As per the socioeconomic characteristics, as given in Table 7.2, 12.8% of men were found to be illiterate, and the remaining 87.2% of them were literate. In the literates' section, 10.6% of men were graduates, 1.8% of them were postgraduates, 24.8% possess the educational qualification of higher secondary or diploma, 23% of them did high schooling, 15.6% of them completed middle school, and 11.4% of men have completed primary school education. The study also shows that 91.7% of men were employed. In the United Kingdom Registrar General Occupational Classification, it is mentioned that men were employed in semi-skilled (33.9%), unskilled (17.3%), and skilled (29.5%) occupations.

The study also shows that 91.7% of men were employed. In the United Kingdom Registrar General Occupational Classification, it is mentioned that men were employed in semi-skilled (33.9%), unskilled (17.3%), and skilled (29.5%) occupations. According to Modified Prasad's classification, 41.8% of men fall under Class I socioeconomic status, 51.7% come under Class II status, 5.7 % in Class III status, and the rest of them in Class IV status. The living standard index seems to be low for 12.1%, medium for 37.4%, and high for 50.5% of the study population.

The audit questionnaire was applied to identify the existence of alcohol addicts, various types of alcoholism, and the prevalence of various types of drinkers such as normal drinkers, current drinkers, and problem drinkers. The participants involved in the study were further analyzed by using MAST for their psychological problems and the prevalence of problem drinkers was assessed. The spectrum of drinkers in this assessment is shown in Figure 7.5.

The study participants whose score is 8 or more under AUDIT were mentioned as alcoholics. In this study, the total number of participants involved was 545. The analysis done helped us

TABLE 7.2
Socioeconomic Characteristics

Characteristics	Number of Participants (Total = 545)	Men (%)
	Educational Qualification	
Uneducated	70	12.8
Schooling (Primary)	62	11.4
Schooling (Middle)	85	15.6
Schooling (High)	125	23
Diploma/Higher secondary	135	24.8
Graduation	58	10.6
Postgraduate	10	1.8
Occupation		
Unemployed	45	8.3
Unskilled	94	17.3
Semi-skilled	185	33.9
Skilled	161	29.5
Semi-professional	50	9.2
Professional	10	1.8
	Socioeconomic Status	
I Class	228	41.8
II Class	282	51.7
III Class	31	5.7
IV Class	4	0.7
V Class	0	0
	Index: Living Standard	
Low	66	12.1
Medium	204	37.4
High	275	50.5

to find that the current drinkers were 326, alcoholics were 210, alcohol dependents were 80, and the problem drinkers were 125. Depending upon the level of risk, alcoholics were classified into three categories namely the full-time drinkers, spree drinkers, and alcohol dependents. The alcohol prevalence of harmful drinkers, binge drinkers, and alcohol dependents is 15.6%, 8.3, and 14.7, respectively as shown in Table 7.3.

The study reports that the major alcoholics were adults and middlemen with 27.6% and 23.8% respectively. The age group (24–34 years) of the harmful drinkers accounted for 35.3%. The age limit is taken to be in the range of 34–44 for binge drinkers (26.7%). Alcohol dependents were highest in the 35–44 years age group as shown in Table 7.4.

During the analysis, the alcohol addicts were also treated for psychosocial troubles being created. The psychosocial problems with alcoholics were further divided into three types, namely behavioral problems experienced by alcoholics and their families, health problems, and social problems as shown in Figures 7.6, 7.7, and 7.8.

Based on behavioral problems analysis, it is found that 93.7% of them are not taking help from anyone to free them from a drinking problem, 73.3% of them are unable to limit themselves from drinking, 72.8% of them believe themselves to be normal drinkers, and 67.4% of them agree on the complaints raised by their parents or wife about their habits. It was also assessed that 56.8% of them could not stop with one and two drinks, whereas 35.4% had hangover drinking habits.

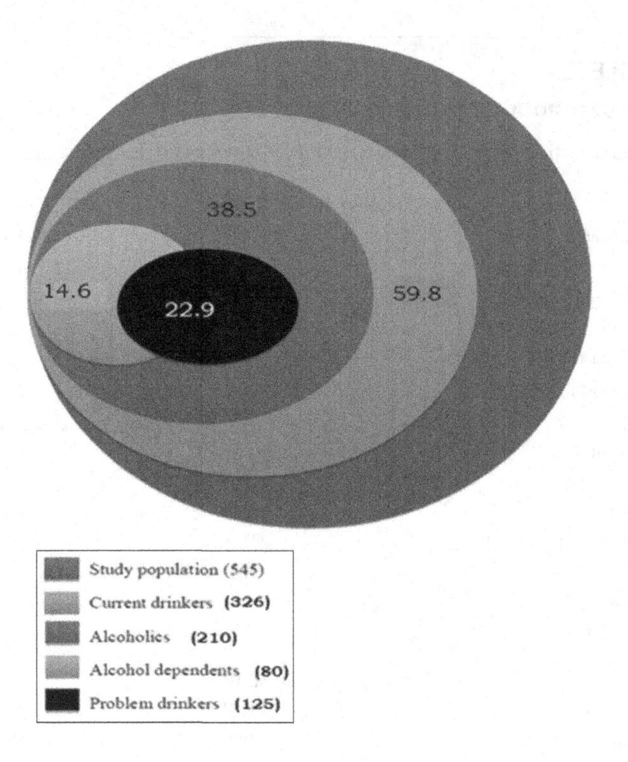

FIGURE 7.5 Spectrum of drinkers in this study.

TABLE 7.3
Alcoholism Prevalence

Problem	Number of Participants (N=320)	Alcohol Prevalence	95% C.I.
Alcoholism	210	38.5	33.8–41.9
Harmful drinker	85	15.6	12.7–18.8
Binge drinker	45	8.3	5.8–10.4
Alcohol dependents	80	14.7	11.6–17.4

TABLE 7.4
Alcoholism Prevalence by Age

	Harmful Drinking		Binge Drinking		Alcohol Dependence		Alcoholism	
Age(Years)	N	%	N	%	N	%	N	%
18–24	21	24.7	3	6.7	5	6.3	29	13.8
25–34	30	35.3	10	22.2	18	22.5	58	27.6
35 44	13	15.3	12	26.7	25	31.2	50	23.8
45–54	9	10.6	8	17.8	15	18.7	32	15.2
55–64	8	9.4	6	13.3	9	11.3	23	11
65 and above	4	4.7	6	13.3	8	10	18	8.6
	85	100	45	100	80	100	210	100

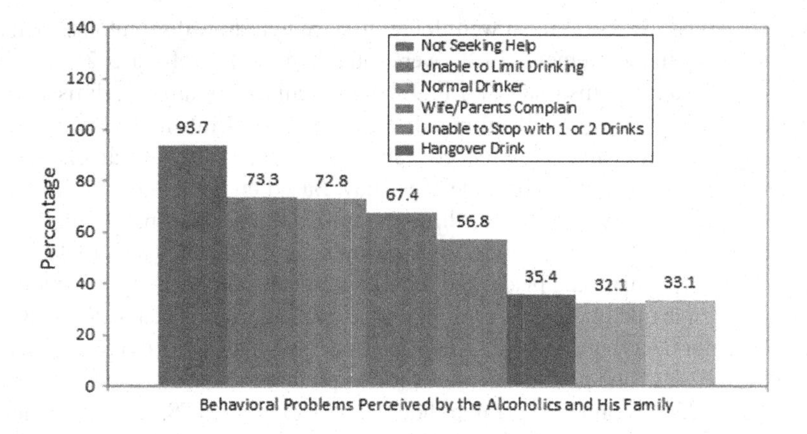

FIGURE 7.6 Prevalence of behavior-based experience by the alcoholics and their families.

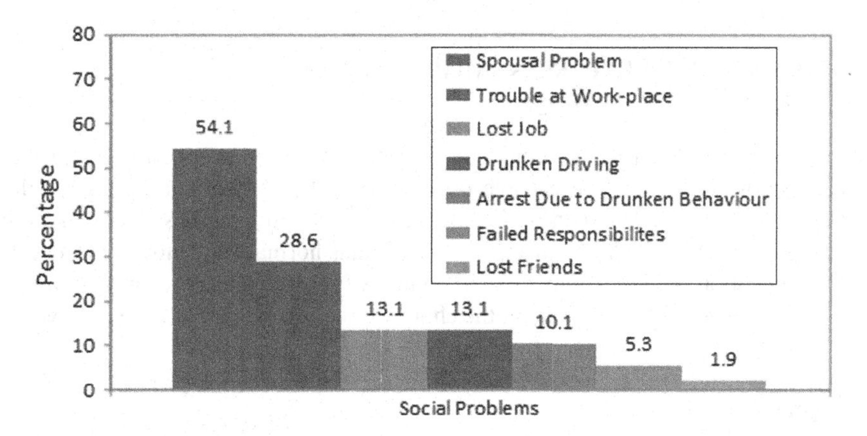

FIGURE 7.7 Prevalence of social problems.

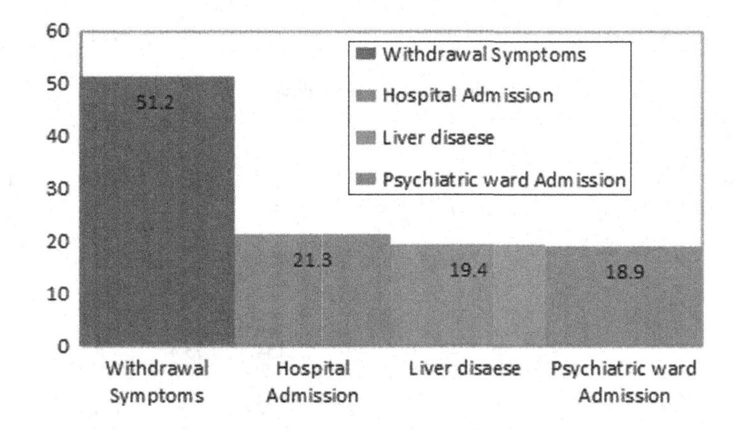

FIGURE 7.8 Prevalence of health problems.

In the overall study, it was evaluated that 54.1% were found to have spousal problems, 28.6% of the drinkers have problems in their workplace, and 1.9% of them lost their friends due to this issue. It was also assessed that 13.1% of them lost their job due to their habit of drinking, 13.1% of them had drunken driving habits and 10.1% of them had been arrested due to drunken driving.

Based on the analysis, 51.5% of them were found to have withdrawal symptoms such as hallucinations, tremors, and delirium tremens; 19.4% were found to have liver disease; 21.3% of them took hospital admission because of this issue; and 18.9% got psychiatric treatment admissions. Based on frequency, type, place, and pattern of drinking, different types of drinkers have been evaluated. As per the assessment, normal drinkers (66.7%) consume less than monthly and alcoholics (61%) consume every week. Problem drinkers consume every day. Based on the number of drinks consumed per day, normal drinkers (40.8%) stop with three to four drinks per day, but the problem drinkers (69.6%) and alcoholics (73.4%) consume five to six drinks per day as shown in Table 7.5.

Depending on the type, drinking place, and tobacco usage during drinking, the pattern of drinking by various types of drinkers was assessed. In the assessment, it has been mentioned that normal drinkers (43.3%) prefer beer, but alcoholics (78.6%) and problem drinkers (85.6%) prefer whisky or brandy. Alcoholics (62.3%) and problem drinkers (68%) prefer to drink at a bar/wine shop, whereas the normal drinkers (25.8%) prefer to drink at home. Alcoholics with 78.6% and problem drinkers with 92% had the habit of tobacco usage while drinking, whereas 38.3% of normal drinkers had the habit of concurrent tobacco usage while drinking as shown in Table 7.6.

7.6 MULTILAYERED PERCEPTRON (MLP) FOR THE PREVALENCE OF ALCOHOLISM

Investigation reveals that intelligent techniques like multilayered perceptron (MLP) trained with radial basis function (RBF) will be capable of predicting the problems associated with various types of alcoholism [17, 44]. The data set is gathered by surveying various places like rehabilitation centers, hospitals, and de-addiction centers. This data is normalized before it is fed as inputs to the MLP. Normalization reduces computational complexity; hence this procedure is carried out as shown in Figure 7.9. The next stage is about the choice of the network architecture for MLP and the

TABLE 7.5
Frequency of Alcohol Consumption

	Normal Drinkers		Alcoholics		Problem Drinkers	
Consumption Characteristics	N (120)	%	N (210)	%	N (125)	%
	Consumption frequency					
Monthly once or less	80	66.7	9	4.3	4	3.2
2–4 times monthly	40	33.3	128	61	54	43.2
2–3 times weekly	0	0	20	9.5	18	14.4
4 times or more weekly	0	0	53	25.2	49	39.2
	No. of drinks per day					
1–2	23	19.2	2	0.9	2	1.6
3–4	49	40.8	31	14.7	16	12.8
5–6	48	40	154	73.4	87	69.6
7–9	0	0	21	10	20	16.0
>10	0	0	2	1.0	0	0
	6 or more drinks per occasion					
No consumption	51	42.5	10	4.8	4	3.2
Less than monthly	49	40.8	17	8.1	9	7.2
Monthly	20	16.7	32	15.2	7	5.6
Weekly	0	0	99	47.1	55	44
Daily or almost daily	0	0	52	24.8	50	40

TABLE 7.6
Drinking Type

Types	Normal Drinkers N (120)	%	Alcoholics N (210)	%	Problem Drinkers N (125)	%
			Varieties of drinks			
Spirits (Whisky, Brandy)	47	39.2	165	78.6	107	85.6
Beer	52	43.3	13	6.2	4	3.2
Others	21	17.5	32	15.2	14	11.2
			Drinking place			
Bars/wine shop	31	25.8	131	62.3	85	68
Friend's home/own home	56	46.7	36	17.1	15	12
Public place	33	27.5	22	10.6	5	4
Working place	0	0	21	10	20	16.0
			Concurrent tobacco use			
Yes	46	38.3	165	78.6	115	92
No	74	61.7	45	21.4	10	8

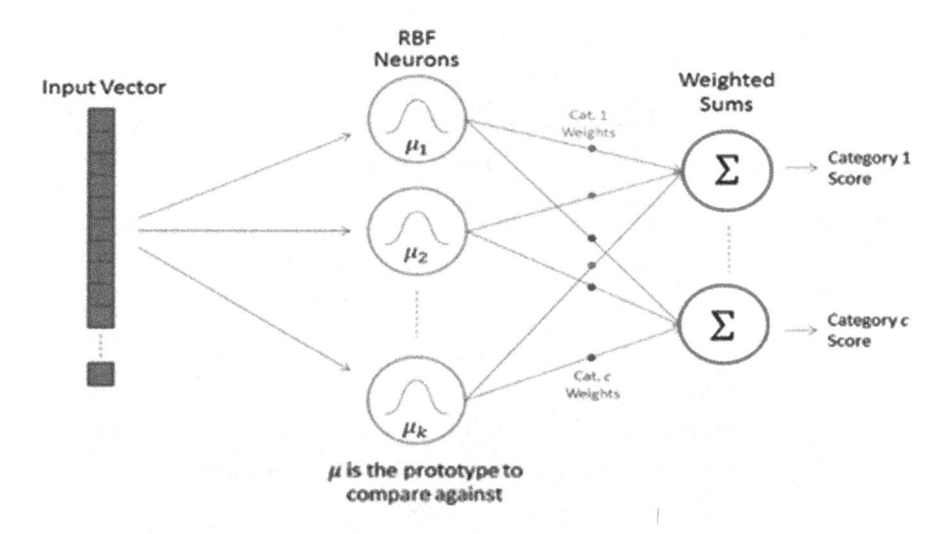

FIGURE 7.9 Multilayered perceptron (MLP) for prevalence of alcoholism.

choice of the training algorithm [30]. Since these intelligent techniques are dependent on optimization of the objective function, they come under the class of optimization algorithms. On analysis, it is understood that the MLP is a two-layered structure as shown in Figure 7.9. Though it is named as a two-layered model, physically it has three layers [1]. The input layer is the first layer, the hidden layer is the second one and the output layer is the third layer.

The input layer simply acts as a buffer, thereby transferring the input values. The inner product of these inputs is calculated and given as inputs to the hidden layer nodes. These nodes in the hidden layer possess a Gaussian activation function, which will process the values of the inner product by substituting them over the Gaussian activation function [10]. This function will facilitate the convergence of the MLP. Thirdly, the output layer uses a sigmoidal activation function, which will facilitate faster convergence so that the actual output matches the target output [35]

- Random centers are chosen from the training set.
- By applying the normalization method, computation of the spread for the RBF function is done.
- Infer the weights by the pseudo-inverse method.

The pattern of health-seeking together with the health care visit reason was found out for alcoholics (Current drinkers). As per current drinkers' analysis, the health care service sought 105 persons with an alcohol-related health problem. In that analysis, 59.0% took treatment in government hospitals but 41.0% went to private hospitals or nursing homes for their drinking problems as shown in Table 7.7.

Among the current drinkers who took health care, 57.1% of them went as an outpatient, whereas 42.9% of them got admitted for their health problems as shown in Table 7.8. Based on the evaluation, 105 drinkers took health care services mainly due to alcohol. Among 105 persons, 35.2% were due to cirrhosis and liver disease, on the road due to accidents were 23%, and 20% suffered injury following the violence, main injury concern is physical violence as shown in Table 7.9.

Based on the analysis, the economic impact of all current drinkers was calculated. Drinking cost and alcohol impact expenditures are considered for the economic impact of drinking. Alcohol cost, travel fare, snacks, and tobacco costs are also included in the cost of drinking. Alcohol impact expenditures include health costs (cost for injuries and hospital admissions), work-related expenditures (including loss of pay and workplace borrowing), and social costs (debts, mortgages,

TABLE 7.7
Health Caring Places

Places	Users	Percentage
Hospital (govt.)	62	59
Hospital (pvt.)	43	41
Sum	105	100

TABLE 7.8
Type of Services for Health

Type of Services for Heath	Users Ever N = 105	Percentage
Outpatient	60	57.1
Inpatient	45	42.9
Sum	105	100

TABLE 7.9
Health Care Seeking Reasons

Health Care Seeking Reasons	No. of Participants N = 105	Percentage
Cirrhosis/Liver disease	37	35.2
Accidents (road)	24	23
Physical assault with others	21	20
Headache and gastritis	18	17.1
Symptoms withdrawal symptoms	5	4.8

gambling, and property damage). In the analysis period of the past 12 months, the expenditures for alcohol-related consequences for a drinker were calculated as 21,058 (twenty-one thousand fifty-eight) Indian rupees as shown in Table 7.10.

An alcohol drinker spent 11,500 (eleven thousand five hundred) Indian rupees on average for his drinks and extra refreshments and also spent 3,273 (three thousand two hundred and seventy-three) Indian rupees for his health-related expenditures in the past one-year evaluation. In the workplace, the expenditures were 14,100 (Fourteen thousand and hundred) Indian rupees and social status cost amounted to 12,650 (twelve thousand six hundred and fifty) Indian rupees.

By using the radial basis function (RBF) and back propagation algorithm (BPA), classification is done to identify the addiction cases as high, medium, and low as shown in Figures 7.10 and 7.11. In connection to the database obtained, a total of 51 data sets were collected about three categories of

TABLE 7.10
Drinking Cost (One Year)

Expenditures	No. of Drinkers	Mean (INR)	Median (INR)	Range (INR)	
				Min.	Max.
Health wise	99	3,273	1,200	50	24,050
Workplace based	147	14,100	12,525	1,100	63,500
Pay Loss	139	13,800	12,525	1,025	63,500
Borrowed expenses out borrowed money	60	3,000	2,525	10,120	12,000
Social-related rxpense	65	12,650	6,250	752	1,10,000
Alcohol-related impact	181	17,600	15,025	52	1,16,500
	0				
Alcohol	322	11,500	8,200	802	54,400
Alcohol only considered	332	6,700	3,675	402	48,450
Food expenses	328	1,800	1,225	101	7,100
Tobacco also included	207	4,067	5,025	101	10,600
Alcohol impact and its expenses	320	21,058	13,400	800	1,30,000
	2200	1,06,548	81,575	15,305	6,40,100

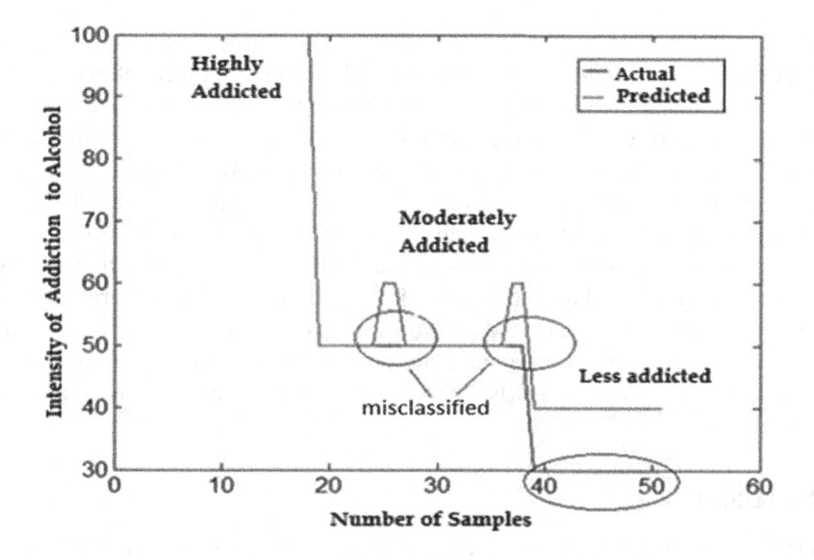

FIGURE 7.10 Prediction of alcohol addiction by FFNN trained with BPA.

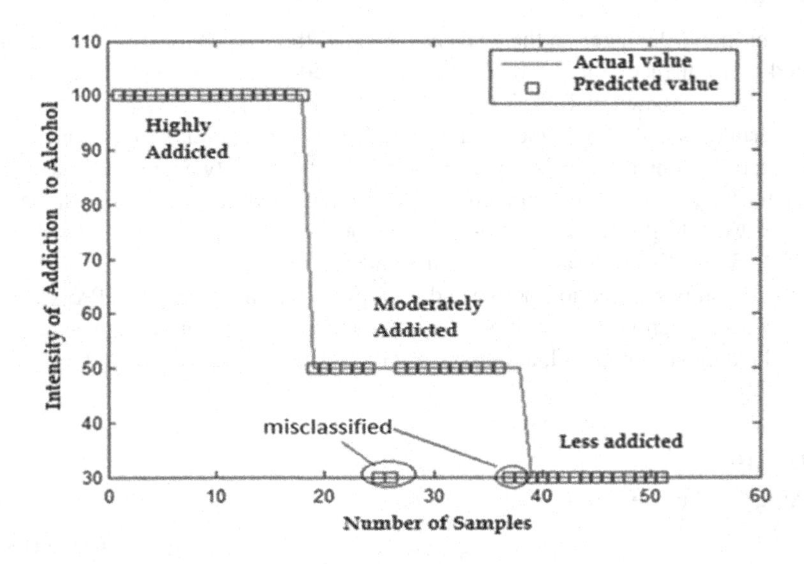

FIGURE 7.11 Prediction of alcohol addiction by FFNN trained with RBF.

alcohol addiction. The first category denotes samples that correspond to less addiction to alcohol, the second category indicates moderate addiction to alcohol, and the third denotes high addiction to alcohol.

The inputs to feed forward neural network (FFNN) include age, gender, height, weight, blood group, level of alcohol content in blood, and blood pressure levels. Seven inputs are used to train the FFNN. All these seven inputs denote the normalized values. There are three outputs for this application: less addiction, moderate addiction, and high addiction to alcohol. The number of nodes in layer (hidden) is finalized using this formula, number of hidden layer nodes = (number of nodes in input layer/2) rounded off to nearest possible integer. On substitution, it is found:

$$\text{No. of hidden layer nodes} = \left(\text{No. of nodes in input layer}/2\right)$$
$$= \left(7/2\right)$$
$$= 3.5 \approx 4$$

During the training process, it is also observed that only for four numbers of nodes in the hidden layer, the network attained convergence, with the lowest value of mean squared error (MSE) of 0.0001. Furthermore, during the training process, optimal values of the learning factor, rate of momentum, and bias values are chosen. To differentiate the representations concerning alcohol addiction and their associated parameters using seven attributes, which signified the importance of BPA and RBF classifier [40], the efficiency metric used is recall and precision, with a score closer to 1. Apart from using the conventional methods for the prediction of alcohol addiction, an intelligent technique for predicting the level of alcohol addiction was developed. The generalized probabilistic methods with the capacity to analyze the data with less computational complexity were found to be used for small-scale analysis in recent studies. The proposed intelligent algorithms were especially dedicated to detecting the alcohol addicts and offering an appropriate remedy so that they get rid of their addiction.

7.7 CONCLUSION

The investigation of alcohol addiction from the data gathered from the de-addiction center. The IoT-based alcohol monitoring on the Blynk app using MQ135 and ESP8266 is designed. The key goal of the work is the identification, interpretation, and understanding of the level of alcohol addiction. The proposed method facilitates properly monitoring and regulating alcohol addicts in de-addiction centers. This kind of data mining approach plays a vital role in reforming the lives of alcohol addicts and saving their lives and future, which is a huge challenge. Therefore, we aimed to focus on tracking and managing alcohol addicts by using intelligent data mining algorithms with related artificial intelligence methods for analysis.

REFERENCES

1. Alsmadi, S., Omar, K. B. and Noah, S. A. (2009) 'Back propagation algorithm: The best algorithm among the multi-layer perceptron algorithm', *International Journal of Computer Science and Network Security*, vol 9, no 4, 378–383,
2. Apostoli, P., et al. (2006) 'Elemental speciation in human health risk assessment', *Environmental Health Criteria*, 234, World Health Organization.
3. Arifin, S. and Chien, I. L. (2007) 'Combined preconcentrator/recovery column design for isopropyl alcohol dehydration process', *Industrial and Engineering Chemistry Research.* https://doi.org/10.1021/ie061446c.
4. Arranz, S., et al. (2012) 'Wine, beer, alcohol and polyphenols on cardiovascular disease and cancer', *Nutrients.* https://doi.org/10.3390/nu4070759.
5. Bartlett, A. (2016) 'Business suit, briefcase, and handkerchief: The material culture of retro masculinity in *The Intern*', *M/C Journal.* https://doi.org/10.5204/mcj.1057.
6. Biswas, S., et al. (2011) 'Spectrum of alcoholic liver disease in tribal alcoholics of Chittagong Hill tracts of Bangladesh', *Journal of Medicine.* https://doi.org/10.3329/jom.v12i1.6925.
7. Brányik, T., et al. (2012) 'A review of methods of low alcohol and alcohol-free beer production', *Journal of Food Engineering.* https://doi.org/10.1016/j.jfoodeng.2011.09.020.
8. Buck, S. and Buck, S. L. (1993) 'Three case studies in the treatment of painted furniture', in *Papers presented at the Wooden Artifacts Group: Specialty Session*, June 4, 1993, *AIC Annual Meeting*, Denver, CO.
9. Chaturvedi, H. K., et al. (2013) 'Correlates of opium use: Retrospective analysis of a survey of tribal communities in Arunachal Pradesh, India', *BMC Public Health.* https://doi.org/10.1186/1471-2458-13-325.
10. Chu, Y., Fei, J. and Hou, S. (2020) 'Adaptive global sliding-mode control for dynamic systems using double hidden layer recurrent neural network structure', *IEEE Transactions on Neural Networks and Learning Systems.* https://doi.org/10.1109/TNNLS.2019.2919676.
11. Dasgupta, A., et al. (2013) 'Alcohol consumption by workers in automobile repair shops of a slum of Kolkata: An assessment with AUDIT instrument', *Nepal Journal of Epidemiology.* https://doi.org/10.3126/nje.v3i3.9188.
12. Dutta, R., et al. (2014) 'A population based study on alcoholism among adult males in a rural area, Tamil Nadu, India', *Journal of Clinical and Diagnostic Research.* https://doi.org/10.7860/JCDR/2014/6308.4411.
13. Endsley, P., Weobong, B. and Nadkarni, A. (2017) 'Psychometric properties of the AUDIT among men in Goa, India', *Asian Journal of Psychiatry.* https://doi.org/10.1016/j.ajp.2017.03.006.
14. Fathima, F., et al. (2015) 'Alcohol consumption among adult males in a village in Bangalore Urban district: Prevalence, harmful use and dependence', *National Journal of Research in Community Medicine.*
15. Filov, I., et al. (2014) 'Relationship between child maltreatment and alcohol abuse -Findings from adverse childhood experience study in Republic of Macedonia', *Open Access Macedonian Journal of Medical Sciences.* https://doi.org/10.3889/oamjms.2014.067.
16. Ganesh, I. (2014) 'Conversion of carbon dioxide into methanol - A potential liquid fuel: Fundamental challenges and opportunities (a review)', *Renewable and Sustainable Energy Reviews.* https://doi.org/10.1016/j.rser.2013.11.045.
17. Hamdani, M., et al. (2020) 'Prediction the inside variables of even-span glass greenhouse with special structure by artificial neural network (MLP-RBF) models', *Journal of Agricultural Machinery.*
18. Hasin, D. S. and Grant, B. F. (2015) 'The National Epidemiologic Survey on Alcohol and Related Conditions (NESARC) waves 1 and 2: Review and summary of findings', *Social Psychiatry and Psychiatric Epidemiology.* https://doi.org/10.1007/s00127-015-1088-0.
19. Hernández-Tobías, A., et al. (2011) 'Natural alcohol exposure: Is ethanol the main substrate for alcohol dehydrogenases in animals?', *Chemico-Biological Interactions.* https://doi.org/10.1016/j.cbi.2011.02.008.

20. Huang, J., et al. (2017) 'Green preparation of a cellulose nanocrystals/polyvinyl alcohol composite superhydrophobic coating', *RSC Advances*. https://doi.org/10.1039/c6ra27663f.
21. Iozzino, L., et al. (2015) 'Prevalence and risk factors of violence by psychiatric acute inpatients: A systematic review and meta-analysis', *PLoS ONE*. https://doi.org/10.1371/journal.pone.0128536.
22. Jabbar, U., et al. (2010) ' Effectiveness of alcohol-based hand rubs for removal of *Clostridium difficile* spores from hands', *Infection Control & Hospital Epidemiology*. https://doi.org/10.1086/652772.
23. Jackson, K. M. and Chung, T. (2011) 'Alcohol use', in *Encyclopedia of Adolescence*. https://doi.org/10.1016/B978-0-12-373951-3.00098-3.
24. Kavi, A., Walvekar, P. and Patil, R. (2019) 'Biological risk factors for coronary artery disease among adults residing in rural area of North Karnataka, India', *Journal of Family Medicine and Primary Care*. https://doi.org/10.4103/jfmpc.jfmpc_278_18.
25. Lhachimi, S. K., et al. (2012) 'Health impacts of increasing alcohol prices in the European Union: A dynamic projection', *Preventive Medicine*. https://doi.org/10.1016/j.ypmed.2012.06.006.
26. Lin, P. H. and Wong, D. S. H. (2014) 'Carbon dioxide capture and regeneration with amine/alcohol/water blends', *International Journal of Greenhouse Gas Control*. https://doi.org/10.1016/j.ijggc.2014.04.020.
27. Malekpour, A., Mostajeran, B. and Koohmareh, G. A. (2017) 'Pervaporation dehydration of binary and ternary mixtures of acetone, isopropanol and water using polyvinyl alcohol/zeolite membranes', *Chemical Engineering and Processing: Process Intensification*. https://doi.org/10.1016/j.cep.2017.04.019.
28. Matar, S., Mirbach, M. J. and Tayim, H. A. (1989) *Catalysis in Petrochemical Processes*. https://link.springer.com/book/10.1007/978-94-009-1177-2.
29. Mitchell, M. C., Teigen, E. L. and Ramchandani, V. A. (2014) 'Absorption and peak blood alcohol concentration after drinking beer, wine, or spirits', *Alcoholism: Clinical and Experimental Research*. https://doi.org/10.1111/acer.12355.
30. Mohd Amiruddin, A. A. A., et al. (2020) 'Neural network applications in fault diagnosis and detection: An overview of implementations in engineering-related systems', *Neural Computing and Applications*. https://doi.org/10.1007/s00521-018-3911-5.
31. Moodie, R., et al. (2013) 'Profits and pandemics: Prevention of harmful effects of tobacco, alcohol, and ultra-processed food and drink industries', *The Lancet*. https://doi.org/10.1016/S0140-6736(12)62089-3.
32. Moral, A. R., et al. (2015) 'Neuromuscular functions on experimental acute methanol intoxication', *Turk Anesteziyoloji ve Reanimasyon Dernegi Dergisi*. https://doi.org/10.5152/TJAR.2015.13471.
33. Nsiewe, N. M., et al. (2018) 'Unusual deaths in two health districts in the east region-Cameroon: A case control study, 2016', *American Journal of Tropical Medicine and Hygiene*.
34. Pires, D., et al. (2017) 'Hand hygiene with alcohol-based hand rub: How long is long enough?', *Infection Control and Hospital Epidemiology*. https://doi.org/10.1017/ice.2017.25.
35. Qian, Y., et al. (2014) 'On the training aspects of Deep Neural Network (DNN) for parametric TTS synthesis', in *ICASSP, IEEE International Conference on Acoustics, Speech and Signal Processing - Proceedings*. https://doi.org/10.1109/ICASSP.2014.6854318.
36. Radhakrishnan, S. and Balamurugan, S. (2013) 'Prevalence of diabetes and hypertension among geriatric population in a rural community of Tamilnadu', *Indian Journal of Medical Sciences*. https://doi.org/10.4103/0019-5359.122742.
37. Santasalo-Aarnio, A., et al. (2011) 'Comparison of methanol, ethanol and iso-propanol oxidation on Pt and Pd electrodes in alkaline media studied by HPLC', *Electrochemistry Communications*. https://doi.org/10.1016/j.elecom.2011.02.022.
38. Sebastian, C. and Suja, M. K. (2019) 'Parental alcoholism-psychosocial problems faced by adolescents', *Indian Journal of Public Health Research and Development*. https://doi.org/10.5958/0976-5506.2019.02393.3.
39. Setzler, B. P., et al. (2012) 'Further development of the isopropanol-acetone chemical heat engine', in *World Renewable Energy Forum, WREF 2012, Including World Renewable Energy Congress XII and Colorado Renewable Energy Society (CRES) Annual Conference*.
40. Subramanian, S., et al. (2021) 'Multilayer perceptron mode and ANN to assess the economic impact and human health due to the alcoholism and its effect in rural areas', *Lecture Notes in Electrical Engineering (LNEE)*.
41. Srinath, R. and Sendilvelan, S. (2017) 'A study on the prevalence of alcoholism among males in rural areas and its impact', *Indian Journal of Public Health Research and Development*. https://doi.org/10.5958/0976-5506.2017.00190.5.
42. Srinath, R. and Sendilvelan, S. (2017) 'Behavioral problems perceived by the alcoholic and his family - A study among males in rural areas', *International Journal of Psychosocial Rehabilitation*, 21(2): 13–19.

43. Tan, A., et al. (2014) 'Flaming alcoholic drinks: Flirting with danger', *Journal of Burn Care and Research*. https://doi.org/10.1097/BCR.0b013e3182a366de.
44. Tavana, M., et al. (2016) 'A hybrid intelligent fuzzy predictive model with simulation for supplier evaluation and selection', *Expert Systems with Applications*. https://doi.org/10.1016/j.eswa.2016.05.027.
45. Thị Tuyết Vân, P. (2018) 'Education as a breaker of poverty: a critical perspective', *Papers of Social Pedagogy*. https://doi.org/10.5604/01.3001.0010.8049.
46. Voas, R. B., Johnson, M. B. and Miller, B. A. (2013) 'Alcohol and drug use among young adults driving to a drinking location', *Drug and Alcohol Dependence*. https://doi.org/10.1016/j.drugalcdep.2013.01.014.
47. Yip, L., et al. (2020) 'Serious adverse health events, including death, associated with ingesting alcohol-based hand sanitizers containing methanol — Arizona and New Mexico, May–June 2020', *MMWR. Morbidity and Mortality Weekly Report*. https://doi.org/10.15585/mmwr.mm6932e1.
48. Zhao, Q., et al. (2013) 'Validation study of 131I-RRL: Assessment of biodistribution, SPECT imaging and radiation dosimetry in mice', *Molecular Medicine Reports*. https://doi.org/10.3892/mmr.2013.1338.

8 Downlink Fronthaul Connectivity for IoT Devices in Rural Areas with Scheduling Approach

Sayanti Ghosh, Sanjay Dhar Roy, and Sumit Kundu

CONTENTS

8.1 INTRODUCTION

Nowadays, the world is converging towards urbanization, and populations of megacities are emerging greater than 10 to 20 million people, so to serve their inhabitants effectively requires large-scale operations and management [1]. Most people enjoy smart villages, towns, suburban, etc., only because of technological advances primarily based on IoT. While technological advances have made smart cities with massive citizens possible, the same development is also possible for the people who live in rural areas. People can live in a "smart home" with all the available facilities, such as a clean village and partially solar panels producing energy for meeting consumption demands. In rural areas, people are connected to their colleagues, i.e. work-from-home (WFH) facility is possible through a high bandwidth communications network. In addition, a high-speed rail system is possible for the workers. Also, kids can enjoy distance learning with virtual reality and advanced technology methods.

Moreover, standard medical management includes health maintenance and protection, even though complicated surgeries are possible via robotics, vocal resonance, and ultra-reliable communication in 5G wireless networks [2]. The concept of "smart everywhere" depends on fast-moving

DOI: 10.1201/9781003217398-8

connectivity between the core network and IoT devices. Also, the expansion of IoT devices can occur in both rural and non-rural areas. In rural areas, people can enjoy their life with the "smart everywhere" concept.

The IoT gateways communicate to IoT devices, but scheduling is necessary to avoid interference from other IoT devices in the same cell. In [3], an IoT-based task scheduling method is considered for cloud computing.

8.1.1 Related Works

This section presents an overview of the related works.

IoT is becoming a profound technology worldwide, and it exists in an ordinary person's everyday life in society. The term "IoT" is like a coin from the two words, i.e., "Internet" and "Things". Madakam et al. [4] report billions of users are served by a standard transmission control protocol or Internet protocol (TCP/IP). Nowadays, millions of private, public, government, academic, and business sectors are linked by electronics, wireless, and optical networking technology, etc. [5]. They are exchanging data, news, and opinions through the internet.

On the other hand, things can be any object or person that can be detectable by the real world. Here, the things may be living things or non-living things. Living things like persons, animals – cow, dog etc. – plants –mango tree, banana tree etc., – and non-living things like a chair, fridge, air-conditioner (AC) tube light, any industry apparatus or home appliances, etc. [6]. IoT devices communicate to the IoT gateway for relaying the information to BS [7]. The IoT gateway acts as a central hub or one of the key elements in this ecosystem [8]. It is used for communication with all sensors and remote connections such as the internet, applications, or users. IoT devices may connect to the IoT gateway using Bluetooth low energy (LE), or Zigbee for short-range wireless communication. Wi-Fi links them to the internet public cloud for long-range wireless communication long-term evolution (LTE) through ethernet local-area network (LAN) or fibre optics wide-area network (WAN) [9]. Kumar et al. [10] have studied IoT becoming an essential aspect of enhancing future technology. Hussein [11] has discussed the current implementation, challenges, and upcoming applications of IoT technologies.

The concept of stochastic geometry was used as early as 1978 for characterizing interference tools in wireless networks [12]. Andrews et al. [13] have considered that the base stations were situated according to the Poisson point process (PPP) and derived the mathematical framework for anticipating the signal to interference noise ratio (SINR) in a downlink cellular network. Pinto et al. [14] have studied the stochastic geometry theory applied and redesigned to cellular systems, cognitive radio, femtocells, relay networks, etc. Jo et al. [15], have studied users' locations as a homogenous Poisson point process, and for each Voronoi cell, the probability distribution of the number of users has been derived. Elsawy et al. [16] have investigated the temporal variation of traffic based on queuing theory in a multi-tier heterogeneous network. Hasan et al. [17] studied human-to-human (H2H) and machine-type communication (MTC) using a random access channel to establish a link with its associated base station (BS).

Zhong et al. [18] have studied the delay of end-to-end communication based on classical queueing theory. Zhang et al. [19] have examined the spatial distribution and the temporal variation for analysing traffic and delay in cellular networks. Luo [20] has studied traffic transmission with delay constraints in heterogeneous cellular networks. Narman et al. [21] have studied the scheduling algorithm using a dynamic approach in heterogeneous and homogenous systems. Kakarla [22] has developed the multipath management algorithm to manage scheduling intelligently.

A few works have been done on IoT reliability at the system level. Behera et al. [23] have proposed modelling the reliability of IoT access networks. The algorithm has been proposed, and the system reliability could be measured using the availability of the program. The algorithm has been tested for a fire alarm system, but it is necessary to measure the scheduling and delay performance in the system. Moore et al. [24] have discussed a set of essential research directions for IoT reliability. The reliability block diagram has been proposed for an end-to-end IoT network in the study of Azghiou et al. [25]. The authors have considered different types of architecture along with their flexibility, scalability, etc. In our proposed IoT access/fronthaul network, we have discussed the network's reliability, such as success probability where the successful transmission happens from the IoT gateway to IoT devices. For the reliability of the network, scheduling is essential for maintaining the interference at the particular IoT device.

8.1.2 Contribution

In previous work [18], authors have considered delay analysis in 5G wireless networks. In our work, IoT access/fronthaul network is investigated for rural areas in a downlink scenario. Currently, rural areas are also being developed according to the upcoming demand for 5G wireless networks. In earlier research works, the authors have not considered this type of network model to the best of our knowledge. In our scenario, we have considered stochastic geometry theory and scheduling approach in an IoT access network. Also, we have investigated the effect of scheduling policies and delay performance in our proposed model.

The main contributions can be summarized as follows:

- An IoT access/fronthaul network is considered, and the performance is evaluated under stochastic geometry theory and scheduling strategies.
- The analytical expression for success probability is developed.
- The area spectral efficiency is measured in each cell.
- Delay in success probability is evaluated for different types of scheduling strategies.

8.1.3 Organization of the Chapter

Section 8.2 discusses the considered system model, which involves the analytical modelling of the success probability, area spectral efficiency, scheduling and delay, and delay success probability. Results are discussed in section 8.3. Finally, the conclusion is made in section 8.4.

8.2 SYSTEM MODEL

In Figure 8.1, a downlink IoT access/fronthaul connectivity can be supplied using suitable technology to each town or village. Fronthaul connectivity refers to a fibre-based connection between the baseband unit and remote radio head in radio access network (RAN) infrastructure. It originated from LTE networks. A flexible fronthaul organization is essential for balancing the throughput, latency, and reliability of 5G applications in an era. However, M number of IoT devices can be connected to N number of IoT gateways. The IoT gateways are working as a BS.

In this system model, we consider N numbers of randomly located IoT gateways, but each cell consists of only one IoT gateway. The positions of the IoT gateways are modelled as a homogenous PPP Φ_N where $(N = 1,\cdots,\mathbb{N})$ with intensity λ_N and $\Phi_1, \Phi_2, \cdots, \Phi_{\mathbb{N}}$ are assumed to be independent. However, we assume that IoT devices are located as a homogenous PPP $\Phi_M = \{x_j\}$ where $j \in (1,\cdots M)$ with intensity λ_M and they are directly connected to the IoT gateways in each cell.

8.2.1 Downlink Signal Transmission

In a downlink IoT access/fronthaul network, the received signal $(y_r(t))$ at the IoT device on a particular cell can be represented as:

$$y_r(t) = \sqrt{P_r} h_r d_r^{-\alpha} s_r(t) + \sum_{u \in \varnothing_I} \sqrt{P_I} h_u d_u^{-\alpha} s_u(t) + W_0 \tag{8.1}$$

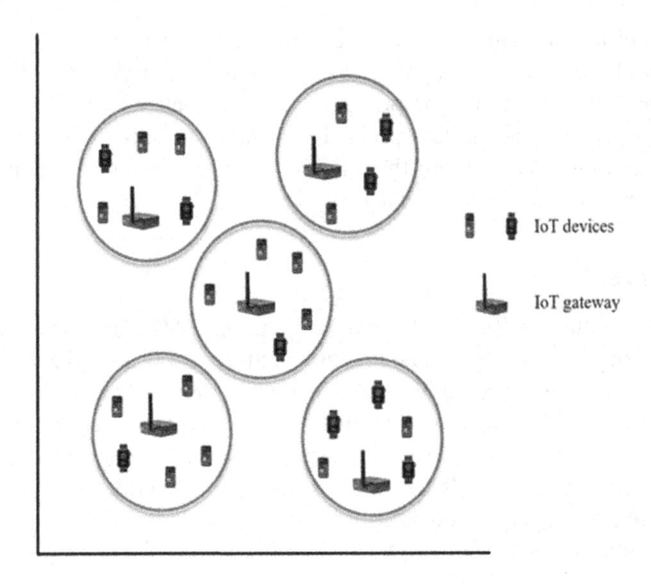

FIGURE 8.1 System model for IoT access network.

where $s(t)$ is the information signal, P_r represents the signal power emitted by the transmitter, d represents a random distance variable between the IoT gateway and IoT device, α is the path-loss exponent, And h_u and h_r represent the Rayleigh fading channel coefficient, and they are also considered as independent and identically distributed. However, the interference is caused by other cells utilizing the same spectrum band. We assume that the $\varnothing_I$ is the interferer users set, and it is distributed according to homogenous PPP over the entire plane $\mathbb{R}^2$. Here, P_I represents the interference power, and W_0 denotes the noise.

8.2.2 Success Probability

In this section, the link-level success probability of the IoT access network is analysed. The success probability depends on the received $SINR(\gamma)$ and a certain $SINR$ threshold (γ_{th}) Value. The success probability defines when the $SINR$ is by a threshold value. The $SINR$ at the IoT device can be represented as:

$$\gamma = \frac{S}{I+N} \tag{8.2}$$

$$\gamma = \frac{P_r |h_r|^2 d_r^{-\alpha}}{\sum_{u\in\varnothing_I} \delta_u P_I |h_u|^2 d_u^{-\alpha} + N} \tag{8.3}$$

where $S = P_r |h_r|^2 d_r^{-\alpha}$, $I = \sum_{u\in\varnothing_I} P_I |h_u|^2 d_u^{-\alpha}$, $P_r = \frac{P_g}{PL_0}$, and $P_I = \frac{P_g}{PL_0}\xi_g$. P_g is the common power of IoT gateway, PL_0 denotes the reference path loss at a distance from the IoT gateway, ξ_g is the interference factor at IoT gateway, and N denotes the noise power. Let δ_u represents whether the IoT gateway is idle $(\delta_u = 0)$ or busy $(\delta_u = 1)$.

However, we assume that the IoT device is located at a distance d_0 from its serving IoT gateway, and this IoT device is also affected by randomly dispersed combined interference. From [26], the link level success probability at an IoT device can be denoted as $\mathbb{P}_S$, and it can be represented as:

$$\mathbb{P}_S = P(\gamma \geq \gamma_{th}) \tag{8.4}$$

$$\mathbb{P}_S = P\left(I \leq \frac{\frac{P_g}{PL_0}}{d_0^{\frac{2}{\alpha}} \gamma_{th}} - N \right) \tag{8.5}$$

$$\mathbb{P}_S = F_I\left(\frac{\frac{P_g}{PL_0}}{d_0^{\frac{2}{\alpha}} \theta} - N \right) \tag{8.6}$$

where F_I represents the cumulative distribution function (CDF) of the interference, and its characteristics function can be expressed as [26]:

$$\Theta_I(n) = \exp\left(-\pi C_\alpha^{-1} q \left(\delta_u \frac{P_g}{PL_0} \xi_g \right)^\alpha \lambda_I |n|^\alpha \left[1 - j sign(n) \tan\left(\frac{\pi\alpha}{2} \right) \right] \right) \tag{8.7}$$

where $C_\alpha = \frac{1-\alpha}{\Gamma(2-\alpha)\cos\left(\pi\alpha/2\right)}$ when $\alpha \neq 1$, and $C_\alpha = \frac{2}{\pi}$ when $\alpha = 1$ [26], and λ_I represents the density of interference users. Here, considering IoT gateway is busy and the probability of $\delta_u = 1$ relies on the scheduling strategy, and assuming $P(\delta_u = 1) = q$.

By applying [27], the CDF at a certain IoT device can be represented as:

$$F_I(y) = \frac{1}{2} - \frac{1}{\pi} \int_0^\infty \frac{1}{n} Im\left[\Theta_I(n) \exp(-jny) \right] dn \tag{8.8}$$

Now, putting Equation (8.8) into Equation (8.6), the link level success probability can be represented as:

$$\mathbb{P}_S = \exp\left(-\frac{d_0^{\frac{2}{\alpha}} \theta N}{\frac{P_g}{PL_0}} \right) \exp\left(-\frac{\pi \lambda_I C_\alpha^{-1} \Gamma(1+\alpha)}{\cos\left(\frac{\pi\alpha}{2}\right)} \left(\frac{\delta_u \frac{P_g}{PL_0} \xi_g}{\frac{P_g}{PL_0}} d_0^{\frac{2}{\alpha}} \right)^\alpha \right) \tag{8.9}$$

8.2.3 Data Rate

Now, we calculate the data rate (R) based on the received *SINR* at the IoT device, and it can be expressed as:

$$R = B \log_2(1+\gamma) \text{ bps / Hz} \tag{8.10}$$

where B denotes the bandwidth and γ is expressed in Equation (8.3).

8.2.4 Area Spectral Efficiency

The average area spectral efficiency (ASE) is defined as the sum of the average data rates/ Hz/ unit area supported by an IoT gateway in an IoT access network. The measurement of ASE is essential to know about the area, which is covered by the single IoT gateway.

$$\text{ASE} = \frac{1}{|a|}\sum_{j=1}^{M} E\left(B\log_2\left(1+\gamma_j\right)\right)\times P\left(\text{IoT device}\right) \tag{8.11}$$

where a denotes the area in each cell.

In our work, we have considered many IoT gateways, but their position is random. So, scheduling is necessary to maintain the interference at the particular IoT device. Also, we need to evaluate the mean delay at the IoT device.

8.2.5 Scheduling and Delay

This section discusses different types of scheduling strategies, i.e., random scheduling, first-in first-out scheduling (FIFO), and round-robin scheduling.

8.2.5.1 Random Scheduling

In this scheduling policy, the active IoT gateway will randomly choose one out of many IoT devices within a cell at each time slot. We consider that each IoT gateway is busy with probability q at each time slot, and the IoT gateway is serving M number of IoT devices. The probability for the IoT device being scheduled and favourably information transmitted in each time slot. It can be represented by ϑ.

The average service rate of the typical IoT device can be expressed as:

$$\vartheta = \frac{q}{M}P\left(\gamma \geq \gamma_{th}\right) \tag{8.12}$$

$$\vartheta = \frac{q}{M}P\left(\frac{P_r\left|h_r\right|^2 d_r^{-\alpha}}{\sum_{u\in\varnothing_I}\delta_u P_I\left|h_u\right|^2 d_u^{-\alpha}+N} \geq \gamma_{th}\right) \tag{8.13}$$

$$\vartheta = \frac{q}{M}\mathbb{P}_{\mathbb{S}} \tag{8.14}$$

In the case of random scheduling, the transmission time slots for IoT devices are independent. So the probability for the successful information transmission in any time slot is also ϑ. According to general retrial policy, Geo/G/1 queue is like a discrete-time single server retrial queue, and based on Geo/G/1 and Bernoulli process, the information arrives per time slot with intensity δ_0 [28]. Now, we get the conditional mean delay $\mathbb{D}_{\mathbb{CM}}$ from [29], and it can be expressed as:

$$\mathbb{D}_{\mathbb{CM}} = \begin{cases} \dfrac{1-\delta_0}{\vartheta-\delta_0} & \text{if } \vartheta > \delta_0 \\ \infty & \text{if } \vartheta \leq \delta_0 \end{cases} \tag{8.15}$$

8.2.5.2 First-In First-Out Scheduling

In this scheduling policy, for each time slot, the fast arriving information will be scheduled by the active IoT gateway. At an IoT gateway, all the queues can be formed as a single large queue. For the large queue, the average service rate can be expressed as:

$$\vartheta = qP\left(\gamma \geq \gamma_{th}\right) \tag{8.16}$$

$$\vartheta = qP\left(\frac{P_r\left|h_r\right|^2 d_r^{-\alpha}}{\sum_{u\in\varnothing_I}\delta_u P_I\left|h_u\right|^2 d_u^{-\alpha}+N} \geq \gamma_{th}\right) \tag{8.17}$$

$$\vartheta = q\mathbb{P}_{\mathbb{S}} \tag{8.18}$$

However, when the probability of more than two IoT devices arrives simultaneously, the large queue is considered to be very small. According to the Bernoulli process, the arrival rate at large queues is $\sum_{k=0}^{M-1}\delta_k$, where δ_k denotes the arrival rate of the kth IoT device. Now, the conditional mean delay is based on FIFO scheduling [18] and can be represented as:

$$\mathbb{D}_{\text{CM}} = \begin{cases} \dfrac{1-\sum_{k=0}^{M-1}\delta_k}{\vartheta-\sum_{k=0}^{M-1}\delta_k} if\ \vartheta > \sum_{k=0}^{M-1}\delta_k \\ \infty if\ \vartheta \le \sum_{k=0}^{M-1}\delta_k \end{cases} \tag{8.19}$$

8.2.5.3 Round-Robin Scheduling

In this scheduling policy [18], M number of IoT devices will occupy M time slots to complete a cycle in each cell. However, the time slot for the typical IoT device is scheduled, and for the specific IoT, M can be considered the period between two scheduled time slots. So, the serving rate for the new typical IoT device can be considered as a new queuing system, and it can be expressed as:

$$\vartheta = qP(\gamma \ge \gamma_{th}) \tag{8.20}$$

$$\vartheta = q\mathbb{P}_{\mathbb{S}} \tag{8.21}$$

Note that, the $\frac{M}{2}$ time slots are needed for the specific IoT device to successfully deliver the information in the first scheduled time slot. Further time slots are needed, and M should be multiplied with an extra number of scheduled time slots. Now, the conditional mean delay for the Round-Robin Scheduling can be represented as:

$$\mathbb{D}_{\text{CM}} = \begin{cases} \dfrac{1-\delta_0}{\vartheta-\delta_0}M - \dfrac{M}{2} & \text{if } \vartheta > \delta_0 \\ \infty & \text{if } \vartheta \le \delta_0 \end{cases} \tag{8.22}$$

8.2.6 Delay Success Probability

The delay success means that the delay requirement of an IoT device can be achieved if it is lesser than the delay requirement φ of the IoT device. Therefore, delay in success probability can be expressed as:

$$\mathbb{S}_{\mathbb{P}} = P(\mathbb{D}_{\text{CM}} \le \varphi) \tag{8.23}$$

Algorithm for delay success probability in an IoT access network
1. GENERATE: IoT devices and IoT gateway within the cell
2. INPUT: θ, N, P_g, PL_0, λ_I, ξ_g, M, δ_0, and φ
3. INITIALIZATION: Count, number of iteration
4. COMPUTE: Success probability i.e. $\mathbb{P}_{\mathbb{S}}$

```
5. Repeat 4 to 8 simulation time
6. CALCULATE: 𝔻CM (for each scheduling strategy)
7. If 𝔻CM < φ
8. Count ← Count + 1, then
9. End
10. COMPUTE 𝕊P = Count / numberofiteration
```

8.3 RESULTS AND DISCUSSIONS

The numerical results using the performance analysis scheme have been shown in this section. More specifically, the success probability, spectral efficiency, delay success probability has been evaluated via simulation. Here, a Monte Carlo simulation is performed in MATLAB to evaluate the results. The values of some network parameters are considered as $P_g = 25$ dB, $PL_0 = 0.2$, $\xi_g = -30\,\text{dB}$, $a = 200\,\text{m}$, $\gamma_{th} = -30\,\text{dB}$, $M = 4$, and $B = 1\,\text{kHz}$ for evaluation of network performances. Figure 8.2 shows the variation in success probability for several values of γ_{th}. The success probability decreases as the γ_{th} increases for a fixed P_g. For a particular γ_{th}, the success probability increases if the common power of the IoT gateway, i.e., P_g increases. As P_g increases, then P_r increases. As a result, *SINR* increases, thus success probability increases.

In Figure 8.3, the average area spectral efficiency of the IoT access network is shown. The average ASE of the considered D2D network is investigated for a = 100 m, 200 m, and 300 m $P_g = 25$ dB, etc. The result of average area spectral efficiency is obtained via simulation and using Equation (8.11). It is found that for particular a, ASE increases as the M increases. If the M increases, then the channel capacity increases, as a result, ASE increases. It is also found that for a specific, ASE decreases as a increases. In particular, for $M = 5$, the area spectral efficiency decreases by 30.77% as a increases from 200 m to 300 m.

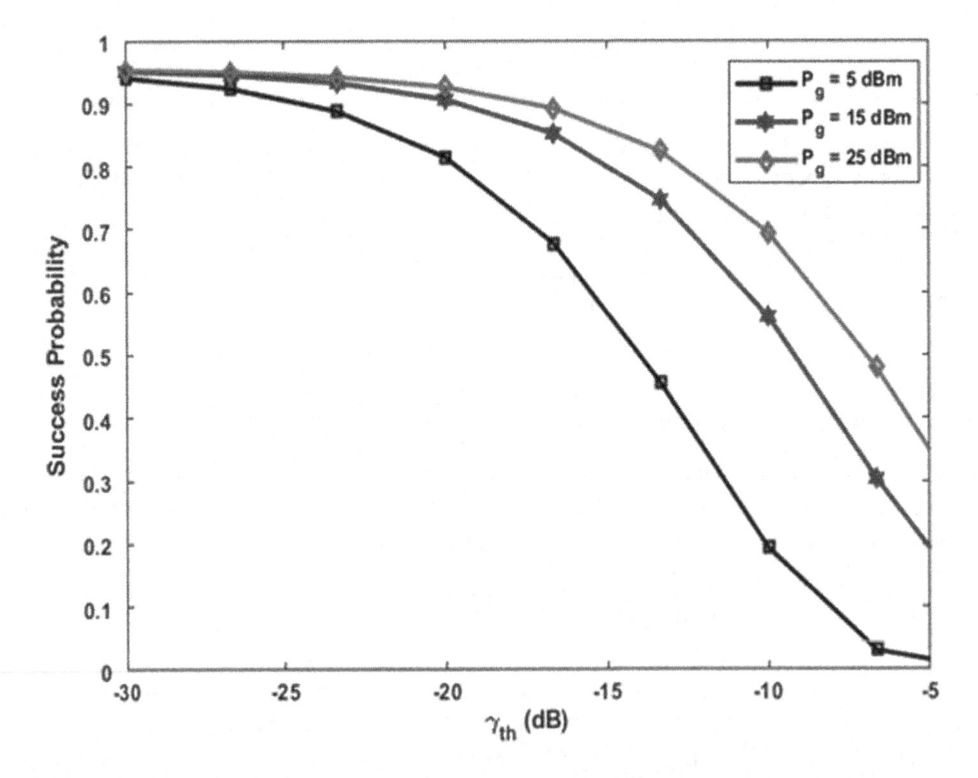

FIGURE 8.2 Variation in success probability for several values of γ_{th} (in dB).

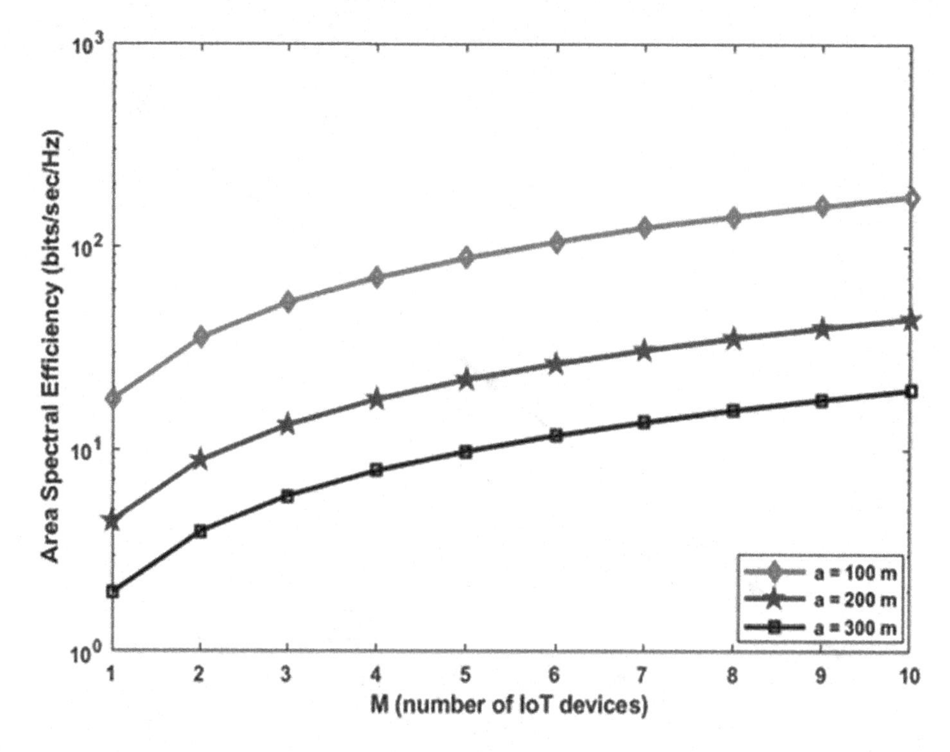

FIGURE 8.3 Impact of M on area spectral efficiency.

Figure 8.4 illustrates the delay in probability as a function of q. Based on the proposed algorithm, the delay success probability is obtained by using Equation (8.23). It is observed as the q increases, the delay in probability increases. This result also shows the scheduling approach on delay in probability. It is shown that the delay in success probability is less for round-robin scheduling as compared to the first-in first-out scheduling and random scheduling. In the case of round-robin scheduling, the conditional mean delay is less than the other scheduling strategies. In contrast, the scheduling time is divided into two slots to deliver the information successfully. Thus, the delay performance is better for round-robin scheduling.

8.4 CONCLUSION

The IoT access/ fronthaul network has been presented in a downlink scenario. In each cell, the randomly located IoT gateways deliver information to the IoT devices. The stochastic geometric theory has been applied to evaluate the performance of the IoT access network. The link-level success probability has been estimated for the proposed network. The area spectral efficiency for each cell has been observed. Accordingly, it has been shown that as the number of IoT devices increases, the area spectral efficiency increases. Moreover, the scheduling approaches have been investigated under the proposed network. Finally, the delay success probability has been shown for the IoT access network. It has been observed that the round-robin scheduling gives better performance than random scheduling and first-in first-out scheduling. Our analysis is helpful in the design of IoT access/ fronthaul network for applications in rural areas and urban areas. In the future, we can improve the performance of our proposed work by considering non-orthogonal multiple access (NOMA). In contrast, NOMA can be used for successive interference cancellation (SIC) and multiple interference cancellation (MIC) schemes. The NOMA technology will be applied in our proposed network; thus, IoT gateways will transmit desired information to the respective IoT devices by cancelling the interference in each cell (Table 8.1).

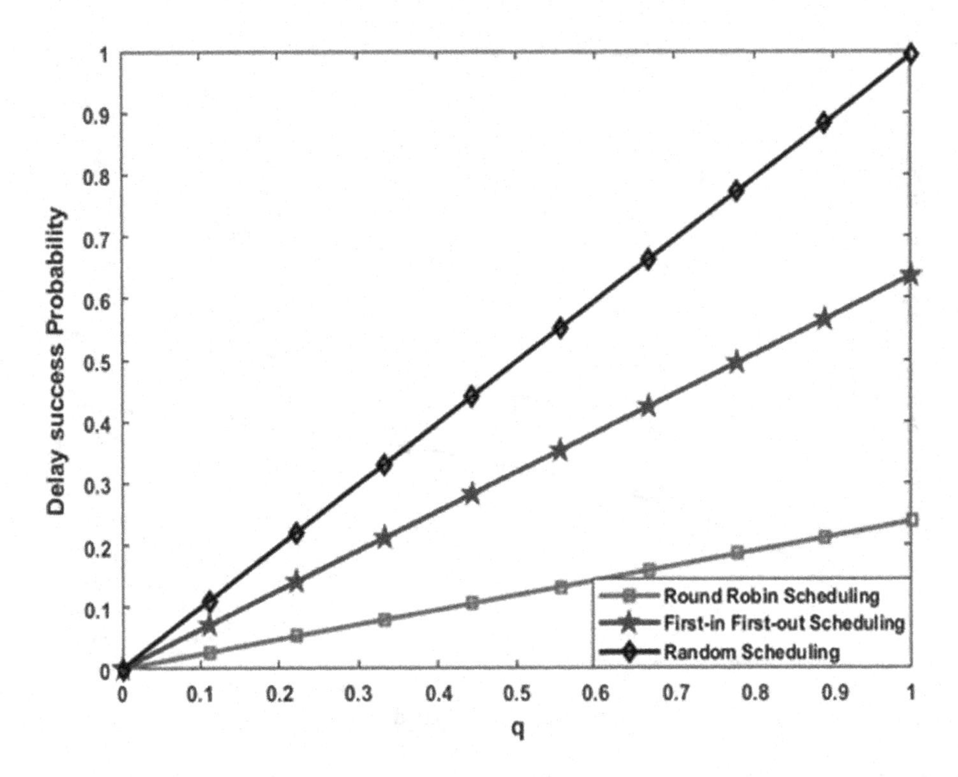

FIGURE 8.4 The delay success probability as a function of q.

TABLE 8.1
Some Important Names and Their Abbreviations and Symbols

Name	Abbreviation and Symbol
Internet of Things	IoT
Radio Access Network	RAN
Base Station	BS
Poisson Point Process	PPP
Success Probability	$\mathbb{P}_S$
Area Spectral Efficiency	ASE
Signal to Interference Noise Ratio	$SINR(\gamma)$
SINR Threshold	γ_{th}
Data Rate	R
Delay Success Probability	$\mathbb{S}_{\mathbb{P}}$

REFERENCES

1. Yaacoub, E. and Alouini, M.S. Efficient fronthaul and backhaul connectivity for IoT traffic in rural areas. *IEEE Internet of Things Magazine*, 4(1), pp.60–66, 2020.
2. Palattella, M.R., Dohler, M., Grieco, A., Rizzo, G., Torsner, J., Engel, T. and Ladid, L. Internet of Things in the 5G era: Enablers, architecture, and business models. *IEEE Journal on Selected Areas in Communications*, 34(3), pp.510–527, 2016.
3. Ma, X., Gao, H., Xu, H. and Bian, M. An IoT-based task scheduling optimization scheme considering the deadline and cost-aware scientific workflow for cloud computing. *EURASIP Journal on Wireless Communications and Networking*, 2019(1), pp.1–19, 2019.

4. Madakam, S., Lake, V., Lake, V. and Lake, V. Internet of Things (IoT): A literature review. *Journal of Computer and Communications*, 3(05), p.164, 2015.
5. Chambers, J. and Evans, J. Informal urbanism and the Internet of Things: Reliability, trust and the reconfiguration of infrastructure. *Urban Studies*, 57(14), pp.2918–2935, 2020.
6. Niranjan, M., Madhukar, N., Ashwini, A., Muddsar, J. and Saish, M. IoT based industrial automation. *IOSR Journal of Computer Engineering (IOSR-JCE)*, 2 pp.36–40, 2017.
7. Haenggi, M., Andrews, J.G., Baccelli, F., Dousse, O. and Franceschetti, M. Stochastic geometry and random graphs for the analysis and design of wireless networks. *IEEE Journal on Selected Areas in Communications*, 27(7), pp.1029–1046, 2009.
8. Gubbi, J., Buyya, R., Marusic, S. and Palaniswami, M. Internet of Things (IoT): A vision, architectural elements, and future directions. *Future Generation Computer Systems*, 29(7), pp.1645–1660, 2013.
9. Zanella, A., Bui, N., Castellani, A., Vangelista, L. and Zorzi, M. Internet of things for smart cities. *IEEE Internet of Things Journal*, 1(1), pp.22–32, 2014.
10. Kumar, S., Tiwari, P. and Zymbler, M. Internet of Things is a revolutionary approach for future technology enhancement: A review. *Journal of Big data*, 6(1), pp.1–21, 2019.
11. Hussein, A.R.H. Internet of Things (IOT): Research challenges and future applications. *International Journal of Advanced Computer Science and Applications*, 10(6), pp.77–82, 2019.
12. Musa, S. and Wasylkiwskyj, W. Co-channel interference of spread spectrum systems in a multiple user environment. *IEEE Transactions on Communications*, 26(10), pp.1405–1413, 1978.
13. Andrews, J.G., Baccelli, F. and Ganti, R.K. A tractable approach to coverage and rate in cellular networks. *IEEE Transactions on Communications*, 59(11), pp.3122–3134, 2011.
14. Pinto, P.C., Giorgetti, A., Win, M.Z. and Chiani, M. A stochastic geometry approach to coexistence in heterogeneous wireless networks. *IEEE Journal on Selected Areas in Communications*, 27(7), pp.1268–1282, 2009.
15. Jo, H.S., Sang, Y.J., Xia, P. and Andrews, J.G. Heterogeneous cellular networks with flexible cell association: A comprehensive downlink SINR analysis. *IEEE Transactions on Wireless Communications*, 11(10), pp.3484–3495, 2012.
16. Elsawy, H., Hossain, E. and Haenggi, M. Stochastic geometry for modeling, analysis, and design of multi-tier and cognitive cellular wireless networks: A survey. *IEEE Communications Surveys & Tutorials*, 15(3), pp.996–1019, 2013.
17. Hasan, M., Hossain, E. and Niyato, D. Random access for machine-to-machine communication in LTE-advanced networks: Issues and approaches. *IEEE communications Magazine*, 51(6), pp.86–93, 2013.
18. Zhong, Y., Quek, T.Q. and Ge, X. Heterogeneous cellular networks with spatio-temporal traffic: Delay analysis and scheduling. *IEEE Journal on Selected Areas in Communications*, 35(6), pp.1373–1386, 2017.
19. Zhang, G., Quek, T.Q., Huang, A. and Shan, H. Delay and reliability trade-offs in heterogeneous cellular networks. *IEEE Transactions on Wireless Communications*, 15(2), pp.1101–1113, 2015.
20. Luo, X. Delay-oriented QoS-aware user association and resource allocation in heterogeneous cellular networks. *IEEE Transactions on Wireless Communications*, 16(3), pp.1809–1822, 2017.
21. Narman, H.S., Hossain, M.S., Atiquzzaman, M. and Shen, H. Scheduling internet of things applications in cloud computing. *Annals of Telecommunications*, 72(1–2), pp.79–93, 2017.
22. Kakarla, A.B. Towards novel multipath data scheduling for future IoT systems: A survey. *arXiv preprint arXiv:2105.07578*, 2021.
23. Behera, R.K., Reddy, K.H.K. and Roy, D.S. Reliability modelling of service oriented Internet of Things. In *IEEE 4th International Conference on Reliability, Infocom Technologies and Optimization (ICRITO) (Trends and Future Directions)*, pp.1–6, 2015.
24. Moore, S.J., Nugent, C.D., Zhang, S. and Cleland, I. IoT reliability: A review leading to 5 key research directions. *CCF Transactions on Pervasive Computing and Interaction*, 2, pp.147–163, 2020, https://doi.org/10.1007/s42486-020-00037-z.
25. Azghiou, K., El Mouhib, M., Koulali, M.A. and Benali, A. An end-to-end reliability framework of the internet of things. *Sensors*, 20(9), p.2439, 2020.
26. Win, M.Z., Pinto, P.C. and Shepp, L.A. A mathematical theory of network interference and its applications. *Proceedings of the IEEE*, 97(2), pp.205–230, 2009.
27. Ilow, J., Hatzinakos, D. and Venetsanopoulos, A.N. Performance of FHSS radio networks with interference modelled as a mixture of Gaussian and alpha-stable noise. *IEEE Transactions on Communications*, 46(4), pp.509–520, 1998.
28. Zhang, F. and Zhu, Z. A discrete-time retrial queue with vacations and two types of breakdowns. *Journal of Applied Mathematics*, 2013, pp.1155, 2013, https://doi.org/10.1155/2013/834731.
29. Falin, G. A survey of retrial queues. *Queueing Systems*, 7(2), pp.127–167, 1990.

9 IoT-Enabled Customizable System for Traffic Management with Real-Time Vehicle Emission Measurement Functionality

Almamun Sheikh, Debabrata Bej and Ashis Kumar Mal

CONTENTS

9.1 INTRODUCTION

A smooth transportation system is a backbone to the economical and sociological growth of a country, whether it is a developed or developing one. India has over 5.9 million kilometers of road networks, one of the largest road networks in the world [1]. The mobility of the transportation system is heavily reliant on better management and control of road networks and traffic. As a result, the traffic management system (TMS) plays an essential role in mitigating the problems posed by modern transportation. TMSs that are appropriate focus on improving traffic efficiency, reducing total travel time, and reducing fuel usage and greenhouse gas (GHG) emissions [2]. Although traffic efficiency is a primary issue for any TMS, close attention to traffic safety should be paid without compromising.

DOI: 10.1201/9781003217398-9

There are many speed-breaking mechanisms, traffic signs, and other roadway features to ensure traffic safety. TMS is an integral part of the intelligent transportation system (ITS). There are many applications of ITS in different modes of the transportation system to address problems like accidents rate, traffic congestion, carbon emissions, and air pollution [3]. We have found that ITS can also effectively optimize reliability, travel speeds, traffic flow, etc. Despite the proven efficiency of ITS, there are still many issues that need to be optimized. In [4], researchers proposed an idea to deal with the problem of sensor placement in intelligent transportation systems (ITS). Gentili and Mirchandani [5] have provided detailed insights regarding sensor placement on traffic networks. Cao et al. [6] proposed a unified framework to reduce traffic congestion. This framework is useful for vehicle rerouting and traffic light control. Shi et al. [7] suggested a method to measure particle number emissions from vehicles driving on the road. Zhang et al. [8] presented a study by remote sensing methodology on worldwide on-road vehicle exhaust emissions. Zhu et al. [9] proposed a novel idea regarding IoT-enabled smart urban traffic control and management. Undoubtedly, ITS is an evolving technology for the betterment of the present transportation system. But the million-dollar question is whether the present transportation infrastructure can utilize the benefits of ITS fully?

Presently installed speed breaking mechanism across Indian roadways is of very primitive type. It causes a lot of road hazards on a day-to-day basis. Although the speed-breaking mechanism (hump, bump etc.) is to provide safety to the vehicle and passengers without causing any damage and discomfort. the traditional speed breakers, although useful for traffic management, are practically a threat to human life and the environment [10]. Speed bumps or breakers are used to slow the vehicles and to enhance road safety. However, sudden strikes of vehicles with speed bumps damage the vehicles and increase the possibility of accidents [11]. These can also highly affect the fuel consumption of the vehicles. Additionally, these can affect the health conditions of the drivers and also the passengers in some cases. Mainly, speed bumps can damage the spine of the traveler and causes back pain. Speed breakers also cause sudden irritation when someone travels in a vehicle [12].

Usually, two types of speed breakers can be seen on Indian roads. One is speed bumps or humps, which utilize vertical deflection to slow down the vehicles [13]. Another one is a barricade deployed on the road by traffic police to slow down over-speed vehicles in a busy traffic zone. The barricade induces a horizontal deflection on the road. There are several types of barricades like fixed railings, Green belts, Lifting barricades, etc.

As speed bumps create vertical deflection on the road, they have a comparatively more chance of strikes to the vehicle than barricades. Chances of vehicle damage are also relatively less for barricades than for speed bumps. Fuel is consumed less for barricade breakers than for speed bumps. Speed is one of the most critical factors for achieving the fuel efficiency of vehicles [14]–[15]. Barricades have less chance of health effects due to the strikes of vehicles at speed bumps very much. Another significant advantage of using barricades as speed breakers is that they can be more visible on the road from long distance. From these benefits of barricades, it can be noted that the barricades can be very much helpful to use as a speed breaker. It may be utilized more in place of the speed bumps. On Indian roads, it is also used but in comparatively fewer numbers than speed bumps. It is very much possible to control the barricade according to the number of vehicles at a time.

Presently, many provisions of automatic mobile barricades based on embedded and IoT systems are available. But most of them are either very complex or oversimplified. In the study of Han [16], the system seems unique to address the tide traffic phenomenon. But the system is complicated and costly for Indian roads. In literature, there are many innovative ideas for mobile barricades [17]–[23], which may address the hazards of their traditional counterparts, as depicted above. Undesirable interruptions like traffic congestion hamper the efficiency of the traffic flow. This problem is getting worse as a large number of vehicles are deploying on roads. Congestions at road junctions and toll gates are occurring on a daily basis. It costs enormous both in terms of time and monetary value to individuals and the country. In literature, researchers have tried to provide solutions to this problem [24]–[26].

As an illustration of India, an electronic toll collection system called 'FASTag' was launched to let people pay their tolls electronically and reduce the toll collection time [27]. This initiative aims to build up a seamless electronic toll collection infrastructure and thereby reduce congestion at toll plazas. Practically the very purpose of this initiative is not achieved yet. Lane congestion at toll plazas is still a common phenomenon. We have also noticed several bumps/humps in the lanes of toll plazas. Although those bumps/humps are indeed helpful in reducing the speed of vehicles, they have many disadvantages, as stated above.

Air pollution due to the emission of vehicles is a significant threat to the environment. Vehicle emissions largely contribute greenhouse gases (GHGs) like CO_2, CO, NO_x, to the environment. These are mainly responsible for global warming and also affect human health. So, to calculate the environmental footprint of an area, measurement of these GHGs is very much essential. In literature, there are many ideas to measure the emission of vehicles. Before the 1990s, dynamometer emission tests were the primarily available means to measure pollutant emissions of vehicles [28]. But as these tests did not provide matching data to the real-world scenario, a portable emission measurement system (PEMS) was adopted later. Macroscopic and microscopic levels are the two families of vehicle emission measurement. The emission factor (EF)-based approach is most commonly accepted for the macroscopic emissions model. Breton [29] proposed a model to estimate traffic flow and vehicle emission. In this model, the author took a Lagrangian model to simulate traffic flow on a complex road network. The main objective of this work was to develop an integrated traffic emission information system (TEIS), which can predict traffic-induced air pollution in real time. But the proposed system seems very complex and costly in the Indian context. Sabiron et al. [30] proposed a framework to estimate pollutant emissions for real-time driving emissions at a microscopic scale and calculate environmental footprint. They have used a smartphone with no additional sensors instead of PEMS to monitor the user's environmental footprint. In the Indian context, this system is also very expensive.

This chapter aims to build a system that detects lane congestion at toll plazas and provides optimum solutions at a low cost. We also tried to replace the bums/humps with movable motorized barricades to ensure road safety and eliminate discomfort due to bumps/humps. Another objective of this chapter is to control the barricade according to the speed of vehicles. We, in this work, have considered two mobile barricades, which will be operated at per speed of the vehicles in a hassle-free manner. In this chapter, we have proposed an idea of collecting vehicle emission data at toll plazas. Whenever a vehicle comes to the toll plaza and pays a toll, a gas sensor placed in the vicinity of the toll gate will measure the emission value in the meantime of toll collection. Our idea is to build an inventory with these available data. We shall match these time-stamped emission data with the available FASTag data to detect a particular vehicle of interest.

The remainder of the article is organized into sections that detail the design methodology. Section 9.2 presents the proposed system. Section 9.3 explains the components and procedures utilized to create the prototype of the proposed approach. Section 9.4 presents the findings and perspectives. Finally, the conclusion has been stated in section 9.5.

9.2 PROPOSED SYSTEM

This section proposes an IoT-enabled system to monitor the vehicle speed, lane congestion parameters, and vehicular emission at the toll plaza. This system will provide a communication backbone to access the available data to the decision-makers (e.g., Transport Managers) to take necessary actions to solve the issues.

9.2.1 Overview of the Proposed System

The overview of the proposed system is presented in Figure 9.1. Two servo motors, three IR sensors and one Gas sensor are used in this proposed system. A NodeMCU Wi-Fi module is used to send our data into a cloud server for storing, monitoring, analyzing, and decision-making purposes.

9.2.2 Aim of the Proposed System

- Count incoming vehicles.
- Measure vehicle speed.

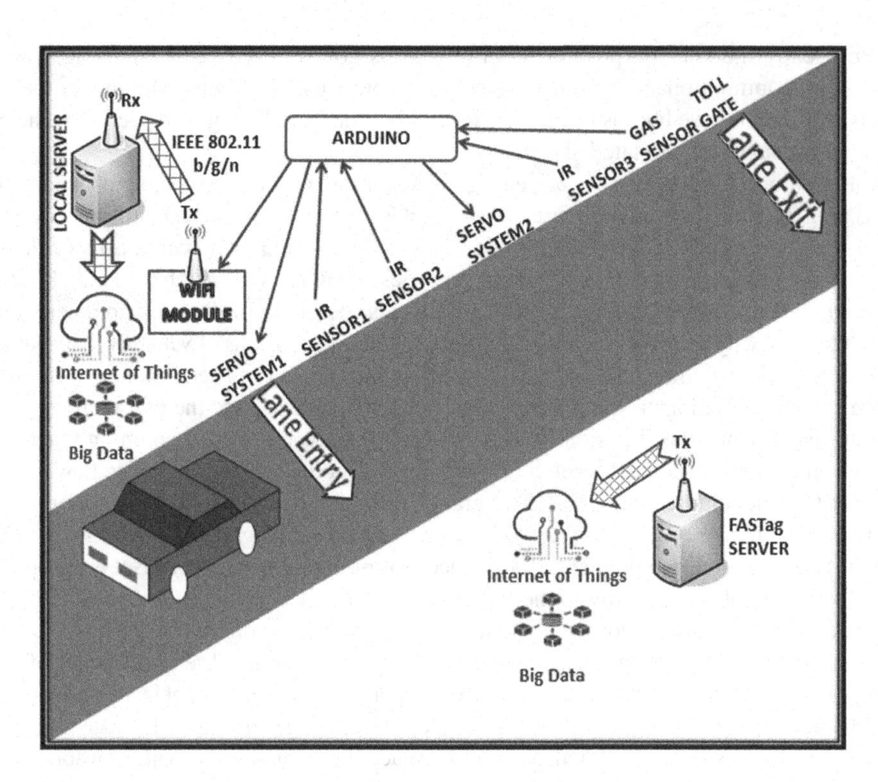

FIGURE 9.1 Overview of the proposed system.

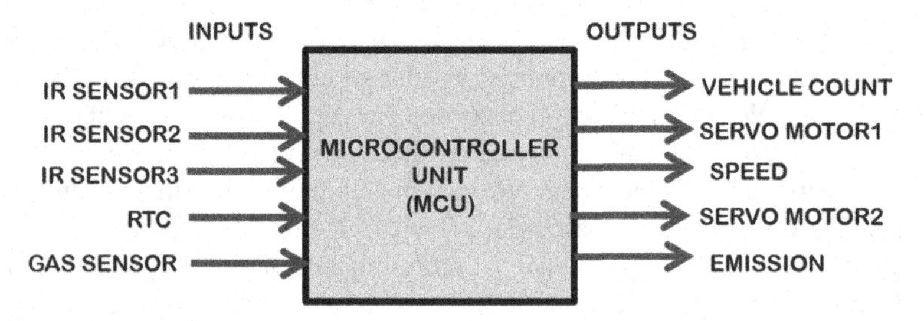

FIGURE 9.2 Block diagram of the proposed system.

- Control speed of the vehicle before entering the Toll plaza zone (using smart barricade).
- Measure vehicular emission.
- Count outgoing vehicle.
- Transmit the data into the cloud.

9.2.3 Block Diagram of the Prototype

The block diagram of the prototype is presented in Figure 9.2. Here, IR sensors and gas sensors are the system's inputs, whereas servo motors are outputs. Arduino Uno is used as the main controller in this model.

9.2.4 Proposed System Architecture

System architecture is presented in Figure 9.3. In this figure, the basic architecture of the system is described. Data comes into Arduino from sensors. Arduino sends this data to NodeMCU via serial communication. NodeMCU transmits this data via the internet into a cloud server where FasTag

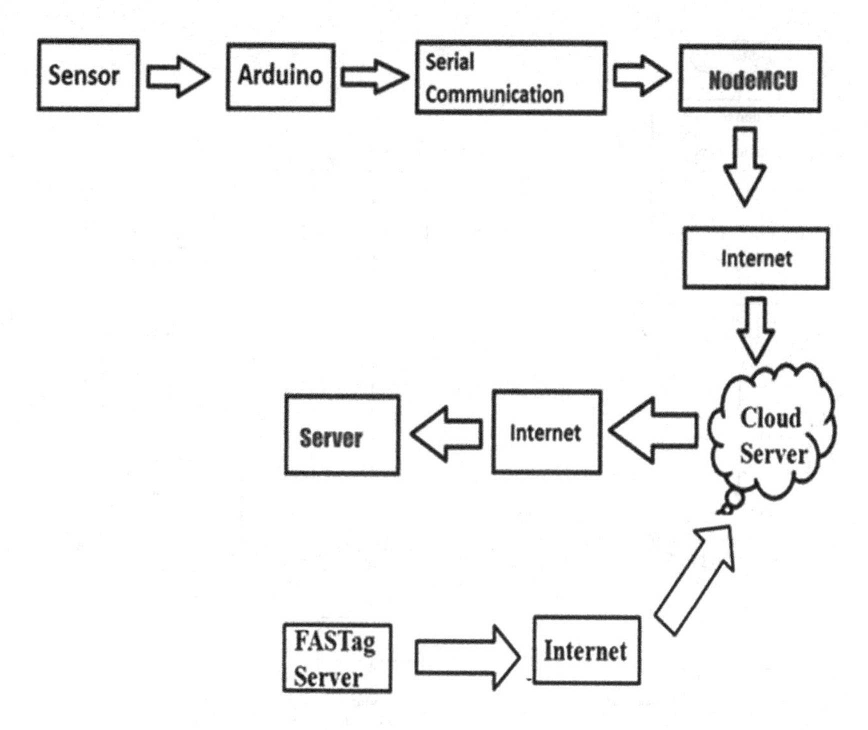

FIGURE 9.3 Proposed system architecture.

data is also synchronized with this data. Then this synchronized data file will be stored on a server for further processing. Here, we propose synchronizing FASTag data of the particular Toll plaza with the system data in the cloud. Time-stamped data of our system and the FASTag data can be compared to detect the vehicle responsible for the emission at that particular instance. In this way, we can detect the polluting vehicle.

9.2.5 Working Principle of the Proposed System (Figure 9.4)

This proposed model works upon the following problem statement:

- Count incoming vehicles and store the data.
-
  i) Detection of the speed of the vehicles.
  ii) Operate servo motors to limit the speed of the vehicles.
-
  i) Count outgoing vehicles and store the data.
  ii) Measure emission of the toll-paying vehicle.
  iii) Detect congestion based on pre-validated conditions.
  iv) Operate servo motorl according to congestion state to prevent further entry of the vehicle into the congested lane.
- Transmit the data into the cloud server using Wi-Fi.

As communication is a vital part of this work, the chapter discusses the available IEEE standard of IoT communication [31] as depicted in Figure 9.5. Here, we have summarized different available protocol stacks for IoT communication. There are I2C, SPI, UART, 1–Wire, GPIO, and other protocols used to communicate boards like Arduino to a system. IoT /M2M protocols for setting up PANS, LANS & WANS can be classified into two primary categories – wired and wireless [32].

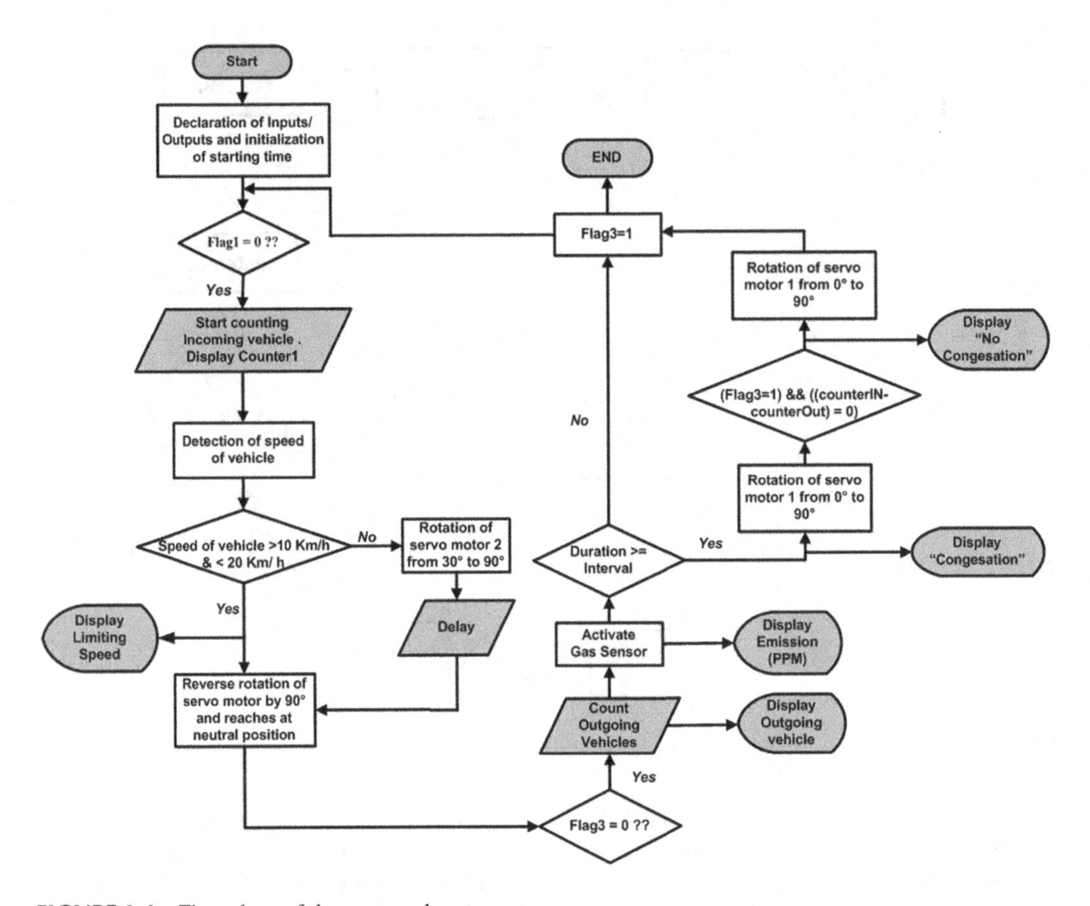

FIGURE 9.4 Flow chart of the proposed system.

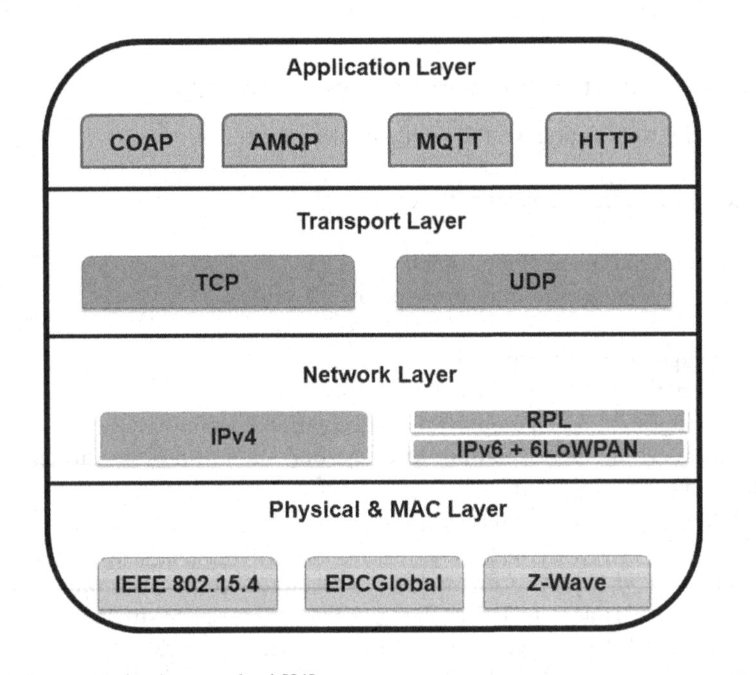

FIGURE 9.5 IoT communication standard [31].

Generally used protocols for wired LANs are ethernet, USB, serial, Firewire (IEEE 1394), MIDI, Thunderbolt, CANbus, Industrial control protocols – BAC net, Modbus, etc. There are IoT /M2M wireless protocols like WiFi-IEEE 802.11 a/b/g/n (range~100m), Wi-Fi Halow-IEEE 802.11 ah, ZigBee 3.0(IEEE 802.15.4), Z-wave, 6LoWPAN, EnOcean (ISO/ IEC 814543-3-10), and many others. We have also found some interesting protocols regarding Low power (LP)WANS like LPWAN, Cellular-2G (GSM), 3G,4G, LTE (Cat 0,1,3), LTE-M, NBIoT,5G, Noncellular LoRaWAN, SigFox, Satellite, etc. Besides these communication protocols, there are many application protocols like HTTP, MQTT, CoAP, WebSockets, etc.

In our work, we have used Wi-Fi communication protocol to send our data to the cloud as this is an available, low-cost technology. But other wireless protocols can also be used. IoT gateway plays a vital role in creating a standard interface that supports the integration of different applications, protocols, and standards. The main advantage of the IoT/M2M gateway is that it is highly customizable. [33] OneM2M is an excellent horizontal integration platform that supports multiple IoT/M2M operations with REST APIs. We have used the HTTPS application protocol in our work because it helps fetch historical data [34].

9.3 COMPONENTS AND TECHNIQUES USED TO DESIGN THE PROPOSED SYSTEM

The specifications have been stated in this section based on the initial experiment. After completion of the initial experiment, we have assembled a prototype of the invention. Following components and techniques have been used to make the prototype: (a) real-time clock (RTC) module, (b) infrared (IR) sensor module, (c) liquid crystal display (LCD) module, (d) rack and pinion mechanism, (e) servo motor, (f) gas sensor, (g) microcontroller unit (MCU), and (h) Wi-Fi module.

9.3.1 PROTOTYPE DEVELOPMENT OF THE SYSTEM

For the development of the prototype, the following modules/components are required:

9.3.1.1 Real-Time Clock Module

This module is used for the purpose of keeping accurate time. DS3231 RTC module has been used for this purpose.

9.3.1.2 Infrared Sensor Module

This module is used to detect the speed of moving vehicles. These sensor modules and RTC modules have been well organized and synchronized to increase fuel efficiency, especially for city vehicles. This module helps the driver of the moving vehicle know the current speed of their vehicle and alert them if the vehicle speed exceeds the limit. Two IR sensors (1 and 2) have been used to detect the vehicle speed and placed 10 cm apart. When a car travels and extends to sensor 1, it has been got started. From this time, a timer has been initiated and continued to record time until the vehicle reaches sensor 2. The distance between sensors 1 and 2 has been considered as 5 meters. Then the speed of the moving vehicle has been computed from a distance between two sensors divided by the traveling time of the moving vehicle from sensor 1 to sensor 2. Sensor 1 and sensor 3 also detect and count incoming and outgoing vehicles, respectively.

9.3.1.3 Liquid Crystal Display Module

This module is used to present the vehicle's speed. It displays all the required information like the number of vehicles entering and exiting a lane, the vehicle moving at high speed, and the vehicle exceeding the speed limit. 16x2" LCD display is used for this purpose.

9.3.1.4 Rack and Pinion Mechanism

Rack and pinion arrangement is used to translate the rotational motion of the motor to linear motion and acts as a linear actuator. A modified rack and pinion arrangement is employed to create the mechanical movement of the barricade. Figure 9.10 shows the modified configuration of the rack and pinion. A servo motor provides the angular displacement (Θ) and torque (T) as per the signal received by the IR sensors based on the vehicle speed. It is further processed by the microcontroller unit (MCU). As per the conditions given, it signals the servo motors to rotate, providing linear motion using the rack and pinion arrangement. Rack and pinion are connected to the barricade. Servo motor is used to provide torque (T) to the pinion and create linear motion to the rack. The rack moves forward/backward according to the directions of the torque provided by the servo motor. Torque (T) provided in a clockwise direction moves rack to the backward, and application of torque in an anti-clockwise direction moves rack to the forward direction.

9.3.1.5 Gas Sensor

We used MQ 135 gas sensor to measure the emission of the vehicle. MQ 135 has the following features, which makes it suitable for our work. It has a wide detecting scope, fast response, and high sensitivity. It is also stable and has a long life. The operating voltage is +5V. It can Detect/Measure NH3, NO_x, alcohol, Benzene, smoke, CO_2, etc. Its analogue output voltage is 0V to 5V; the digital output voltage is 0V or 5V (TTL Logic). Preheat duration is 20 seconds. It can be used as a digital or an analogue sensor.

9.3.1.6 Microcontroller Unit

We have used Arduino Uno Rev.3 as the microcontroller for our work. Arduino Uno is an inexpensive 8 bit microcontroller board based on ATmega328P [35]. It has a USB programming interface and software environment or integrated development environment (IDE).

9.3.1.7 NodeMCU

In our work, we have used the NodeMCU Wi-Fi module to establish wireless connectivity to the cloud. It can cover up to 300 m range. This development board is based on ESP8266 [36]. It integrates GPIO, PWM, I2C, 1-Wire, and ADC all in one board. This board is the most inexpensive IoT development board with inbuilt Wi-Fi connectivity. NodeMCU is an open-source Lua-based firmware for the ESP8266 Wi-Fi SOC from Espressif. An on-module flash-based SPIFFS file system has been implemented in this module. It also supports Arduino IDE for programming.

9.3.1.8 Programming Tools/Software

Arduino IDE/ C++ is used here. Arduino integrated development environment (IDE) supports C/C++ languages. This software interface is required for programming and uploading code to the board. In this work, we have used Arduino IDE 1.8.13. In Figure 9.6, a system model has been presented.

9.4 PROTOTYPE DESIGNING STEPS

Arduino Uno has been used as the central control unit of the system. RTC module, IR sensor modules 1, 2, and 3, and gas sensor (MQ135) have been used as inputs of the Arduino. LCD screen and servo motors have been used as the outputs of Arduino. Timing information, which is provided by the RTC module, helps the microcontroller to keep accurate timing information. IR sensor modules help the microcontroller to identify the high-speed vehicle and take necessary actions on that. The microcontroller detects vehicle speed using an IR sensor and represents that on an LCD screen. It displays the information as vehicle entry and exits the lane, indicates high-speed vehicles and limiting speed. Arduino Uno also controls the movement of the servo motor as per the signal received from the IR sensor modules based on the vehicle speed.

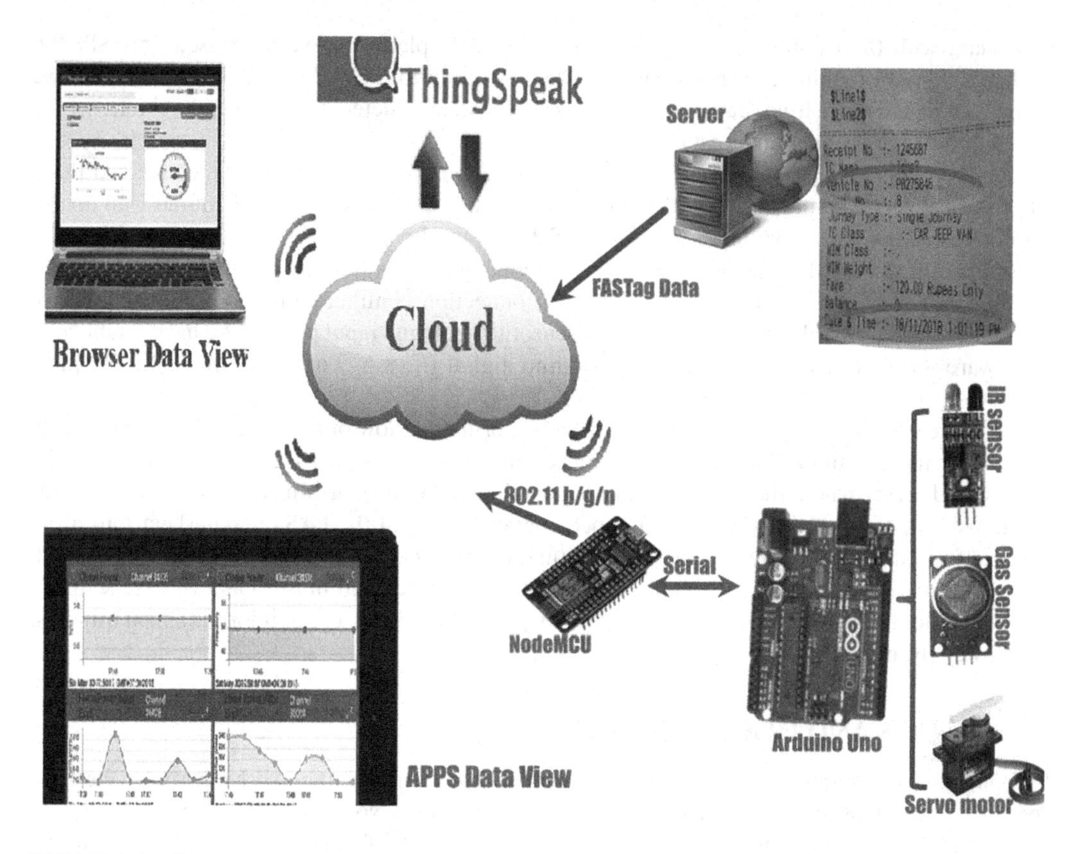

FIGURE 9.6 System model.

A flow chart of the prototype of the system has been presented in Figure 9.4. Initially, the servo motor rotates by 30° and indicates the neutral position. IR sensors are arranged so that a time delay is measured, the distance of 10 cm between the two sensors was scaled to 5 m, and the speed was calculated. If the speed was found between 60 to 80 km/h, then the servo motors were rotated by 60° from 30° to 90°, and the vehicle's speed is presented on the LCD screen as "High speed" before increasing the barricade level. Then the barricade level was raised to control the speed of that vehicle. After the vehicle's passing, the barricade returns to the neutral position by the reverse rotation of 60° of the servo motor, and at that time, Θ will be 30°. If the vehicle speed is below 20 km/h, the LCD module displays the message as "Limiting speed" to notify the traveler that he is going within the limit. Then the servo motor has been rotated by 90° from the neutral position (30°) to 120°. Then it again shifts to the neutral position after the passing of the vehicle. These speeds have been considered as an example. However, these speeds can be further adaptable by the slight changes in code as per the requirement of the traffic conditions. IR sensor 3 detects the vehicle at the place of the toll collecting office. It prevents false information regarding vehicle emissions. The gas sensor works as long as the IR sensor 3 detects any vehicle. IR sensor 3 also keeps track of the departing vehicle from the lane. If IR sensor 3 detects any vehicle for more than a specific time period, it will signify the congestion state of the particular lane. A suitable delay has been provided by calculating the stopping distance of the vehicle. Whenever a congestion state arises, Arduino would command the servo motor 1, placed at the entry of the lane, to restrict vehicle entry into this particular lane. The system will guide the incoming vehicle to the available lanes to move in. The method, in turn, would reduce the average delay time.

The timing information was made available by the RTC module, as mentioned previously. It is essentially required to time-stamp the emission value accurately. We propose an idea to integrate these data with the existing FASTag data into a big data platform. We have used an ESP8266 NodeMCU Wi-Fi module to send serial data from Arduino to a cloud server. In this chapter, we propose to match these time-stamped data and FASTag data to detect the particular vehicle, which has caused the emission at that instance.

Details of the wiring connections are provided in Figure 9.7. In this work, we connected three IR sensors as inputs to the digital (PWM) pins 0, 8, and 9, respectively, of the Arduino Uno board. We connected two DC servo motors to digital (PWM) pins 10 and 13. We connected the SDA and SCL pins of the DS3231 module to the A4 and A5 analogue input pins, respectively. We connected one LCD 16X2 to the Arduino board with this connection configuration RS=12, EN=11, d4=5, d5=4, d6=3, d7=2. We also connected one gas sensor to analogue input pin A0. We have established a software serial communication between Arduino digital I/O-s 6, 7 and NodeMCU Tx, Rx pins, respectively.

In Figure 9.8. we have presented the basic data/information flow of the system. Here sensor data are coming into Arduino. Then this serial data is transmitted via NodeMCU Wi-Fi module into the local/ cloud server where the suitable data file is archived. We convert this raw data into a spreadsheet. We will synchronize this time-stamped spreadsheet with the FASTag datasheet into a big data platform like Hadoop, etc. After that, the final data file containing synchronized time, speed, pollutant emission, vehicle details, and congestion will be processed in this platform. We will use these data files to make an inventory. This inventory will provide historical information on minutes, hours, weekly, monthly, or yearly basis (Figures 9.9 and 9.10).

9.5 RESULTS AND DISCUSSIONS

In Figure 9.11, we can see that serial communication between Arduino and NodeMCU. We have sent this serial data into a local/cloud server via internet and NodeMCU Wi-Fi connectivity. In Figure 9.12, we have presented a web server where the required information has been displayed. We have used the HTTPS application protocol for web server communication. Figure 9.12, we have presented a web server where the required information has been displayed. We have used the HTTPS application protocol for web server communication.

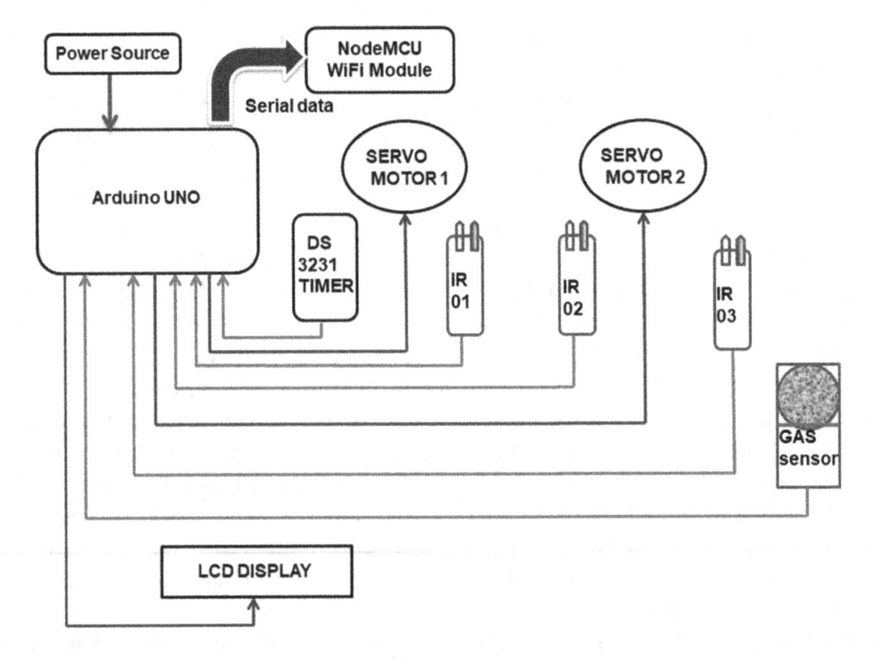

FIGURE 9.7 Wiring connections of the system.

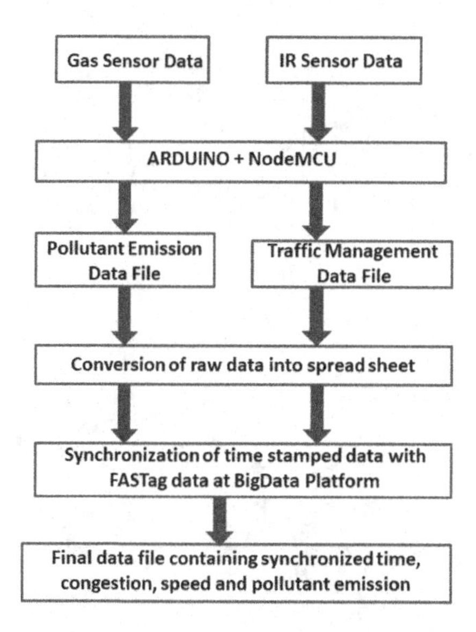

FIGURE 9.8 Dataflow of the system.

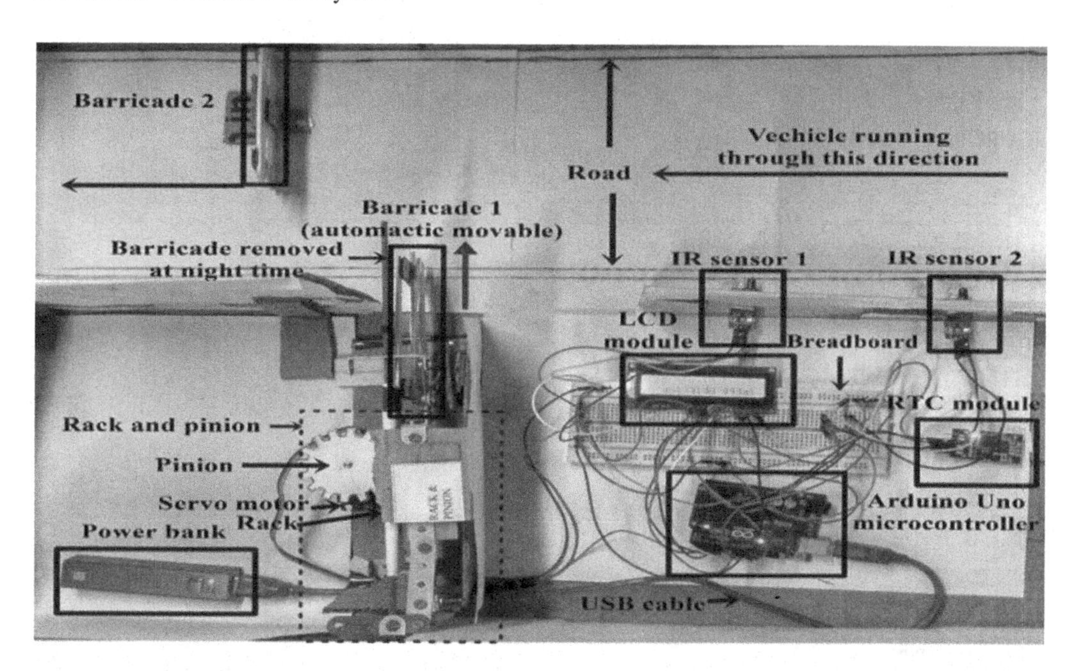

FIGURE 9.9 Picture of the prototype of the smart barricade system.

We have established an API communication with IoT application ThingSpeak to convey the information to the end-user. We have presented this information in Figure 9.13. Willing users can subscribe for services like notifications regarding emission, congestion, or other related information for their journey. Figure 9.14 presents an instance of such notification.

In Figure 9.15, we can see the measured speed of the vehicles. We have operated the servo motors as per the measured speed. If the speed is within the limit, then servo motors permit the vehicle to pass through the lane without any restrictions; otherwise, they will block the vehicle from reducing its speed within the limit. In the study of Hussain et al. [37], IR sensor-based vehicle speed measurement reliability has been discussed.

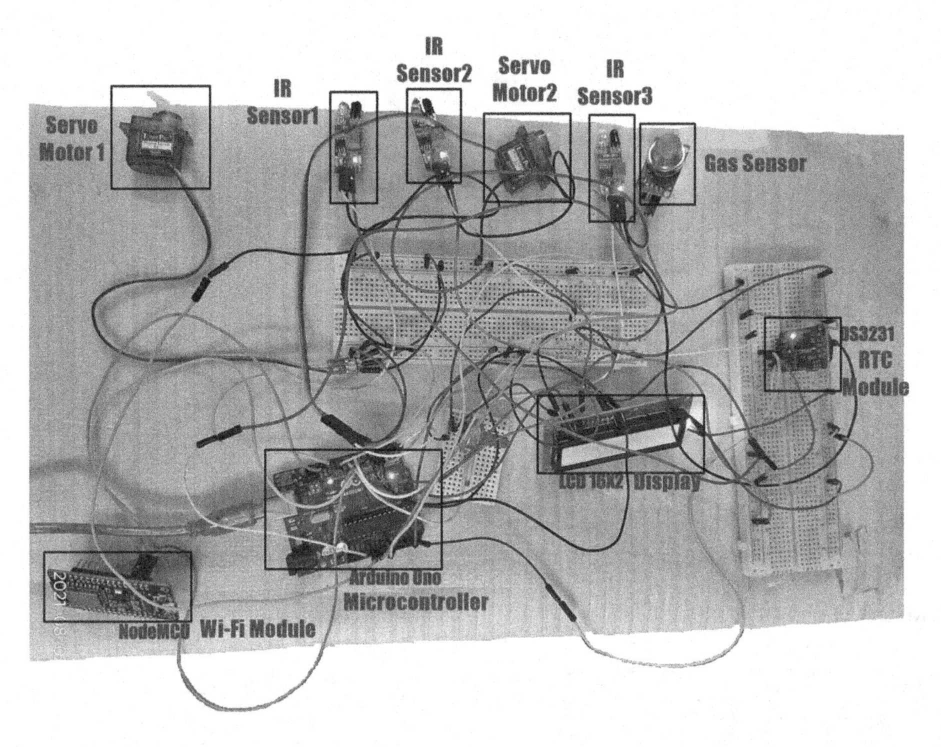

FIGURE 9.10 Picture of the prototype.

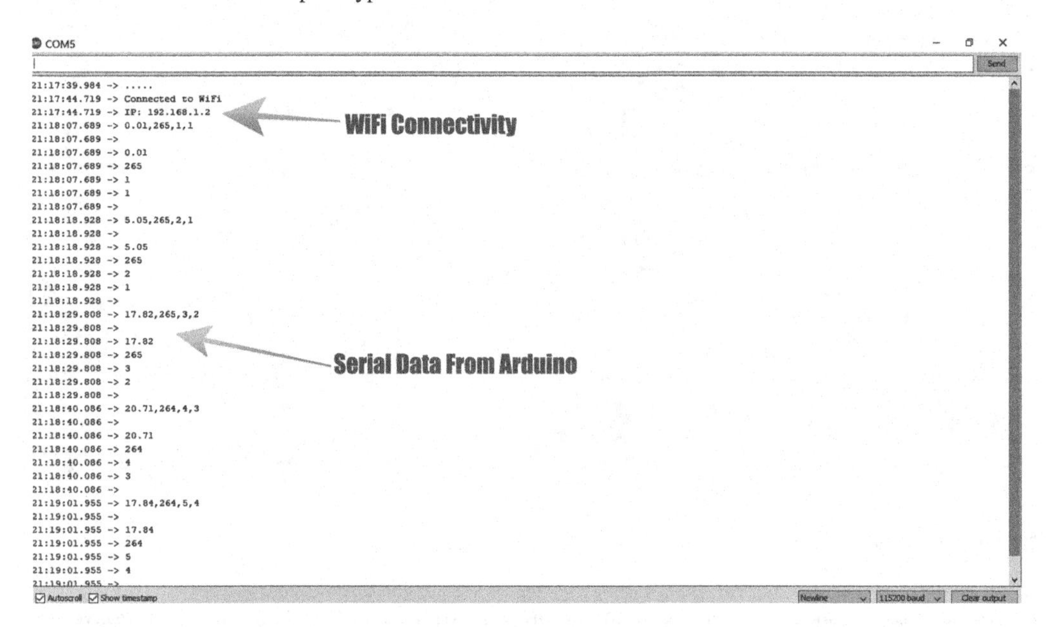

FIGURE 9.11 NodeMCU serial monitor.

We obtained an emission profile from this system. This emission profile in Figure 9.16 depicts the status of air pollution at the toll plaza at a specific time. We can fetch historical data of emissions on an hourly, daily, monthly, or yearly basis.

A vehicle's total fuel consumption in a journey is fuel consumed at running condition and fuel consumption at idle state. Therefore, we can write,

Total fuel consumption | = | fuel consume at running + consume at idle state.

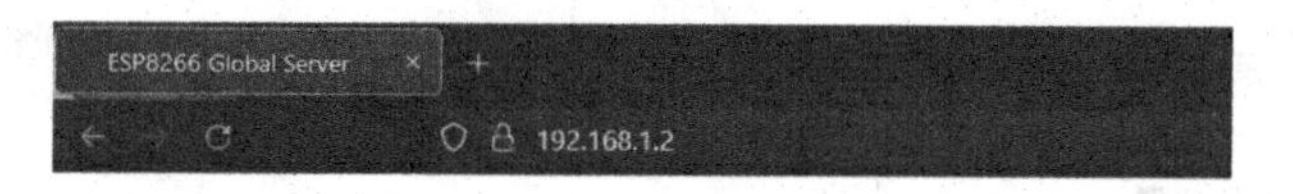

FIGURE 9.12 Web server information.

From [3], we obtain the equation of Total Fuel Consumption is as follows:

$$\text{Total Fuel Consumption} = \sum_{i}^{n} S_i v_i + f_c \sum_{j}^{m} t_j \tag{9.1}$$

where, S_i |=| length of road section i, v_i |=| mean speed of road section S_i,
f_c = Fuel consumption per second while vehicle at idle, and t_j |=| idle time at point j.

Our prototype model has tried to minimize this idle time significantly, thereby reducing the vehicle's total fuel consumption. For our work, we have used a two-lane toll plaza model. In Figure 9.17, we can observe that our proposed model can reduce the minimum time interval for a vehicle to pass the lane (average saturation headway time) than that of the presently installed system.

From the study of Shinde et al. [38], and Figure 9.17, we notice that the average saturation headway is around 30 seconds. This prototype demonstrates a reduction of the average saturation headway around nine seconds for similar lane segments, i.e., nearly 30% reduction in average idle time. Around 46,326 traffic (PCU/day) passes through a toll plaza [39]. Therefore, reduction in this average saturation headway has a significant impact on total fuel consumption, journey time, and the emission of vehicle pollutants. This nine-second reduction in idle time can save fuel economy by around Rs. 3,381,798 yearly for a single toll plaza with 46,326 traffics per day (considering petrol price Rs. 100/liter) [40]. This fuel economy is equivalent to 106257.54 kg of CO_2 (Carbon footprint) in a year [41].

Table 9.1 depicts some possible techniques and technologies that are useful to reduce fuel consumption of vehicles. This chapter discusses the possible improvement of fuel reduction by the proposed IoT system. In Table 9.1, we can see that techniques and technologies for upgrading the existing mechanical properties of vehicles and civil properties of the highways can improve fuel efficiency of vehicles. This chapter discusses the upgradation of the existing speed-breaking mechanism, which has the potential benefit of fuel reduction for vehicles. Table 9.1 also signifies that techniques and technologies to avoid unnecessary idling and intelligently management of highways, viz. lanes can effectively reduce fuel consumption of vehicles. In this chapter, Table 9.1 is used to signify the possible techniques and technologies (highlighted with green color) that have been implemented in this chapter to reduce fuel consumption.

From Table 9.1, we can say that this proposed system is helpful to reduce fuel consumption by optimizing three critical attributes of an intelligent traffic system (ITS). In this chapter, we have proposed to replace the existing civil infrastructure with a speed reduction mechanism, i.e., speed bumps/humps, with smart barricades. Our proposed system is helpful to avoid unnecessary idling and stop-and-go timing of vehicles; thereby, fuel reduction is achieved. This system is also beneficial for the intelligent management of highways.

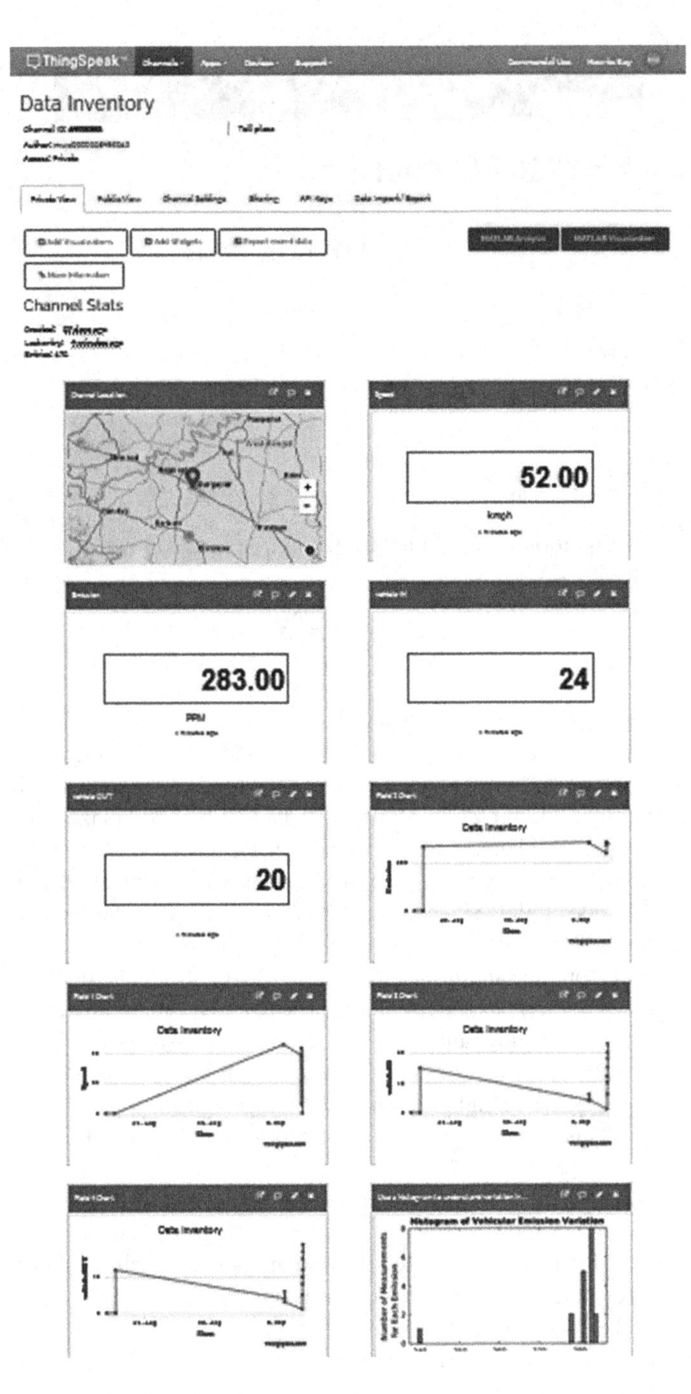

FIGURE 9.13 Information in ThingSpeak.

9.6 CONCLUSION

In this chapter, we have proposed some intricate features like speed measurement, smart barricades, vehicle flow density measurement by counting incoming and outgoing traffic, and pollutant emission measurement in a low-cost manner. This system is helpful to curb air pollution by reducing the stop-and-go times of vehicles as we have omitted the traditional bumps/humps for a speed-reducing mechanism. This proposed model also eliminates the discomfort and other disadvantages of these

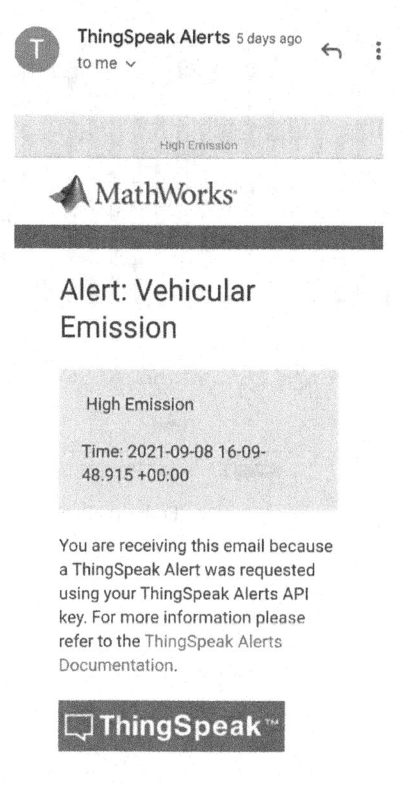

FIGURE 9.14 Alert notification via email.

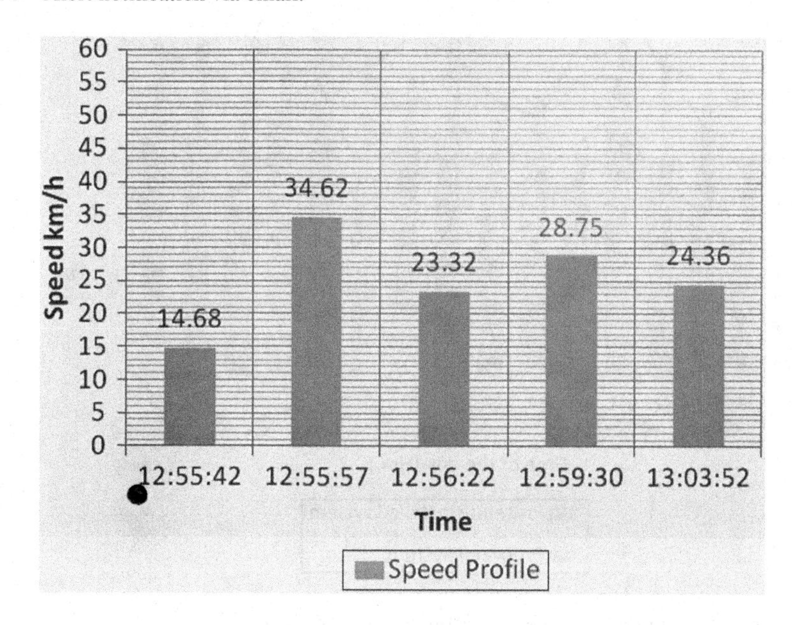

FIGURE 9.15 Speed profile of the system.

humps/bumps. This chapter can also reduce congestion at the toll plaza lane. Users can avoid their journey when congestion is high or choose an alternate travel route to avoid waiting in the queue. Therefore, this system is indeed successful in improving fuel efficiency and reduction of air pollution. Other than that, the concerned authority may serve notice to the polluting vehicle if its average emission on a monthly basis exceeds the limiting value of pollution. For practical implementation of

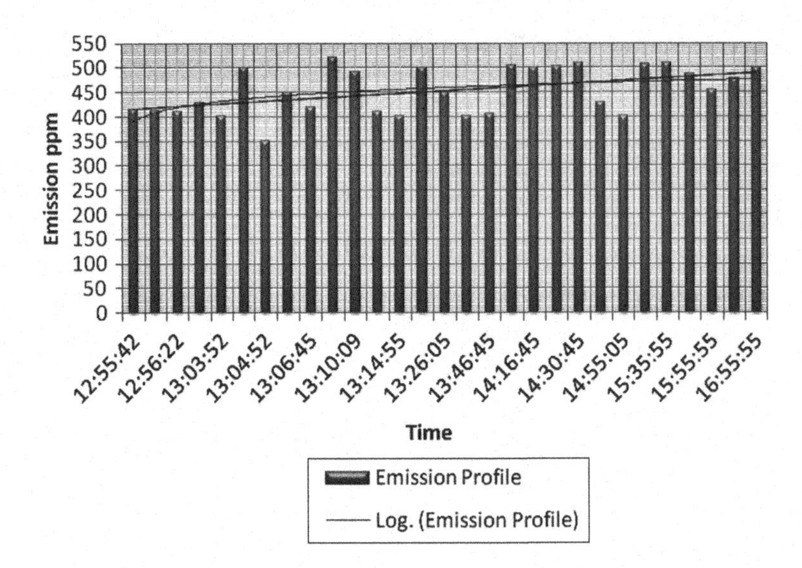

FIGURE 9.16 Emission profile.

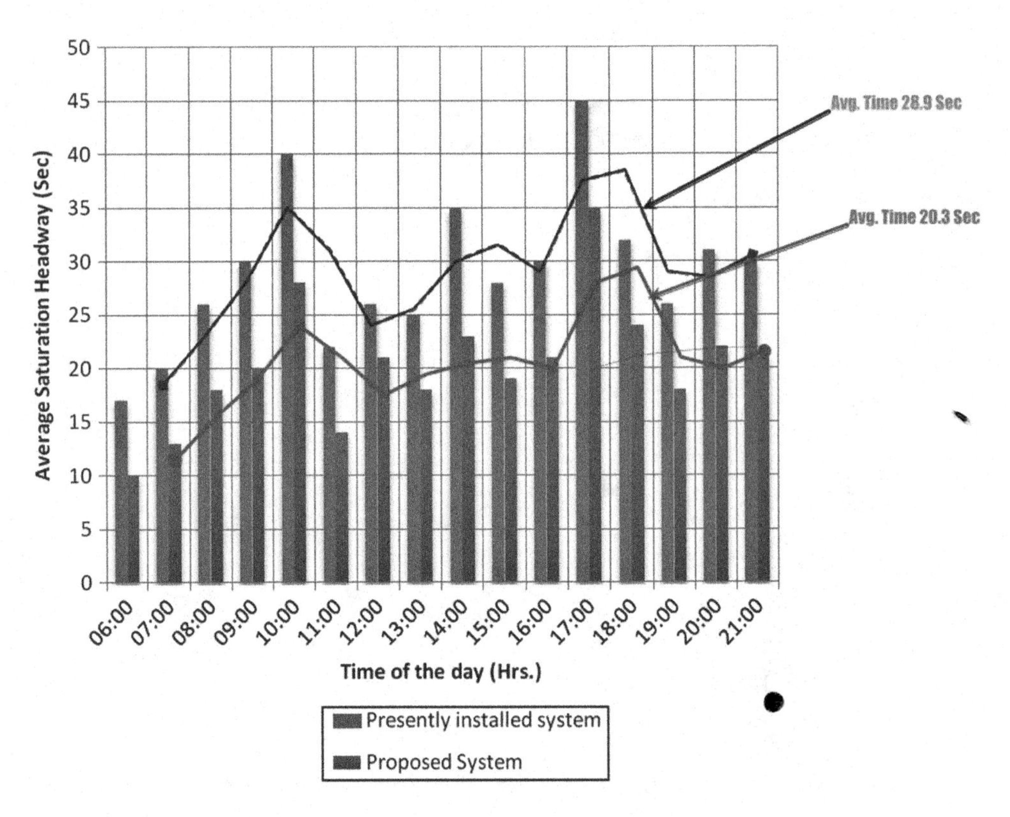

FIGURE 9.17 Average saturation headway vs. time of the day.

this system, we need to consider the points: (a) the power to drive the barricades, and (b) the requirement of multiple processing units. These two points will shape our future course of the chapter for this research.

This chapter discusses some future scopes of the present work that includes processing of large datasets in big data platform like Hadoop to efficiently detect the polluting vehicle, implementation

TABLE 9.1
Fuel reduction of vehicle (Techniques and Technologies)

Reduction Parameter	Reduction Type	Attribute	Techniques	Technologies	Proposed System
Fuel reduction	Reduction of fuel consumption for green driving	Vehicles	Improvement of fuel efficiency of vehicle by upgrading mechanical properties	Upgrading mechanical properties	
		Roadways	Improvement of highways	Upgrading civil properties	Yes
	Reduction of fuel by intelligent driving	Green driving behavior	Maintain optimum tire pressure		
			Adjust drive technique		
			Maintain the ride		
			Get rid of weight and reduce the drag		
			Avoid unnecessary idling		Yes
			Use latest-technology car		
		Traffic flow	Intelligent management of highways	Lane Electronic toll collection Traffic Traffic light	Yes

[3]

of appropriate machine learning algorithm to improve lane congestion problem in multiple lane scenario, customization of IoT gateway to improve system performance, latency, etc.

REFERENCES

1. Basic road statistics of India (2016–17). Ministry of Road Transport and Highways. Available: https://morth.nic.in/sites/default/files/Basic%20_Road_Statics_of_India.pdf [accessed on 2 October 2021].
2. de Souza, A. M., Brennand, C. A. R. L., Yokoyama, R. S., Donato, E. A., Madeira, E. R. M., & VillasL. A., (2017). Traffic management systems: A classification, review, challenges, and future perspectives. *International Journal of Distributed Sensor Networks*, 13(4), https://doi.org/10.1177/1550147716683612.
3. Nasir, M. K., Md Noor, R., Kalam, M. A., & Masum, B. M. (2014). Reduction of fuel consumption and exhaust pollutant using intelligent transport systems. *The Scientific World Journal*, 2014, https://doi.org/10.1155/2014/836375.
4. Castillo, E., Jimenez, P., Menendez, J. M., & Conejo, A. J. (2008). The observability problem in traffic models: Algebraic and topological methods. *IEEE Transactions on Intelligent Transportation Systems*, 9(2), 275–287, https://doi.org/10.1109/TITS.2008.922929.
5. Gentili, M., & Mirchandani, P. B. (2012). Locating sensors on traffic networks: Models, challenges and research opportunities. *Transportation Research Part C: Emerging Technologies*, 24, 227–255, https://doi.org/10.1016/j.trc.2012.01.004.
6. Cao, Z., Jiang, S., Zhang, J., & Guo, H. (2016). A unified framework for vehicle rerouting and traffic light control to reduce traffic congestion. *IEEE Transactions on Intelligent Transportation Systems*, 18(7), 1958–1973, https://doi.org/10.1109/TITS.2016.2613997.
7. Shi, J. P., Harrison, R. M., Evans, D. E., Alam, A., Barnes, C., & Carter, G. (2002). A method for measuring particle number emissions from vehicles driving on the road. *Environmental Technology*, 23(1), 1–14, https://doi.org/10.1080/09593332508618430.
8. Zhang, Y., Stedman, D. H., Bishop, G. A., Guenther, P. L., & Beaton, S. P. (1995). Worldwide on-road vehicle exhaust emissions study by remote sensing. *Environmental Science & Technology*, 29(9), 2286–2294, https://doi.org/10.1021/es00009a020.
9. Zhu, F., Lv, Y., Chen, Y., Wang, X., Xiong, G., & Wang, F. Y. (2019). Parallel transportation systems: Toward IoT-enabled smart urban traffic control and management. *IEEE Transactions on Intelligent Transportation Systems*, 21(10), 4063–4071, https://doi.org/10.1109/TITS.2019.2934991.

10. Pau, M., & Angius, S. (2001). Do speed bumps really decrease traffic speed? An Italian experience. *Accident Analysis & Prevention*, 33(5), 585–597, https://doi.org/10.1016/S0001-4575(00)00070-1.
11. Zaidel, D., Hakkert, A. S., & Pistiner, A. H. (1992). The use of road humps for moderating speeds on urban streets. *Accident Analysis & Prevention*, 24(1), 45–56, https://doi.org/10.1016/0001-4575(92)90071-P.
12. Munjin, M. A., Zamorano, J. J., Marré, B., Ilabaca, F., Ballesteros, V., Martínez, C., ... & García, N. (2011). Speed hump spine fractures: Injury mechanism and case series. *Clinical Spine Surgery*, 24(6), 386–389, https://doi.org/10.1097/BSD.0b013e3182019dda.
13. Tiwari, G. (2009). Indian case studies of traffic calming measures on national and state highways. *Transportation Research and Injury Prevention Program*. http://tripp.iitd.ac.in/assets/publication/TRIPP97-20151.pdf
14. Shamshirband, S., Anuar, N. B., Kiah, M. L. M., & Patel, A. (2013). An appraisal and design of a multi-agent system based cooperative wireless intrusion detection computational intelligence technique. *Engineering Applications of Artificial Intelligence*, 26(9), 2105–2127.
15. Haworth, N., & Symmons, M. (2001). Driving to reduce fuel consumption and improve road safety. In *Proceedings of the Australasian Road Safety Research, Policing and Education Conference* (Vol. 5). Monash University.
16. Han, Y. (2014). Research on the performance of mobile barricades based on fuzzy-AHP method. *Sensors & Transducers*, 167(3), 9.
17. Hossam-E-Haider, M., & Rokonuzzaman, M. (2015, February). Design of a efficient energy generating system using speed breaker for Bangladesh. In *2015 5th National Symposium on Information Technology: Towards New Smart World (NSITNSW)* (pp. 1–5). IEEE, https://doi.org/10.1109/NSITNSW.2015.7176393.
18. Manitha, P. V., Anandaraman, S. S., Manikumaran, K., & Aswathaman, K. (2017, August). Design and development of enhanced road safety mechanism using smart roads and energy-optimized solar street lights. In *2017 International Conference on Energy, Communication, Data Analytics and Soft Computing (ICECDS)* (pp. 1650–1654). IEEE, https://doi.org/10.1109/ICECDS.2017.8389727.
19. Hossain, M. N., Hoque, K. A., Ullah, S. M. R., & Islam, M. M. (2014, April). RFID based virtual speed breakers: Perspective Bangladesh. In *2014 International Conference on Electrical Engineering and Information & Communication Technology* (pp. 1–5). IEEE, https://doi.org/10.1109/ICEEICT.2014.6919147.
20. Raskar, C., & Nema, S. (2021). Modified fuzzy-based smart barricade movement for traffic management system. *Wireless Personal Communications*, 116(4), 3351–3370, https://doi.org/10.1007/s11277-020-07856-4.
21. zer-Ming, J., Tzeng, S. C., Yang, B.-J., & Li, Y.-C. (2017). *Design Manufacture and Performance Test of the Speed Breaker System*. IEEE.
22. Dewangan, A., & Saikhedkar, N. K. (2018). *Experimental Analysis of Different Types of Speed Breakers*. IEEE.
23. Karuppaiah, A, Gansh, S., Dileepan, T., & Jayabharathi, S. (2019). *Fabrication and Analysis of Automatic Speed Breakers*. IEEE.
24. Zafar, N., & Ul Haq, I. (2020). Traffic congestion prediction based on estimated time of arrival. *PloS one*, 15(12), e0238200, https://doi.org/10.1371/journal.pone.0238200.
25. Nguyen, T. B. (2017). *Evaluation of Lane Detection Algorithms Based on an Embedded Platform*, https://d-nb.info/1214649149/34.
26. Zheng, Z. (2014). Recent developments and research needs in modelling lane changing. *Transportation Research Part B: Methodological*, 60, 16–32, https://doi.org/10.1016/j.trb.2013.11.009.
27. Berlin, M. A., Selvakanmani, S., Umamaheswari, T. S., Jausmin, K. J., & Babu, S. (2021). Alert message based automated toll collection and payment violation management system using smart road side units. *Materials Today: Proceedings*, https://doi.org/10.1016/j.matpr.2021.01.217.
28. Falcocchio, J. C., & Levinson, H. S. (2015). *Road Traffic Congestion: A Concise Guide* (Vol. 7). Cham: Springer, https://doi.org/10.1007/978-3-319-15165-6.
29. Breton, L. A. G. (2000). Real-time on-road vehicle exhaust gas modular flowmeter and emissions reporting system. *U.S. Patent No. 6,148,656*. 21 November.
30. Sabiron, G., Thibault, L., Dégeilh, P., & Corde, G. (2018, June). Pollutant emissions estimation framework for real-driving emissions at microscopic scale and environmental footprint calculation. In *2018 IEEE Intelligent Vehicles Symposium (IV)* (pp. 381–388). IEEE, https://doi.org/10.1109/IVS.2018.8500435.
31. Nóbrega, L., Gonçalves, P., Pedreiras, P., & Pereira, J. (2019). An IoT-based solution for intelligent farming. *Sensors*, 19(3), 603, https://doi.org/10.3390/s19030603.

32. Introduction to LANs, WANs, and other kinds of area networks. Available: https://www.lifewire.com/lans-wans-and-other-area-networks-817376 [accessed on 2 October 2021].
33. OneM2M-The IoT standard. Available: http://www.onem2m.org/ [accessed on 2 October 2021].
34. IoT messaging protocols. Available: http://www.eejournal.com/archives/articles/20150420-protocols/ [accessed on 2 October 2021].
35. Arduino UNO R3. Available: https://docs.arduino.cc/hardware/uno-rev3 [accessed on 2 October 2021].
36. NodeMCU documentation. Available: https://nodemcu.readthedocs.io/en/release/ [accessed on 2 October 2021].
37. Hussain, T. M., Saadawi, T. N., & Ahmed, S. A. (1993). Overhead infrared sensor for monitoring vehicular traffic. *IEEE Transactions on Vehicular Technology*, 42(4), 477–483, https://doi.org/10.1109/25.260764.
38. Shinde, M. S., Pokharkar, H., Shinde, Y., & Kashid, P. (2019). Traffic congestion at toll plaza: A case study of Khed-Shivapur, Pune. *International Research Journal of Engineering and Technology (IRJET)*, 6(10), 877–881.
39. Toll Plaza Information by National Highways Authority of India (NHAI). Available: https://tis.nhai.gov.in/TollInformation.aspx?TollPlazaID=4545 [accessed on 2 October 2021].
40. Krivoshapov, S. I., Nazarov, A. I., Mysiura, M. I., Marmut, I. A., Zuyev, V. A., Bezridnyi, V. V., & Pavlenko, V. N. (2020, December). Calculation methods for determining of fuel consumption per hour by transport vehicles. *In IOP Conference Series: Materials Science and Engineering* (Vol. 977, No. 1, p. 012004). IOP Publishing.
41. Carbon footprint calculator. Available: https://www.fleetnews.co.uk/costs/carbon-footprint-calculator/ [accessed on 2 October 2021].

10 Development of Fuel Cell-Based Energy Systems for 3-ph Power Development and Internet of Things Devices

Parth Sarathi Panigrahy, B. Sai Reddy, M. R. Harika, and B. Arun Kumar

CONTENTS

10.1 INTRODUCTION

Approximately, 46% of electric power that is produced globally originates from fossil fuel combustion, and has an eco-friendly effect. Also, these available fossil fuels are not long lasting as the increasing population uses up all the available resources faster than ever. Thus, for the sustainable generation of electricity, there is a need for alternative solutions, which are reliable, high-quality, and cheap; and reduce harmful emissions such as greenhouse gases and toxic wastes.

Fuel cells can be applied as they provide higher efficiency, have excellent load performances, and lower emissions. In past, fuel cells were extensively used in on-site power production, and on vehicles like buses and trucks. Many investigators, makers, power corporations, and supervisory authorities have recently functioned to develop a spread of different cell kinds and strategize the arrangement, which can back these fresh technologies. Such attempts involve the advancement in the latest resources, inexpensive making procedures, and the development of advanced devices for providing fuel and air. State of art power electronic equipment also contributes toward effective methods of governing the cell productivity and efficient methodologies for scheme study and helps in optimization. The upcoming era for the fuel cells is anticipated to be decent acquiring state of art strategies like teamwork by various countries supporting the joint energy necessity due to which, it would able to the limit the application of fossil fuels [1-2].

DOI: 10.1201/9781003217398-10

Broadly Internet of Things (IoT) apparatuses are driven by electrical grids. Improved IoT tools are anticipated to endorse care, like accident escaping using assistance along with automated dynamic backing systems. For instance, Yang et al. established a reliable monitoring healthcare setup [4]. Further, an IoT system is developed by Pereira et al. [5] for accessing the photovoltaic plant condition applying Raspberry Pi. A proposition by Suma et al. was made for condition monitoring setup by means of various sensors in the application of smart agriculture [6]. Understanding all the facts, the project shows the simulation model of a proton exchange membrane fuel cell-based three-phase inverter where three-phase power development is aimed and the DC output is targeted to assist the uninterrupted power supply for IoT devices. On provision of the application of IoT apparatus those can work all through disasters like cyclone area, the fuel cell-based independent energy system is attempted instead of the frequently applied energy systems which failed at those times.

Covering all the needs, a three-phase supply is developed using a PEMFC-based fuel cell and also the steady output is aimed to feed the IoT supply system through a DC-DC converter. This work shows that the power supply to very remote places like Top Mountain places or islands is possible not only in single phase but also in three phase. The steady output is aimed to feed the IoT supply system through a DC–DC converter. Using the DC–DC converter, the constant 5V will be supplied to the IoT system. However, the chapter focuses primarily on the three-phase power development wherein the uninterrupted supply can easily be given to IoT devices.

10.2 PRESENTED WORK

The proposed model can be clearly explained in four stages: (1) Obtaining DC output from the fuel cells; (2) boosting up the obtained DC output using boost converter; (3) DC–DC converter [2] to bring the steady output to level of 5 V; (4) inversion of DC to three-phase AC power.

In the first step, the running of a fuel cell is done. During this process, the electrons move from cathode to anode. Hence, a very minute amount of electricity is generated. This generated DC output is used in further stages. In the second stage, the obtained DC output from the fuel cells can be given to the boost converter by which the obtained DC output voltage from a fuel cell could be boosted up for further use and then in third stage, the constant voltage is aimed to bring the voltage level to 5V, which will be fed as a power supply system for the IoT device. The final stage includes the inversion of the boost converter output DC voltage to three-phase AC power where the boost converter can be used in the application of IoT or can be connected to the load according to our necessity. The systematic flow of the presented work is displayed in the block diagram as shown in Figure 10.1.

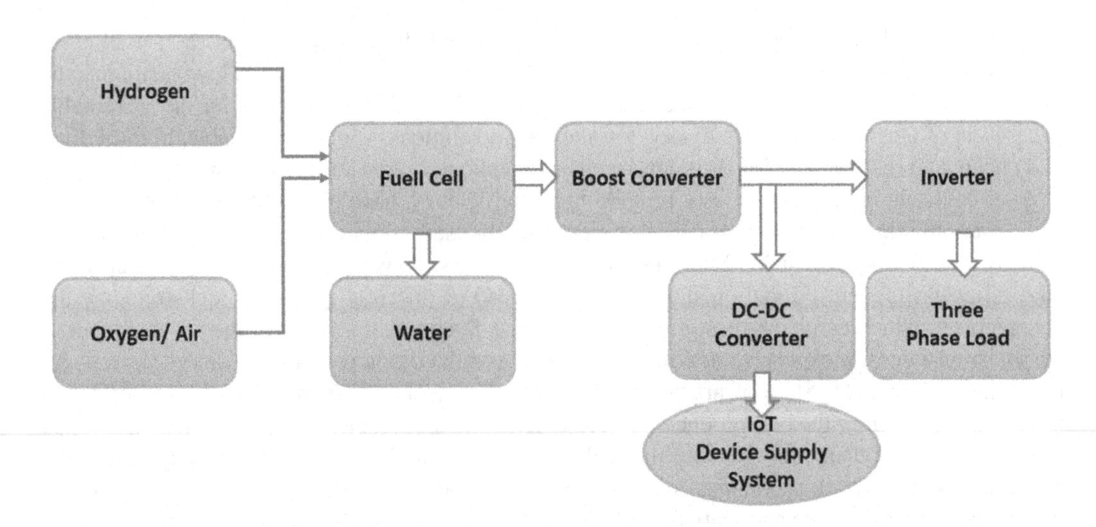

FIGURE 10.1 Schematic of the proposed work.

10.3 ACQUAINTANCE WITH FUEL CELLS

Chemical energy is converted into electrical energy by the application of the fuel cell. Having hydrogen as fuel, fuel cells produce water from the chemical reaction. Fuel cell promises a unique source for producing electrical energy when compared with other energy resources such as conventional and nonconventional energy resources. As ignition is evaded, these cells yield energy having insignificant contaminants. Yet, contrasting to storage battery, uninterrupted refill of the reductant and oxidant occurs for such cells to perform nonstop tasks. The process of producing electrical energy doesn't show an effect on the environment and is eco-friendly.

Fuel cell generally comprises large fuel types and different oxidants. However, fuel cells are considered for utmost attention, as these cells apply hydrogen and air for reductant and oxidant, respectively.

Extensively in a power system, a fuel cell is made using many constituents:

1. Unit cells: Here the phenomenon of electrochemical process occurs.
2. Stacks: Here each cell is electrically joined to form a single unit as per the required output.
3. Balance of plant: This includes constituents those offer feed stream conditioning, temperature supervision, & electrical power conditioning.

There are different electrolytes used for different applications. For example, an alkaline fuel cell applies potassium hydroxide as alkaline electrolyte.

10.3.1 UNIT CELL

These are the powerhouse of a fuel cell, which converts chemical energy contained in a fuel to electrical energy. The generic physical structure of a fuel cell consists of an anode and cathode electrodes on either side of the container and the unit cell is filled with electrolyte. In these cells, fuel is served uninterruptedly at the anode, which is a –ve electrode, and frequently oxygen out of air, which acts as oxidant, is supplied constantly at the cathode. Due to electrochemical reactions, an electric current is produced at the electrodes, which is fed to the loads. These cells are similar to battery but differ in various aspects. The battery halts storing electrical energy until the chemical properties exhaust.

10.3.2 FUEL CELL STACKING

Fuel cell is constructed with building blocks of unit cells and they are arranged in a modular form into a stack in which voltage and current is extracted. Normally, the stacking comprises electrically joined several unit cells in a cascade fashion through conductive connections. Common stacking systems are planar-bipolar stacking, Stacks with Tubular Cells.

10.3.3 BALANCE OF PLANT

Real-world fuel cell units need some additional subunits and constituents, which are termed as balance of plant (BoP). In combination with the stack, the total unit is called a fuel cell unit. Accurate BoP organization is mainly influenced by the type of fuel cell, the kind of fuel chosen, and finally where it is going to be applied. Further, features of BoP are governed by particular operational situations along with the necessity of each cell and stack design.

The fuel cell unit maintains its proficiency in any situation like off-design circumstances. The competence of different such units can be varied up to 50% of efficiency using a simple unit too. Lesser the size of the unit larger the productivity, which relates to those given by fuel cell units in developing situations. Characteristics of fuel cells include: effective methods of energy transformation, unmovable constituents in the energy converter system, suppleness for fuel, fast load observing proficiency [2]. A generic view of proton exchange membrane F.C and F.C Stack is presented in Figure 10.2.

Table 10.1 depicts the fuel cell stack parameters and fuel cell nominal parameters that are used in the present work, as the fuel cell parameters in the simulation part of a fuel cell. Fuel cell stack is the combination of the arrangement of fuel cells in an array and interconnecting them for producing a unique output voltage. The developed MATLAB model for fuel cell and V-I Characteristics of a fuel cell are presented as shown in Figures 10.3 and 10.4, respectively. As the fuel flow rate increases, the power and current produced from the fuel cell will increase; if the voltage magnitude is reducing, prompt the current value deduced. The fuel source constants are presented as follows.

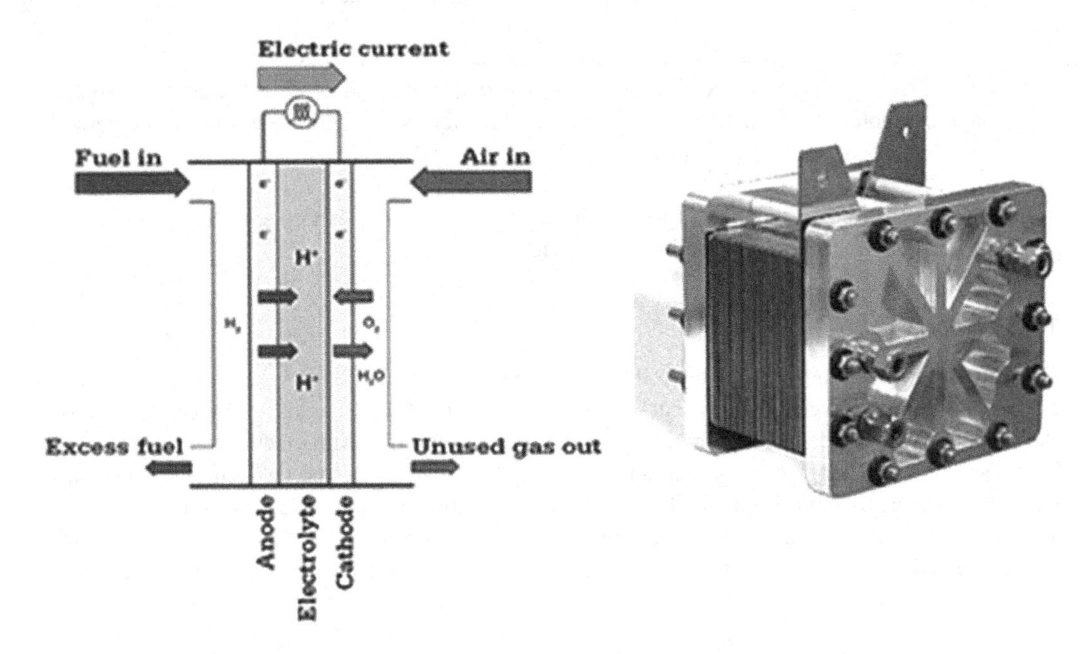

FIGURE 10.2 Proton Exchange Membrane F.C and F.C Stack. [3].

TABLE 10.1
Fuel Cell Stack Parameters and Fuel Cell Nominal Parameters

S No.	Fuel Stack Parameters	Fuel Cell Nominal Parameters
1	Input sources are of fuel and air. Fuel Fr: Hydrogen H_2. Output ports are of *m*, line (+ve), line (−ve).	StackPower: Nominal=1259.96 W, Maximal=2000 W
2	Present Model: PEMFC – 1.26 KW –24Vdc	Fuel Cell Resistance=0.061871 ohms
3	PEMFC: Proton Exchange Membrane Fuel Cell	Nerst Voltage of one cell[En]=1.115 V
4	Voltage at 0 A and 1 A [V_0(v), V_1[v]]: [42,35]	Nominal utilization:
5	Nominal operating point [Inom(A), Vnom(V)]: [52,24.23]	Hydrogen (H_2)=99.92%
6	Maximum operating point [Iend(A), Vend(V)]: [100,20]	Oxidant (O_2)=1.813%
7	Number of cells: 42	Nominal consumption:
8	Nominal stack efficiency (%): 46	Fuel=15.22 slpm
9	Nominal air flow rate (lpm): 2400	Air=36.22 slpm
10	Nominal supply pressure [fuel (bar), Air (bar)]: [1.5, 1]	Exchange current [i0]=0.027318A
11	Nominal composition (%) [H_2 O_2 H_2O (Air)]: [99.95,21,1]	Exchange coefficient [alpha]=0.308

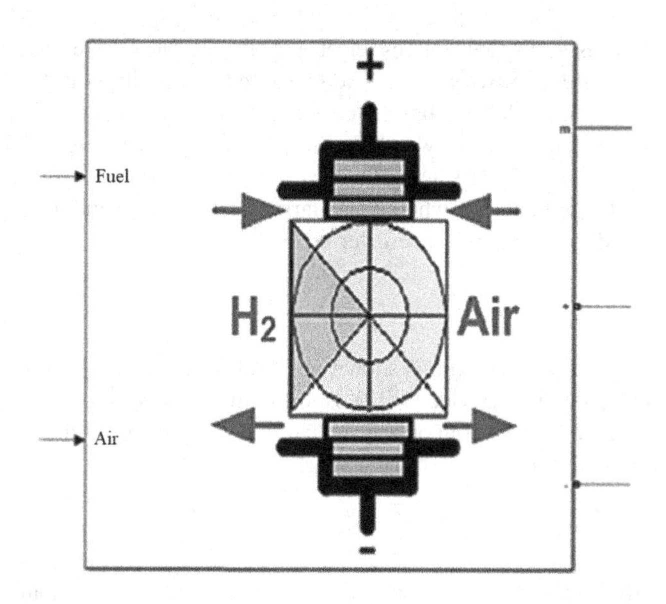

FIGURE 10.3 PEMFC model of fuel cell.

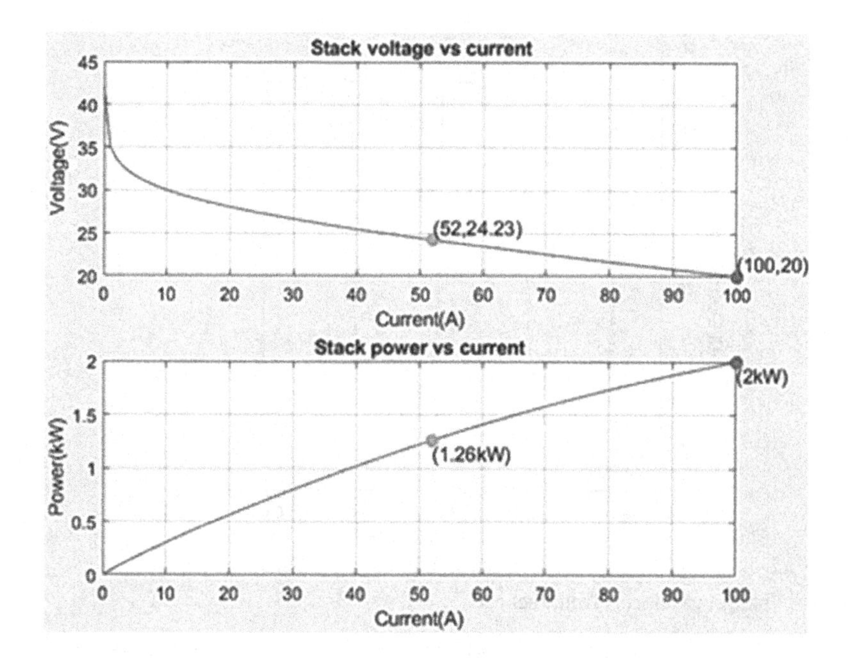

FIGURE 10.4 V-I Characteristics of fuel cell.

10.3.3.1 Fuel Source Constants

- *Fuel flow rate(Hydrogen):*

$$60000*8.3145*(273+95)*400*u(1)/(2*96485*(3*101325)*0.919*0.995)$$

which is equal to 1.36908036 atomic mass units.

- *Air flow rate(Oxygen/Air):*

$$60000*8.3145*(273+95)*400*u(1)/(2*96485*(3*101325)*0.5057*0.21)$$

which is equal to 11.7884115 atomic mass units.

Using hydrogen and air as input fuel sources, electricity is generated from the electrolysis process in which water is produced as a by-product. The generated electricity is in the form of fixed DC voltage, where in the given model, we have used PEMFC 1.26 KW, 24Vdc. The obtained output voltage waveform of the fuel cell is shown in Figure 10.5. The peak voltage of the resulted output DC waveform is 45.67 volts and the stack efficiency is found to be 16%. This voltage obtained is sufficient to smaller DC applications, whereas for large electricity, essential applications boosting the obtained voltage is done using a boost converter.

10.4 PYROLYSIS

A circuit diagram of the boost converter is shown in Figure 10.2. It mainly consists of an inductor, diode, capacitor, and a switching device [7–12]. Boost converter operation can be explained using two stages with turning off and turning on the switching device in a given period of time, which is controlled by the timing circuit.

10.4.1 Stage 1

As shown in Figure 10.6, when the switching device is turned on, the shortest path will exist between the positive voltage source terminal and negative voltage source terminal, Diode will be in reverse

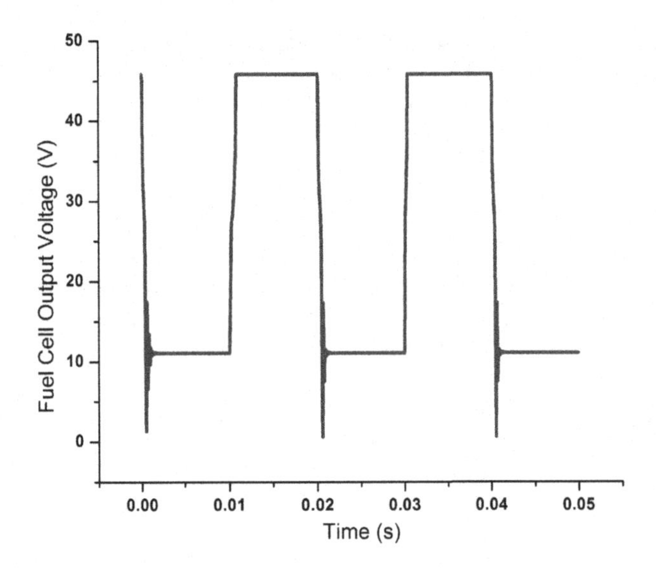

FIGURE 10.5 Voltage waveforms from fuel cell.

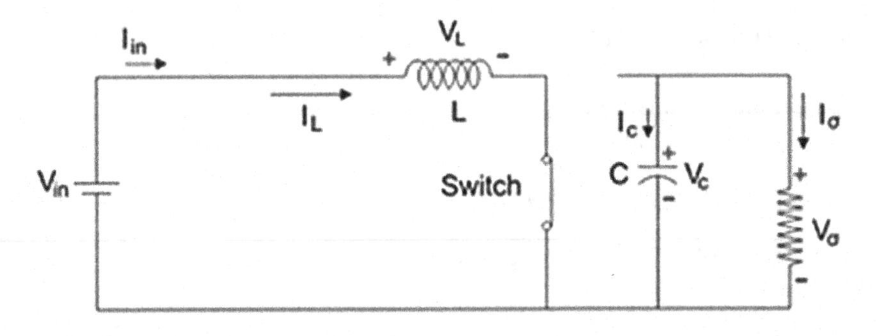

FIGURE 10.6 Switch is on and diode is off.

bias. The inductor tends to charge during this condition. During this condition, input voltage is equal to the voltage across the inductor ($V_{In} = V_L$).

10.4.2 Stage 2

When the switching device is turned off, the current will flow through the inductor, diode, and load as shown in Figure 10.7. During this conduction, the inductor will be having reverse polarity, unlike stage 1. The output voltage is increased by conjunction of inductor discharging voltage with the source voltage ($V_{Out} = V_{In} + V_L$) and current remains in the same direction. Relationship between output voltage and input voltage is given as $V_0 = V_{In}$ (1/ (1–D)).

In the present work, different required parameters considered for the simulation of the boost converter are depicted in Table 10.2. Regarding switches, it is very clear that a snubber circuit becomes in series with parallel combination of MOSFET and internal diode. By providing a gate signal, the current passes through the MOSFET. This works like bidirectional resistance (R_{on}). With the no-gate pulse, the antiparallel diode conducts the current due to negative current.

The output voltage has been increased by twice that of input voltage with considering the appropriate inductor value and we have achieved the stepping up of fuel cell output voltage with constant magnitude. Ripples in the output waveforms are reduced by considering an appropriate capacitor value in the circuit. The obtained constant voltage with its transient is given in Figure 10.8, where a steady voltage is obtained with a magnitude of 148.6 volts. On provision of the application of IoT apparatus those can work all through disasters like cyclone area, the fuel cell-based independent energy system is attempted instead of the frequently applied energy systems, which failed at those times. In this study, the proton exchange membrane as a fuel stack parameter performs superior to others in terms of their operation time and output power. The steady output as shown in Figure 10.8 is aimed to feed the IoT supply system through a DC–DC converter. Using the DC–DC converter,

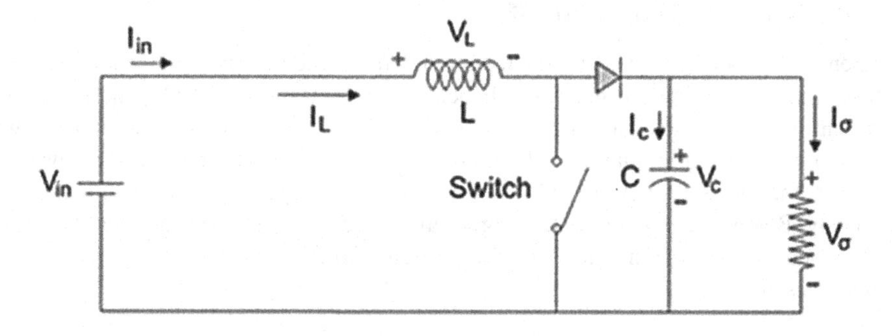

FIGURE 10.7 Switch is off and diode is on.

TABLE 10.2
Boost Converter Parameters

S. No.	Parameters	Values
1	Inductor	$100*10^{-6}$ H
2	Capacitor	$1000*10^{-6}$ F
3	Diode resistance	0.001Ω
4	Forward voltage V_f (V)	0.8 V
5	Snubber resistance Rs (Ohms)	500Ω
6	Snubber capacitance Cs (F)	$250*10^{-9}$ F

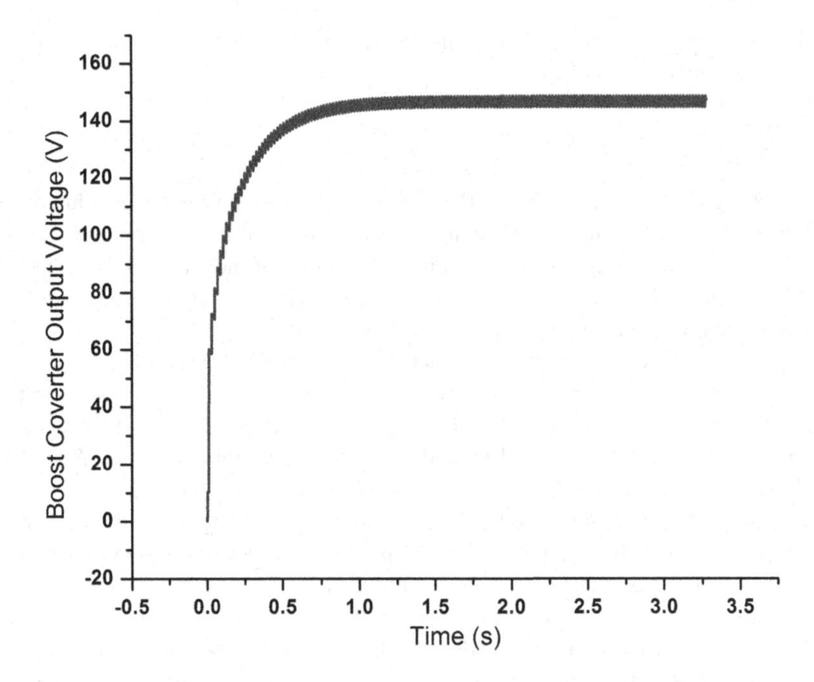

FIGURE 10.8 Voltage waveform.

the constant 5V will be supplied to the IoT system. However, primarily, the three-phase power development is focused in the paper wherein uninterrupted supply can be easily given to IoT devices.

10.5 THREE-PPHASE FULL BRIDGE

Advancement and application in switching technology make the inverter application extensive [13–16]. A three-phase full bridge inverter is a device that converts a fixed DC quantity into a three-phase alternating quantity. By changing the frequency of turning on and off the switch (6-switches), we can obtain an alternating quantity. There are two types of operating modes in inverter: 1200 mode and 1800 mode of operation and it depends on the triggering of the number of switches simultaneously. Below are the parameters considered for designing of an inverter. The developed MATLAB-based three-phase inverter is shown in Figure 10.9.

Parameters used:

- Switch:
  Insulate gate bipolar transistor (IGBT)
  Implements an IGBT device in parallel with a series RC snubber circuit.
  In on-state, the IGBT model has internal resistance (Ron) and inductance (Lon).
  For most applications, Lon should be set to zero.
  In off-state, the IGBT model has infinite impedance [17–20].
- Resistance = 0.001 Ohms
- Snubber resistance = 1*105 Ohms
- Forward Voltage = 1 V
- Pulse generator: 50 Hz, amplitude = 1

The aforementioned figures depict the output waveforms of a three-phase full bridge inverter with turning off and on switches simultaneously in the given period of time. The respective line and phase voltages V_a, V_b, V_c obtained from the inverter are shown in Figures 10.10 and 10.11. Since we

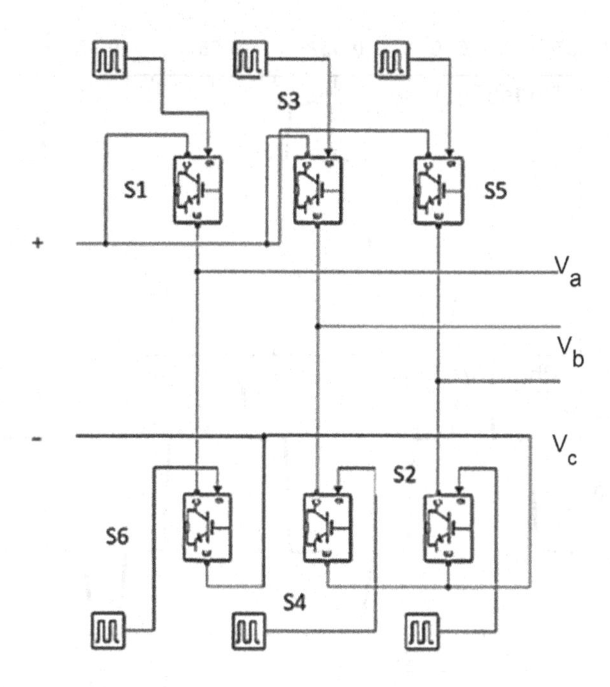

FIGURE 10.9 Simulated model of 3-ph inverter in MATLAB.

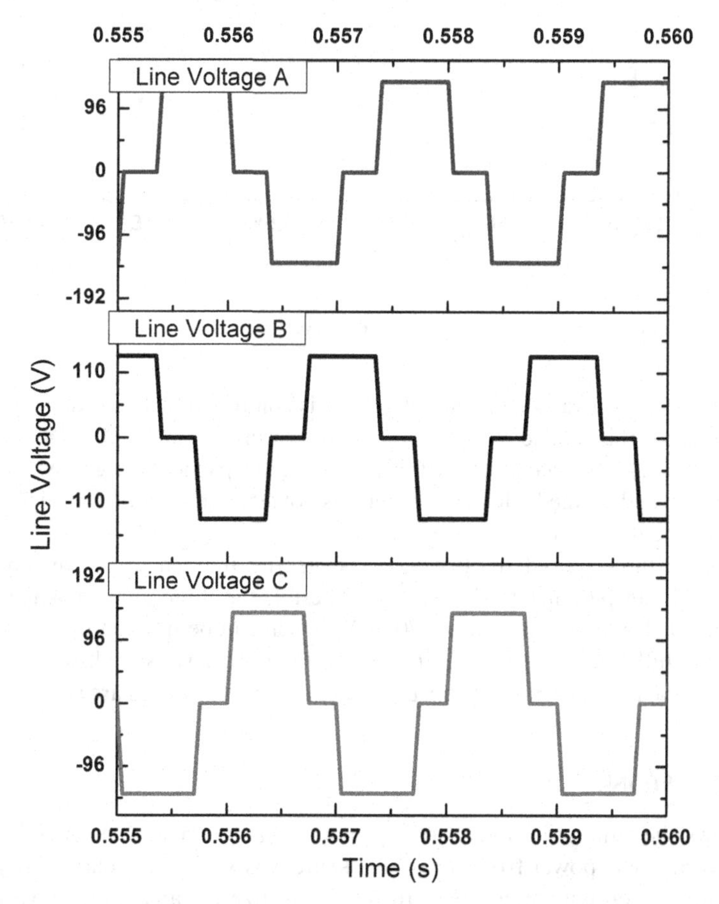

FIGURE 10.10 Obtained line voltage waveform from inverter.

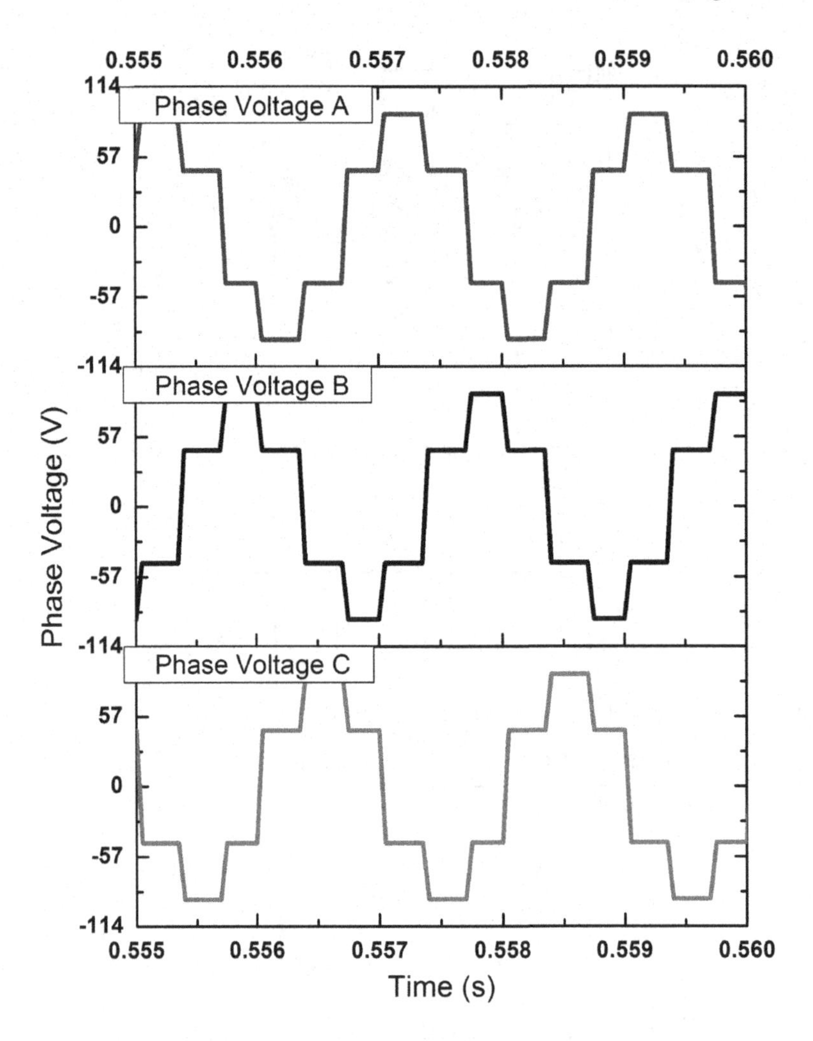

FIGURE 10.11 Obtained phase voltage waveform from inverter.

have used 1200 mode of operation, the output voltage is controlled by two switches simultaneously, in 120° mode inverter, the voltage of only two output terminals connected to DC supply is defined at any time of cycle [21]. The voltage of the third terminal of a particular leg in which neither switch is conducting is not well defined. Hence, for analysis context, we designed a balanced three-phase load for operating the inverter effectively.

Depending upon the required frequency, the switching frequency can be moduled with the changing timing circuit parameters. In the output result, the three-phase voltage is obtained as shown in Figure 10.11 with r.m.s. value of 70.71 V, which can be utilized in isolated power areas like remote places, hilly areas, top mountains, etc. A three-phase resistive load is connected across the output to draw the real power and corresponding current wave forms are shown in Figure 10.12.

10.6 CONCLUSION

The report shows the simulation model of a proton exchange membrane fuel cell-based three-phase boost-inverter. The power from renewable sources is similar to solar energy; wind energy has extra deviations in output voltage. So a fuel cell is utilized as an additional source for electrical energy generation, which gives a stable output. In this project, the concept of boost-inverter

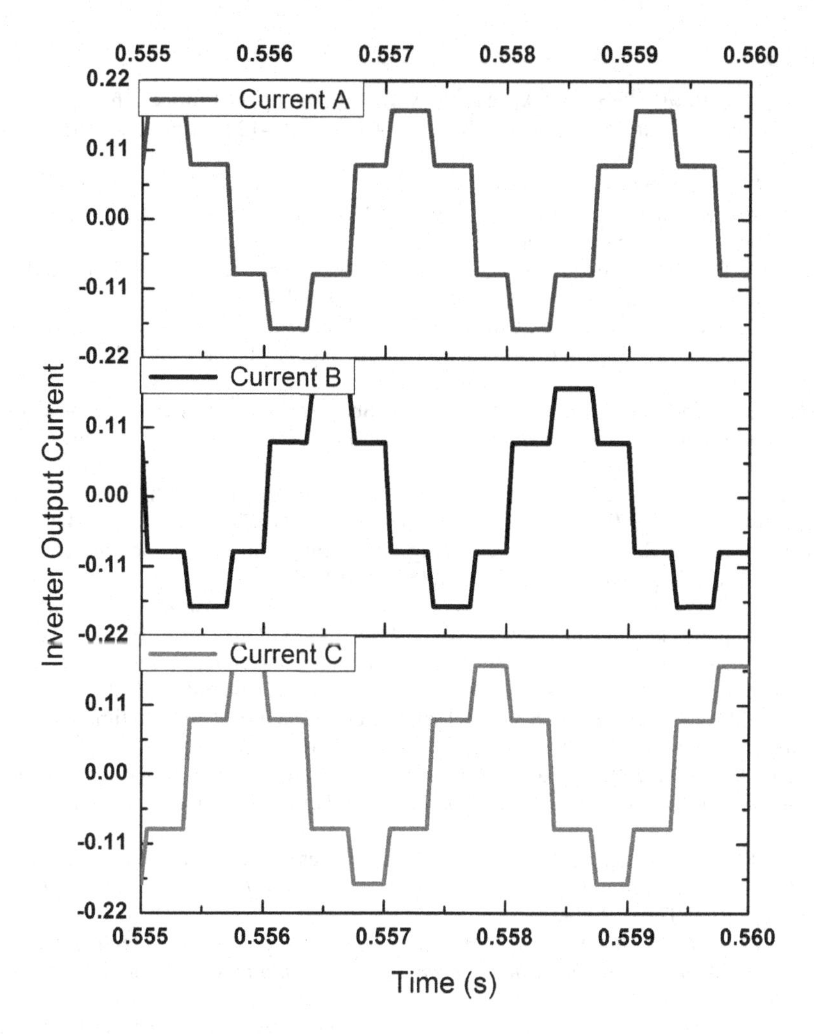

FIGURE 10.12 Obtained inverter current waveform.

is used. This means the electrical energy obtained by the fuel cell is given as input to the boost converter to boost up the DC electrical energy and the inversion of DC to three-phase AC is done using an inverter, which takes the input from the output of the boost inverter and the three-phase electrical energy can be extracted. The switching of boost converter and inverter is done using the gate pulse generating technique. Simulation results are presented, which depict the efficiency of the model.

Two objectives are focused on in the present work. Three-phase supply is developed using a PEMFC-based fuel cell, and also the steady output is aimed to feed the IoT supply system through a DC–DC converter. This work shows that the power supply to very remote places like top mountain places or islands is possible not only in a single phase but also in three phase. The output power level needs to be improved. It was found that uninterrupted operation is possible even in such harsh environments. Although the application of PEMFC is costlier, still due to its large power density per volume, it becomes an attractive choice for three-phase power development. These results indicate the possibility of uninterrupted power supply for militant islands in a security environment also. Furthermore, Using DC–DC converter, the constant 5V will be easily supplied to the IoT system. However, primarily, the three-phase power development is focused on in the paper wherein uninterrupted supply can be easily given to IoT devices.

REFERENCES

1. Ortiz-Rivera EI, Reyes-Hernandez AL, Febo RA. Understanding the history of fuel cells. In *2007 IEEE Conference on the History of Electric Power*, 2007, pp. 117–122, https://doi.org/10.1109/HEP.2007.4510259.
2. Sangwine S. *Electronic Components and Technology*, Third Edition. CRC Press, 2007, 73.
3. *Fuel Cells Proton-Exchange Membrane Fuel Cell Membrane Electrode Assembly, Angle, Hydrogen png*. https://www.pngegg.com/en/png-ejmzh.
4. Yang Z, Zhou Q, Lei L, Zheng K, Xiang W. An IoT-cloud based wearable ECG monitoring system for smart healthcare. *Journal of Medical Systems*, 2016, 40(12): 1–11.
5. Pereira RIS, Dupont IM, Carvalho PCM, Jucá SCS. IoT embedded linux system based on Raspberry Pi applied to real-time cloud monitoring of a decentralized photovoltaic plant. *Measurement*, 2018, 114: 286–297.
6. Suma N, Samson SR, Saranya S, Shanmugapriya G, Subhashri R. IOT based smart agriculture monitoring system. *International Journal on Recent and Innovation Trends in Computing and Communication*, 2017, 2017: 177–81.
7. Filsecker F, Alvarez R, Bernet S. Comparison of 4.5-kV press pack IGBTs and IGCTs for medium-voltage converters. *IEEE Transactions on Industrial Electronics*, 2013, 60(2): 440–449.
8. Hualong Y, Lu T, Ji S, et al. Active clamping circuit threshold voltage design for seriesconnected HVIGBTs. *Proceedings of the CSEE*, 2016, 36(5): 1357–1365.
9. Meng Q, Yan M, Pan Q, et al. Research on a insulated gate bipolar transistor snubber circuit for the high power neutral point clamped three-level inverter. *Proceedings of the CSEE*, 2016, 36(3): 755–764.
10. Sano K, Takasaki M. A surgeless solid-state DC circuit breaker for voltage-source-converterbased HVDC systems. *IEEE Transactions on Industry Applications*, 2014, 50(4): 2690–2699.
11. Xu Y, Zhao C, Xu Y, et al. Research on IGBT module electrical model and real time simulation. *Journal of North China Electric Power University*, 2016, 43(2): 8–16.
12. Shiggekane H, Kirihata H, Uchida Y. Developments in modern high power semiconductor devices. In *Proceedings of the 5th International Symposium on Power Semiconductor Devices and ICs*, 1993, 16–21.
13. Panigrahy PS, Chattopadhyay P. Cascaded signal processing approach for motor fault diagnosis. *COMPEL - The International Journal for Computation and Mathematics in Electrical and Electronic Engineering*, 2018, 37(6): 2122–2137.
14. Panigrahy P, Santra D, Chattopadhyay P. Decent fault classification of VFD fed induction motor using random forest algorithm. *Artificial Intelligence for Engineering Design, Analysis and Manufacturing*, 2020, 34(4): 492–504.
15. Panigrahy P, Chattopadhyay P. Tri-axial vibration based collective feature analysis for decent fault classification of VFD fed induction motor. *Measurement*, 2021, 168: 108460.
16. Panigrahy PS, Mitra S, Konar P, Chattopadhyay P. FPGA friendly fault detection technique for drive fed induction motor. In *2016 2nd International Conference on Control, Instrumentation, Energy & Communication (CIEC)*, 2016, 299–303.
17. Meng J, Ma W, Zhang L, et al. EMI evaluation of power converters considering IGBT switching transient modeling. *Proceedings of the CSEE*, 2005, 25(20): 16–20.
18. Hefner AR. Analytical modeling of device-circuit interactions for the power insulated gate bipolar transistor (IGBT). *IEEE Transactions on Industry Applications*, 1990, 26(6): 995–1005.
19. Hefner AR, Blackburn DL. An analytical model for the steady-state and transien characteristics of the power insulated-gate bipolar transistor. *Solid-State Electronics*, 1988, 31(10): 1513–1532.
20. Budihardjo I, Lauritzen PO. The lumped-charge power MOSFET model, including parameter extraction. *IEEE Transactions on Power Electronics*, 1995, 10(3): 379–387.
21. Bryant AT, Liqing L, Santi E, et al. Modeling of IGBT resistive and inductive turn-on behavior. *IEEE Transactions on Industry Applications*, 2008, 44(3): 904–914.

11 Fuzzy Logic-Based IoT Technique for Direct Torque Control of Induction Motor Drive

Aurobinda Bag and Bibhuti Bhushan Pati

CONTENTS

11.1 INTRODUCTION

More than half of the total electricity consumed in industry is by electric motors. Among them, the three-phase induction motor is used about 80% for industrial control. It has replaced the DC motor for its simple construction, reliability, low cost and easy maintenance. Though it has several advantages, the dynamics of the induction machine are complex. However, the advanced control of torque and flux is necessary for an induction motor. Therefore, scalar control like the V/F control strategy for induction machines keeps the flux of the induction machine constant. But this control technique is suitable where the speed variation is not large. In the early days, Direct Torque Control (DTC) for induction machine drive has been considered to exhibit a very fast and superior dynamic response of torque. Furthermore, DTC for induction machine drive has been considered a surrogate to the field-oriented control (FOC) algorithm [1, 2]. In the FOC technique, rotor flux has been taken as the reference frame. The DTC scheme abandons the stator current control philosophy. The DTC scheme directly controls the flux itself. DTC scheme consists of a hysteresis controller, voltage source inverter (VSI), flux and torque estimator [3]. It utilizes the band of hysteresis controller for controlling the flux and torque directly of the machine with taking into account the errors resulting among the calculated values and the actual values for the torque and the flux. Also, the inverter states are directly controlled for the reduction of the torque error and the flux errors under the predetermined band value [4, 5]. In [6], rotor flux and back EMF-based speed estimators are used. The calculated speed is used as feedback for the vector control system.

Further, some improved technique has been implemented in the following literature. In the study of Malla et al. [7], a fuzzy controller, along with the space vector modulation (SVM) technique, has been applied to VSI, which is dramatically reducing the torque ripple. The DTC for induction machines has been implemented extensively in industries for variable speed drive, which is

DOI: 10.1201/9781003217398-11

explained by Vignesh et al. [8]. In the study of Ouanjli et al. [9], DTC strategy with improved technique has been proposed for a DFIM, which is powered by two-level VSI.

Korkmaz et al. [10] proposed the implementation of SVM integrated with a fuzzy logic on a DTC induction machine, with the objective of reducing the ripple in torque. Ouanjli et al. [11] proposed various modern techniques for improving the performance of DTC control. Ravindrakumar et al. [12] proposed an improved DTC using a fuzzy controller called Fuzzy Direct Torque Control (FDTC). Bindal and Kaur [13], in their study, applied the DTC integrated with a fuzzy logic controller to the induction machine for controlling the rotor speed and fluctuations in the rotor torque.

The DTC scheme using a conventional controller [14–16], [17, 18] and having variable switching frequency causes more ripples in torque and flux errors [19], leading to the introduction of current harmonics and acoustic noise that degrade the control output. This effect is more prominent in the region of low speed. These ripples are mostly affected by the magnitude of the hysteresis band. But if the hysteresis band is reduced, then the inverter switching frequency is increased. To eliminate this, an intelligent controller, i.e., fuzzy-based IoT technique, is used in the direct torque control of induction motor drive.

11.2 BASIC DTC PRINCIPLE

In the DTC scheme, as shown in Figure 11.1 [4], the flux error, ϵ_{φ}, and torque error, ϵ_{τ}, are given as input to two comparators of the hysteresis band. With respective digitized outputs such as change in magnetic flux $\Delta\varphi$, change in mechanical torque $\Delta\tau_e$ and the position of stator flux, S_N creates a digital word. The digitized output picks out the corresponding voltage vector from the given switching table. Then the output of the switching table, the pulses S_a, S_b, S_c, is used to control the power switches of the voltage source inverter (VSI). The torque hysteresis controller used is of three levels and that of flux having two levels for the DTC of induction machine. Furthermore, a flux estimator and a torque estimator are used for the estimation of actual flux and torque. The actual estimated value of torque and flux is compared with the predetermined value of flux and torque and is given to hysteresis comparators [4, 5, 20]. Thus, the stator flux and the torque are controlled directly and also independently by selecting properly the switching configuration of VSI.

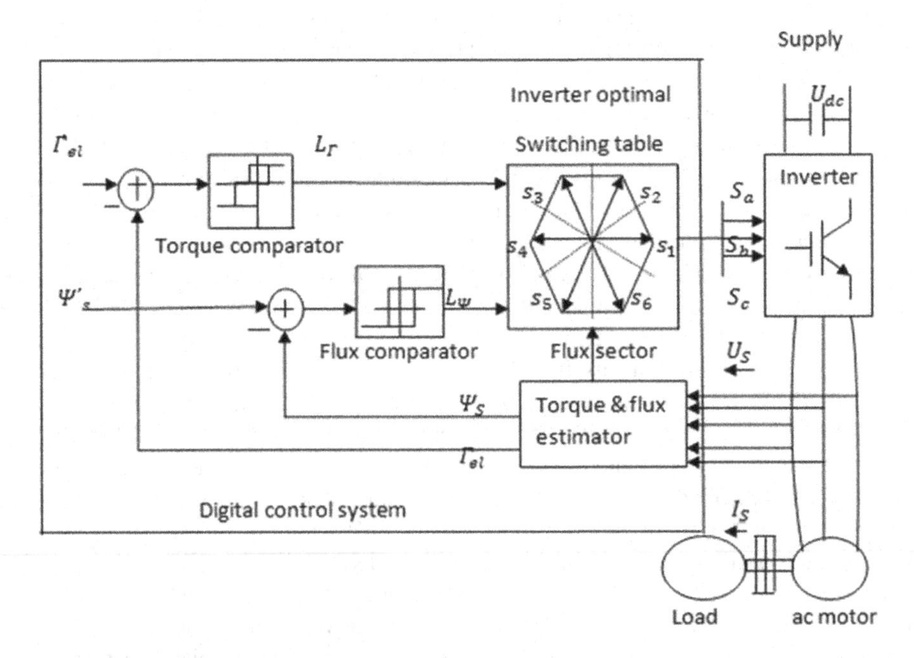

FIGURE 11.1 Block diagram for DTC of induction machine.

11.2.1 Three-Phase Voltage Source Inverter

In a voltage-fed three-phase inverter, there exists six non-zero voltage vectors (i.e. $v_1, v_2, \ldots, v_6$) and also two zero voltage vectors (i.e. v_0, v_7) that are in respect of $(C_1, C_2, C_3) = (111)/(000)$ as seen from Figure 11.2 [4, 5].

11.2.2 Direct Flux Control

In the case of DTC for an induction machine, a circular path is required to follow by the stator flux in the way of keeping its magnitude at a fixed value within its band of hysteresis [3]. If the status of flux error is equal to 1 that specifies the upper band touched by the stator flux. So it is necessary to increase the actual stator flux. Furthermore, it is necessary to reduce the actual stator flux, if the status of flux error is equal to 0. The aforesaid action is performed using a two-level hysteresis comparator as shown in Figure 11.3. The resulted digital flux error output is presented in the condition stated in Equations (11.1) and (11.2).

$$\text{if } |\Psi_s| \leq |\Psi_{sref}| - \left|\frac{\Delta\Psi_s}{2}\right|, \text{ then } d\Psi = 1 \tag{11.1}$$

$$\text{if } |\Psi_s| \geq |\Psi_{sref}| + \left|\frac{\Delta\Psi_s}{2}\right|, \text{ then } d\Psi = 0 \tag{11.2}$$

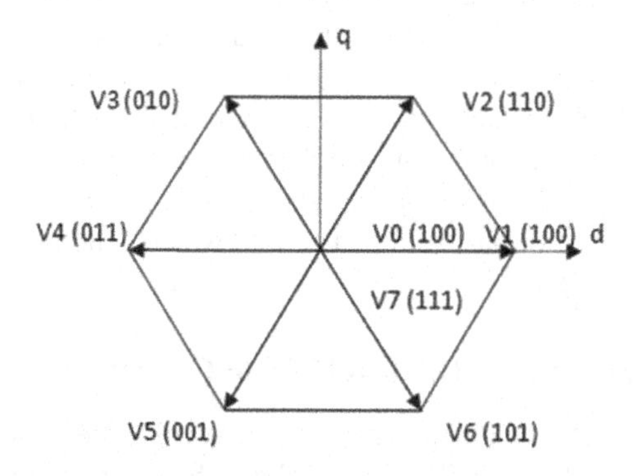

FIGURE 11.2 Partition of d, q plane into six angular sectors.

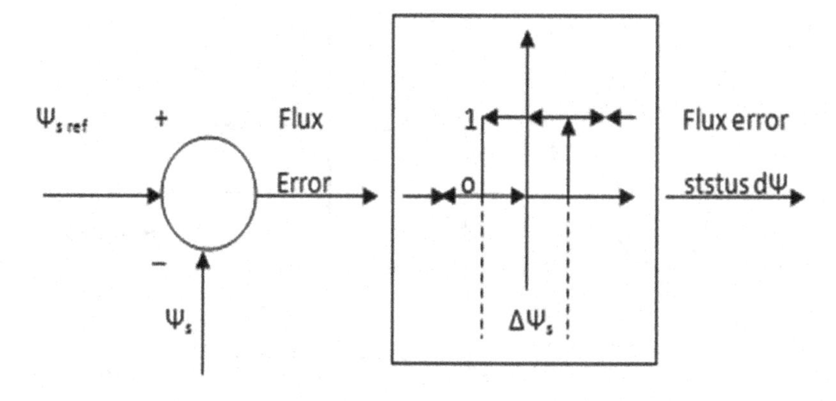

FIGURE 11.3 Two-level hysteresis comparator for flux error.

11.2.3 Direct Torque Control

In the case of the DTC for the induction machine drive, the voltage vectors are picked out to restrict the electromagnetic torque within the band of the hysteresis controller, during each switching period. To perform the aforesaid work, a hysteresis comparator of three levels has been implemented in Figure 11.4. In order to increase the torque, the $d\tau_e$ is made equal to 1. Furthermore, if it is required to decrease the torque, then $d\tau_e$ is made equal to –1, and if there is no change required, then $d\tau_e$ is made equal to 0. The resulting $d\tau_e$ for anticlockwise rotation of stator flux is based on the conditions stated in Equations (11.3) and (11.4). Furthermore, the resulting $d\tau_e$ is based on conditions as given in Equations (11.5) and (11.6), for clockwise rotation of the stator flux [3].

$$\text{if}\left|\tau_e\right| \le \left|\tau_{eref}\right| - \left|\frac{\Delta\tau_e}{2}\right|,\ \text{then}\ d\tau_e = 1 \tag{11.3}$$

$$\text{if}\left|\tau_e\right| \ge \left|\tau_{eref}\right|,\ \text{then}\ d\tau_e = 0 \tag{11.4}$$

$$\text{if}\left|\tau_e\right| \ge \left|\tau_{eref}\right| + \left|\frac{\Delta\tau_e}{2}\right|,\ \text{then}\ d\tau_e = -1 \tag{11.5}$$

$$\text{if}\left|\tau_e\right| \le \left|\tau_{eref}\right|,\ \text{then}\ d\tau_e = 0 \tag{11.6}$$

11.2.4 Selection of Switching Table

In the DTC induction machine strategy, the respective voltage vectors are selected such that the torque error and flux error are restricted within the predetermined band of the hysteresis comparator. The chosen optimum voltage vectors are sufficient to fulfil the required torque and flux value, which is tabulated in the look-up table as viewed from Table 11.1. In Table 11.1 if a change in flux, $\Delta\ \varphi$ is 1, then there are three conditions for change in torque, $\Delta\ \Gamma$ i.e., $\Delta\ \Gamma = 1$, 0 and –1. Also for $\Delta\ \varphi = 0$, there are three conditions for change in torque, $\Delta\ \Gamma = 1, 0, -1$. Accordingly, for each of the six conditions, a voltage vector has been picked out, which generates the required pulse for the switching of VSI.

11.3 PRINCIPLE OF FUZZY DIRECT TORQUE CONTROL

The torque error signal is sent to the cloud, and the same is collected using Bluetooth. The collected data has been sent as input to the fuzzy logic controller. This strategy enhances the DTC induction motor drive as a remote-controlled operation.

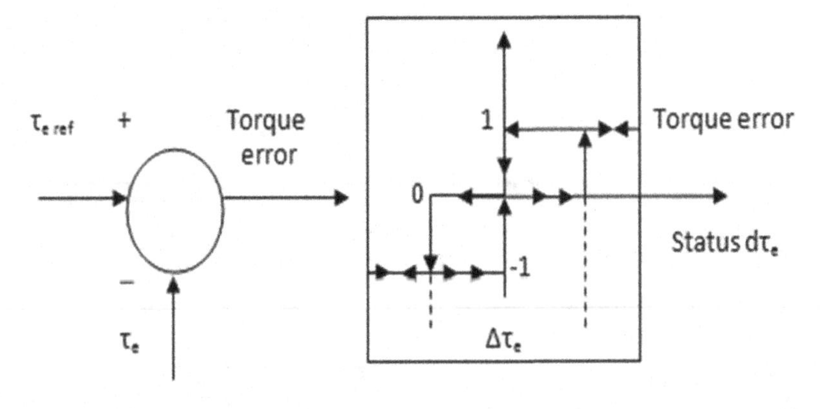

FIGURE 11.4 Three-level hysteresis comparator for torque.

TABLE 11.1
Switching Table for DTC of Induction Machine

	Sector						
Flux	**Torque**	**1**	**2**	**3**	**4**	**5**	**6**
$\Delta\varphi = 1$	$\Delta\Gamma = 1$	V_2	V_3	V_4	V_5	V_6	V_1
	$\Delta\Gamma = 0$	V_7	V_0	V_7	V_0	V_7	V_0
	$\Delta\Gamma = -1$	V_6	V_1	V_2	V_3	V_4	V_5
$\Delta\varphi = 0$	$\Delta\Gamma = 1$	V_3	V_4	V_5	V_6	V_1	V_2
	$\Delta\Gamma = 0$	V_0	V_7	V_0	V_7	V_0	V_7
	$\Delta\Gamma = -1$	V_5	V_6	V_1	V_2	V_3	V_4

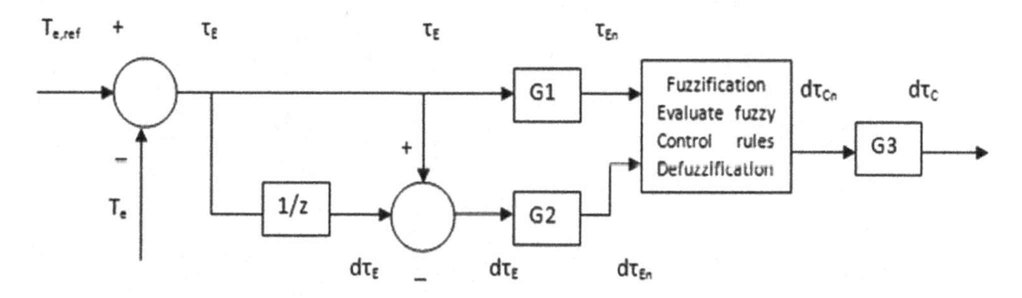

FIGURE 11.5 Fuzzy PI controller block diagram.

TABLE 11.2
Fuzzification of Input and Output

Linguistic Term	**Positive Big**	**Positive Medium**	**Positive Small**	**Zero**	**Negative Small**	**Negative Medium**	**Negative Big**
Symbol	PB	PM	PS	Z	NS	NM	NM
Fuzzy Subset	+3	+2	+1	0	−1	−2	−3

The fuzzy logic controller is designed to have two fuzzy-state variables and one control variable Figure 11.5. The two-state variables are: the torque error signal, $\tau_E = \tau_{e,\mathrm{ref}} - \tau_e$ = Reference Torque – Actual Torque, the rate of change of torque error signal, $d\tau_E = \tau_E(t) - \tau_E(t - \Delta t)$.

The inputs, i.e. torque error and change in torque error, are made normalized using the input normalization gains G_1 and G_2, and the same is delivered to the hysteresis controller.

Normalized torque error $\tau_{,En} = G_1.\tau_E$; $d\tau_{En} = G_2.d\tau_E$; $d\tau_{Cn} = G_3.d\tau_C$, where G_1 is defined as normalization gain of torque error τ_E, G_2 as normalization gain for the rate of change of torque error, $d\tau_E$. Furthermore, G_3 is defined as the un-normalization gain for the change of control signal $d\tau_C$.

The controller output is defined as normalized change for the control signal $d\tau_{Cn}$. The actual change of control signal $d\tau_C$ is picked out with output un-normalization gain G_3. In the case of the said controller, the input has been divided into seven numbers of fuzzy subsets. The selected normalized inputs are specified from −3 to 3. Table 11.2 depicts seven fuzzy subsets. According to the seven fuzzy subsets, 49 rules are assigned for obtaining the required response, which is summarized in Table 11.3. The membership function plots are shown in Figures 11.6 to 11.8.

TABLE 11.3
Decision Table for Fuzzy Control Rule

τ_E \ $d\tau_E$	−3	−2	−1	0	+1	+2	+3
−3	0	0	−3	−3	0	0	0
−2	−3	−2	−3	−1	−2	0	0
−1	−2	−2	−3	−3	0	1	0
0	−2	−1	−3	0	0	1	0
+1	−1	−1	0	0	0	2	0
+2	−1	0	−3	1	0	2	0
+3	0	1	−3	−3	0	3	0

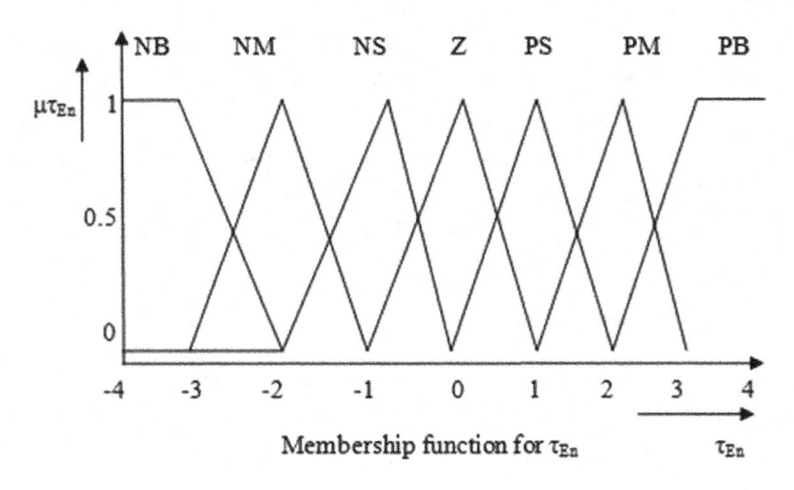

FIGURE 11.6 Membership function for τ_{En}.

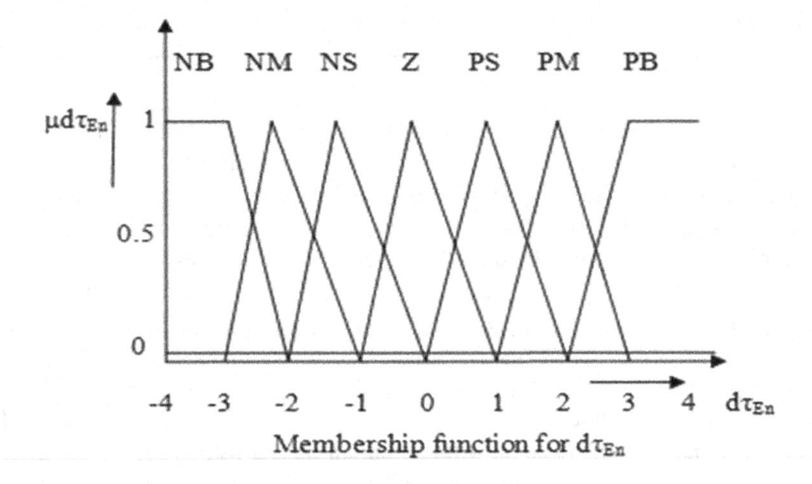

FIGURE 11.7 Membership function for $d\tau_{En}$.

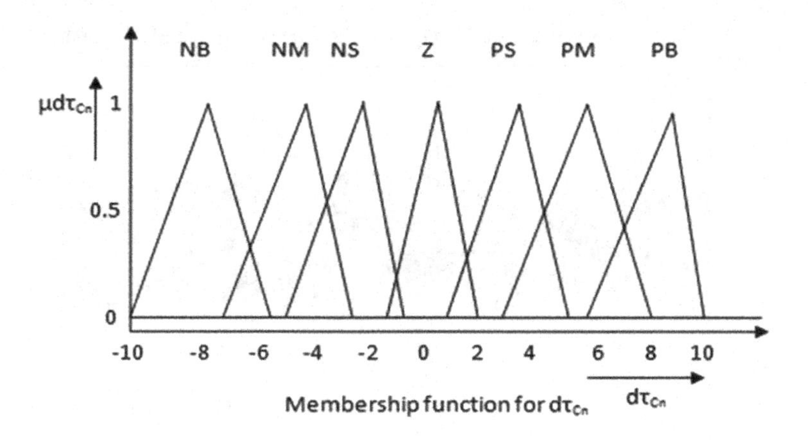

FIGURE 11.8 Membership function for $d\tau_{Cn}$.

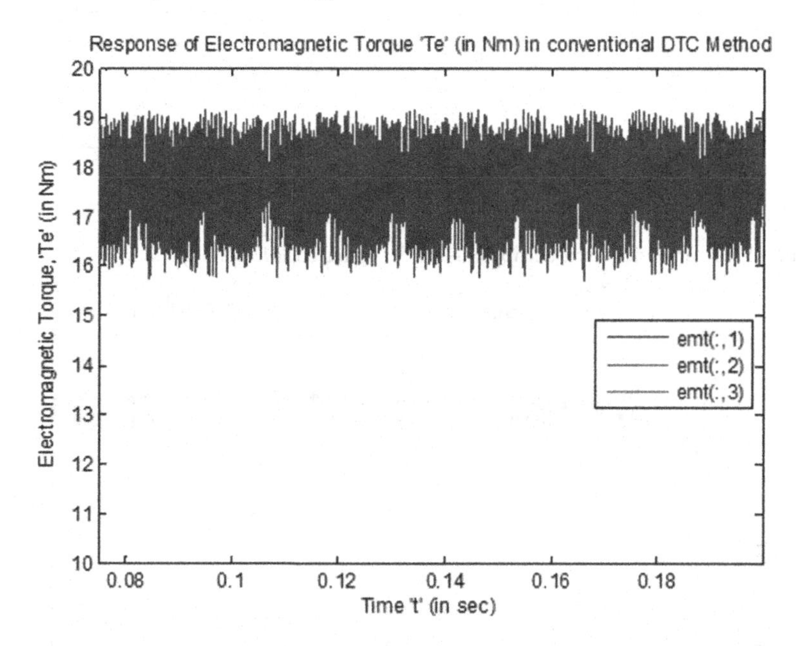

FIGURE 11.9 Electromagnetic torque ripple using conventional PI controller.

11.4 SIMULATED OUTPUT AND DISCUSSIONS

The control technique is implemented in this work on the induction machine, and the digital simulation is carried out using MATLAB/Simulink. The selected induction motor for the implementation of the proposed controller has the following parameters: nominal power, $P_N = 3$ HP; nominal voltage, $U_N = 220$ V; nominal frequency, $F_N = 60$ Hz, stator resistance, $R_S = 0.435\Omega$; rotor resistance, $R_r = 0.816\Omega$; number of poles, $P = 2$; stator inductance, L_S = rotor inductance; $L_r = 2$ mH; mutual inductance, $L_m = 69.31$ mH; inertia constant, $J = 0.089$ kg.m^2; friction coefficient = 0.005 N.m/s; sampling time, $T_s = 2$ μs.

In Figures 11.9 and 11.10, the ripples in electromagnetic torque have been shown for DTC induction motor drive using PI controllers and fuzzy logic-based IoT technique, respectively. From the obtained result, it is observed that in the fuzzy-based IoT technique, the DTC method contains less ripple as compared to the PI-based DTC method [3, 4, 5].

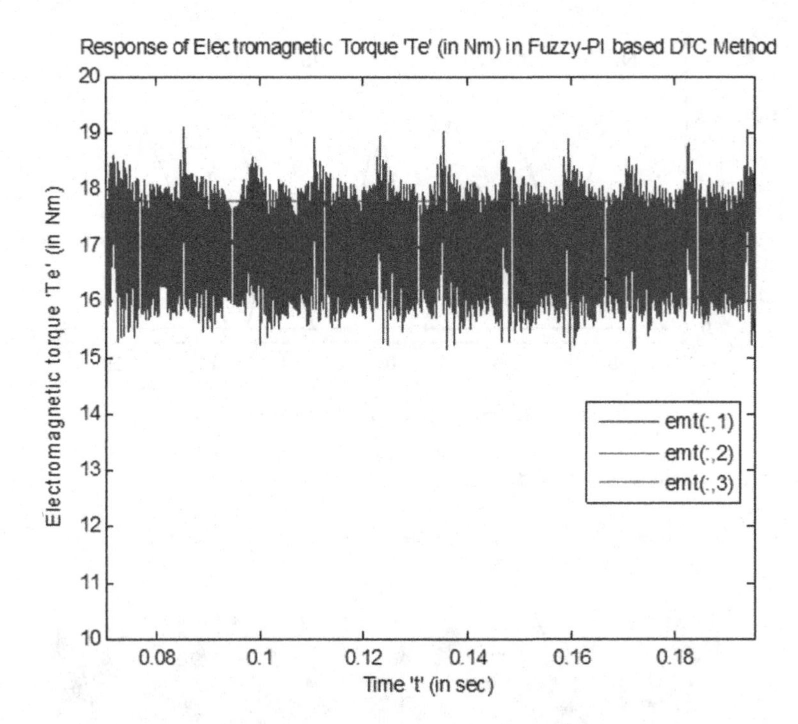

FIGURE 11.10 Electromagnetic torque ripple using fuzzy-based IoT technique.

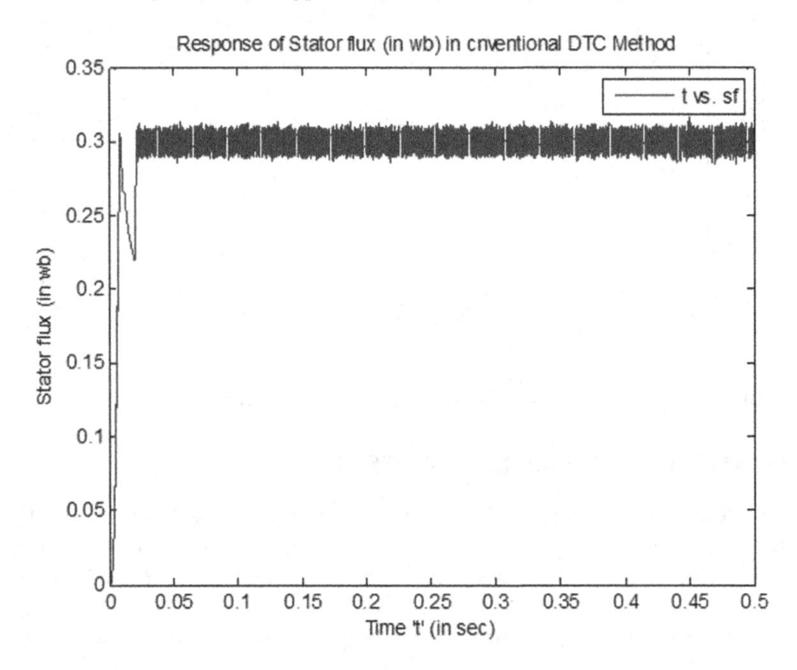

FIGURE 11.11 Stator flux ripple using conventional PI controller.

The stator flux ripples for DTC induction motor drives using the PI controller and fuzzy logic-based IoT technique can be observed from Figures 11.11 and 11.12, respectively. Fewer ripples in flux can also be noticed. Furthermore, flux locus for DTC induction motor drive for PI controller and fuzzy-based IoT technique is shown in Figures 11.13 and 11.14, respectively. In this locus, flux error is minimized in the fuzzy-based IoT technique.

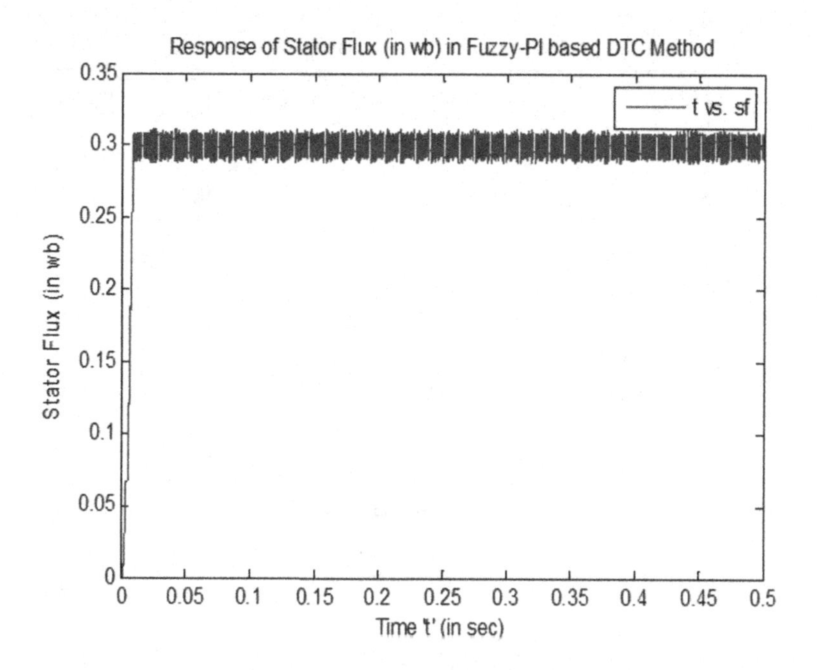

FIGURE 11.12 Stator flux ripple using fuzzy-based IoT technique.

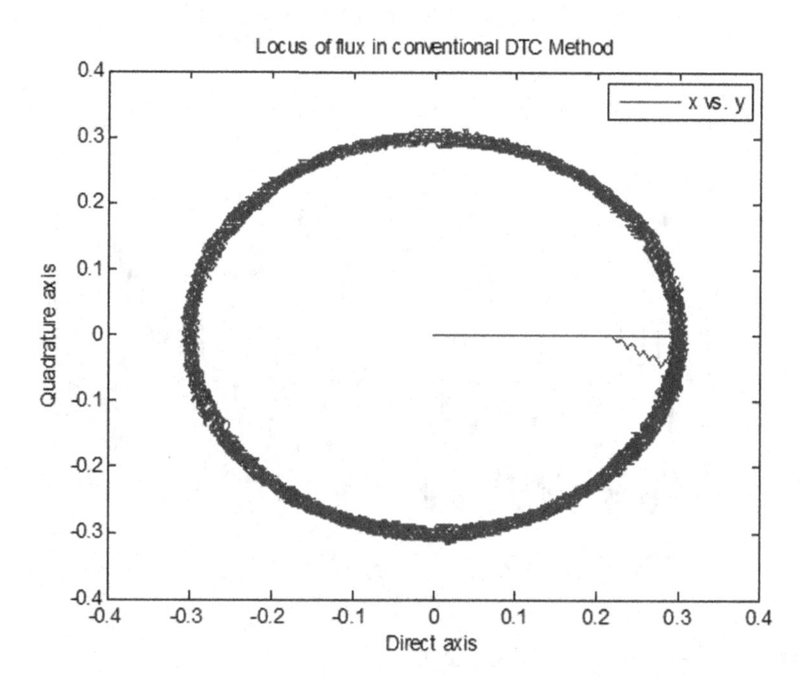

FIGURE 11.13 Flux locus using conventional PI controller.

The resulted stator current from the DTC for induction machines using a PI controller and fuzzy-based IoT technique is represented in Figures 11.15 and 11.16, respectively. The response of rotor speed using a PI controller and fuzzy-based IoT technique are shown in Figures 11.17 and 11.18, respectively. Lastly, DC bus voltage for DTC of induction machines is presented in Figures 11.19 and 11.20, respectively.

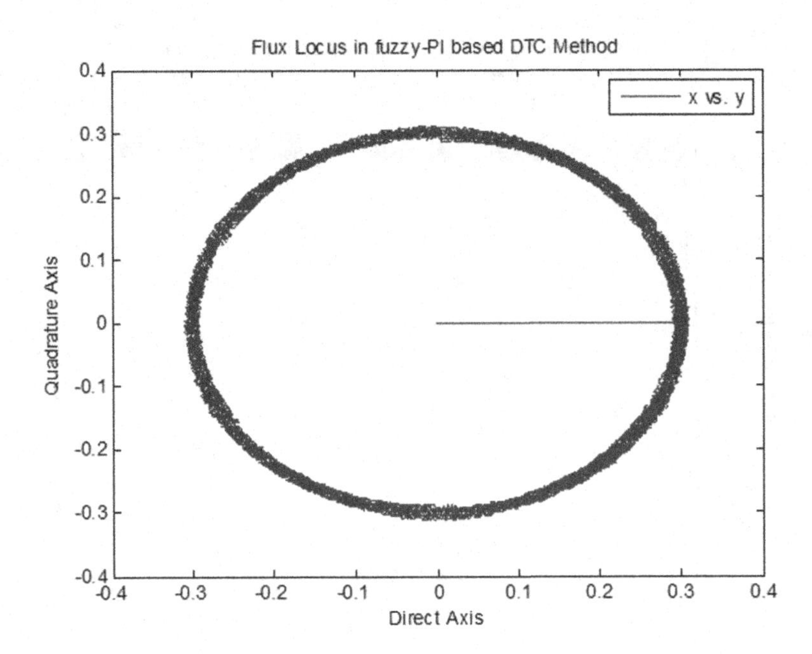

FIGURE 11.14 Flux locus using fuzzy-based IoT technique.

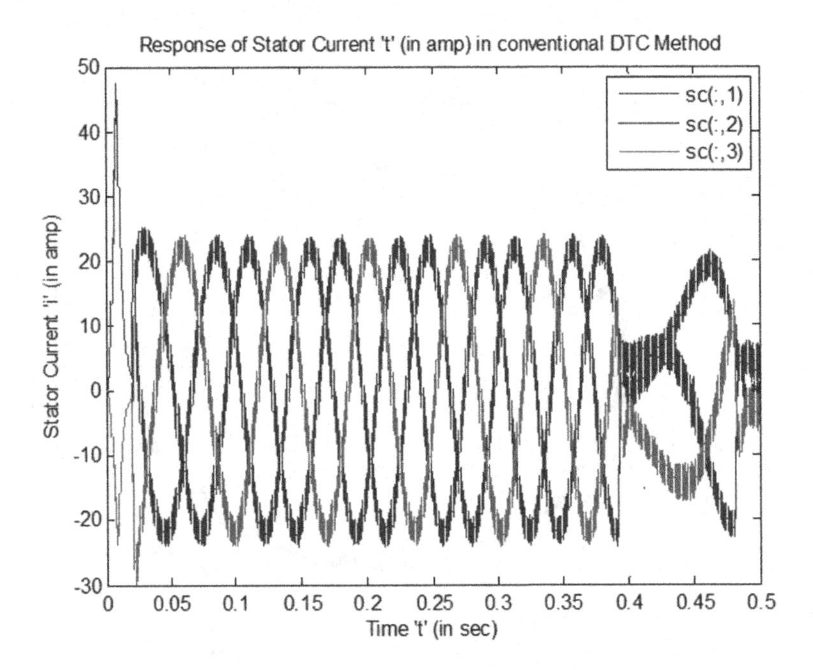

FIGURE 11.15 Stator current using conventional PI controller.

Also from the waveform of flux response and locus of flux, the fuzzy-based IoT method gives a better result. So as fuzzy-based IoT method reduces ripples in flux and torque. In a fuzzy logic controller, the magnitude of torque error is divided into seven sub-sections. But in a conventional PI controller whatever the torque error magnitude, it takes the same control action.

So using the fuzzy logic controller and integration with the IoT technique, the effective reduction of flux and torque error can be possible. Furthermore, as ripple causes higher acoustic noise,

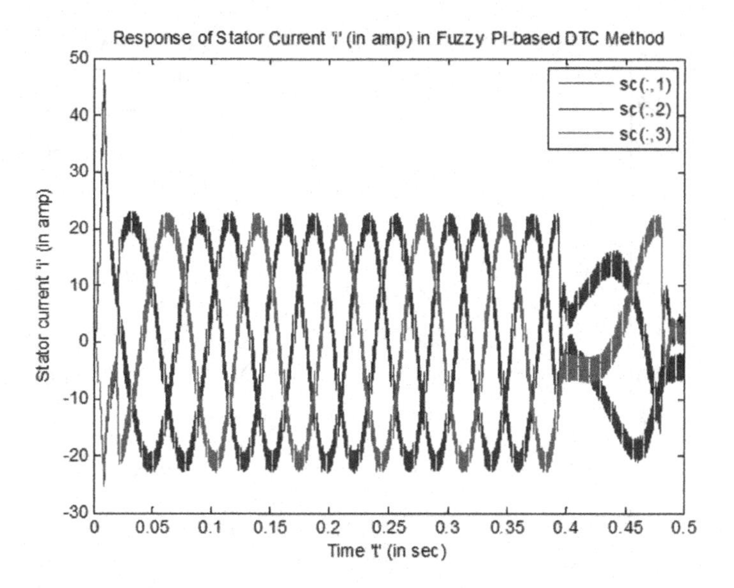

FIGURE 11.16 Stator current using fuzzy-based IoT technique.

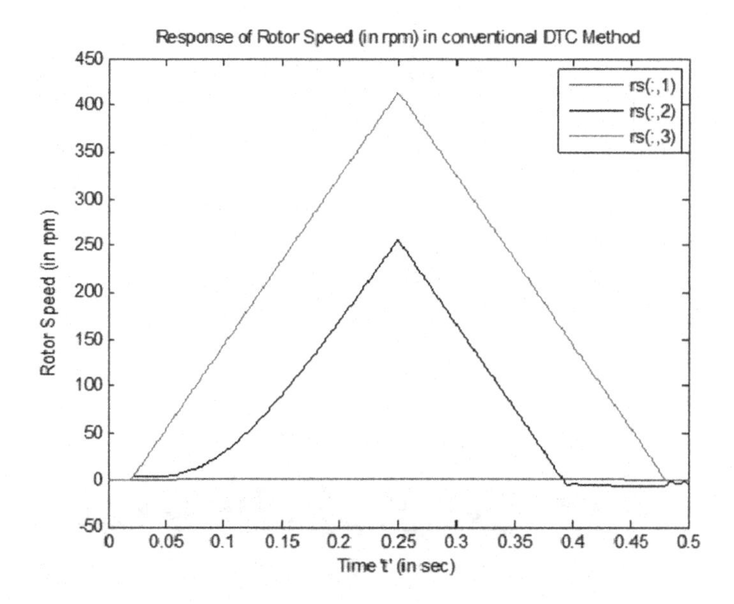

FIGURE 11.17 Rotor speed using conventional PI controller.

component failure and harmonic loss, this method is superior as compared to the conventional PI method [20, 21].

11.5 CONCLUSION

In this work, a fuzzy logic-based IoT technique is implemented for DTC of induction machines and the same has been simulated using MATLAB/Simulink software. Then fuzzy-based IoT technique for induction machines is compared with the conventional PI-based DTC for induction machines. From the obtained result, it is observed that the conventional PI-based DTC method contains more

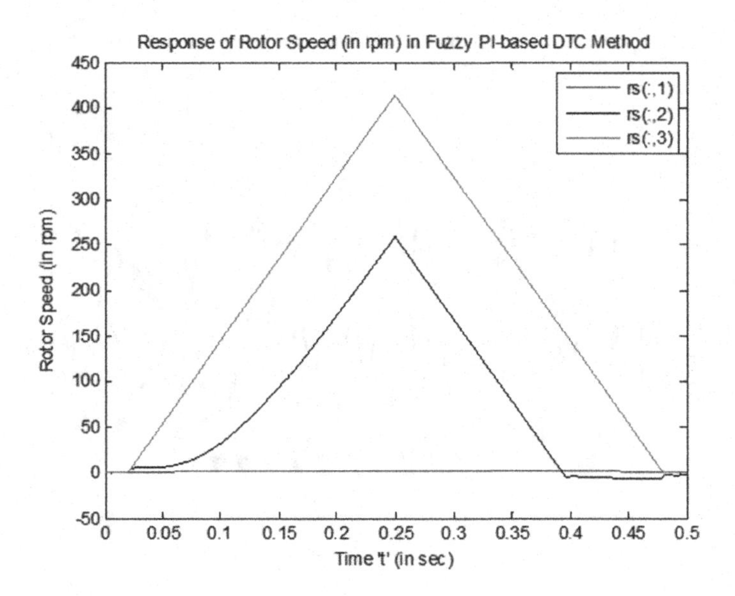

FIGURE 11.18 Rotor speed using fuzzy-based IoT technique.

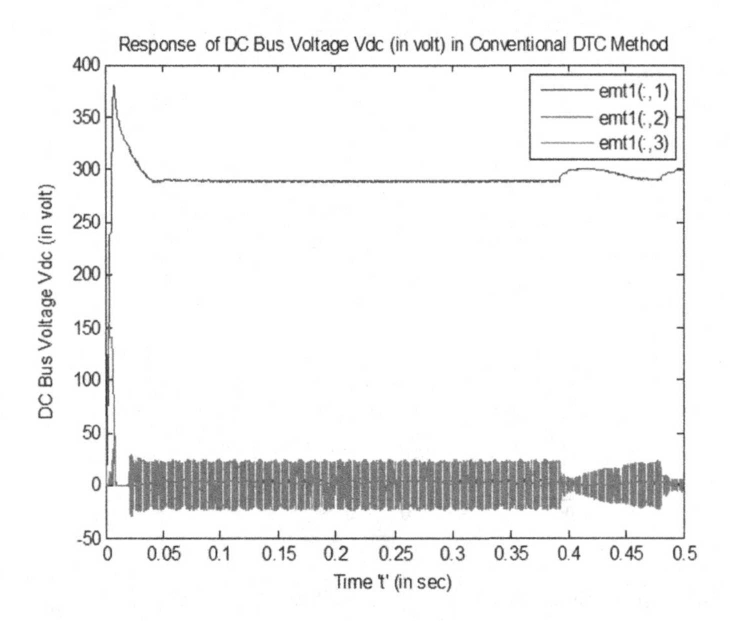

FIGURE 11.19 DC bus voltage using conventional PI controller.

flux and torque ripples. This method causes higher acoustical noise which affects the accuracy of speed estimation and harmonic losses. This is not desirable under normal operating conditions. To overcome the above disadvantage, an intelligent controller like a fuzzy logic controller is used. The fuzzy logic controller is integrated with the IoT technique for effective reduction of ripple for flux and torque especially at the low-speed region.

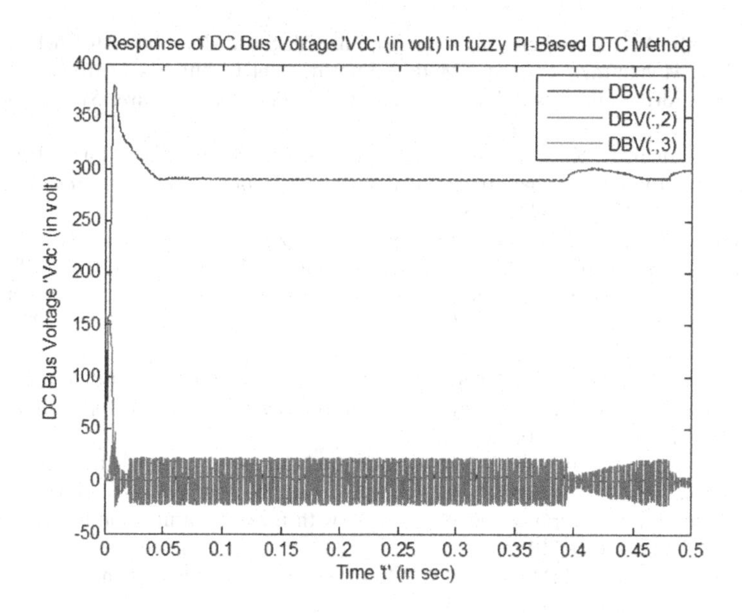

FIGURE 11.20 DC bus voltage using fuzzy-based IoT technique.

REFERENCES

1. Toshihiko Noguchi, Seiji Kondo, and Isao Takahashi, "Field-oriented control of an induction motor with robust on-line tuning of its parameters", *IEEE Transactions on Industry Applications*, vol. 33, no. 1, pp. 35–42, 1997, doi: 10.1109/28.567074.
2. G. Kang and K. Nam, "Field-oriented control scheme for linear induction motor with the end effect", *IEE Proceedings - Electric Power Applications*, vol. 152, no. 6, pp. 1565–1572, 2005.
3. NurHakimah Ab Aziz and Azhan Ab Rahman, "Simulation on Simulink AC4 model (200hp DTC induction motor drive) using fuzzy logic controller", in *2010 International Conference on Computer Applications and Industrial Electronics (ICCAIE 2010)*, Kuala Lumpur, Malaysia, December 5–7, 2010.
4. R. Toufouti, S. Meziane, and H. Benalla, "Direct torque control for induction motor using fuzzy logic", *Laboratory of Electrical Engineering University Constantine Algeria ACSE Journal*, vol. 6, no. 2, pp. 19–26, 2006.
5. Fatiha Zidani and Rachid Nait Said, "Direct torque control of induction motor with fuzzy minimization torque ripple", *Journal of Electrical Engineering*, vol. 56, no. 7–8, pp. 183–188, 2005.
6. Soufien Gdaim, Abdellatif Mtibaa, and Mohamed Faouzi Mimouni, "Direct torque control of induction machine using fuzzy logic technique", in *10th International Conference on Sciences and Techniques of Automatic Control & Computer Engineering*, pp. 1898–1909, 2016.
7. Jagan Mohana Rao Malla, Manoj Kumar Sahu, and P.K. Subudhi, "DTC-SVM of induction motor by applying two fuzzy logic controllers", in *2016 International Conference on Electrical, Electronics, and Optimization Techniques (ICEEOT)*, pp. 4941–4945, 2016.
8. C. Vignesh, S. Shantha Sheela, E. Chidam Meenakchi Devi, and R. Balachandar, "Direct torque control of induction motor using fuzzy logic controller", *International Refereed Journal of Engineering and Science*, vol. 3, no. 2, pp. 56–61, 2014.
9. Najib Ouanjli, Saad Motahhir, Aziz Derouich, Abdelaziz El Ghzizal, Ali Chebabhi, and Mohammed Taoussi, "Improved DTC strategy of doubly fed induction motor using fuzzy logic controller", *Energy Reports*, vol. 5, pp. 271–279, 2019.
10. Fatih Korkmaz, Ismail Topaloglu, and Hayati Mamur, "Fuzzy logic based direct torque control of induction motor with space vector modulation", *International Journal on Soft Computing, Artificial Intelligence and Applications*, vol. 2, no. 5/6, pp. 31–40 2013.

11. Najib El Ouanjli, Aziz Derouich, Abdelaziz El Ghzizal, Saad Motahhir, Ali Chebabhi, Youness, El Mourabit, and Mohammed Taoussi, "Modern improvement techniques of direct torque control for induction motor drives-a review", *Protection and Control of Modern Power Systems*, vol. 4, no. 1, pp. 1–12, 2019.
12. K.B. Ravindrakumar, K. Karthick, D. Sivanandakumar, and S. Sivarajan, "Fuzzy based approach for direct torque control of three phase induction motor", *International Journal of Scientific & Technology Research*, vol. 8, no. 10, pp. 1687–1693, 2019.
13. R.K. Bindal and I. Kaur, "Design and development of fuzzy controller model with DTC on induction motor", *International Journal of Electrical Engineering*, vol. 11, no. 1, pp. 17–29, 2018.
14. C. Lascu, I. Boldea, and F. Blaabjerg, "A modified direct torque control for induction motor sensorless drive", *IEEE Transactions on Industry Applications*, vol. 36, no. 1, pp. 122–130, 2000, doi: 10.1109/28.821806.
15. Jun-Koo Kang and Seung-Ki Sul, "New direct torque control of induction motor for minimum torque ripple and constant switching frequency", *IEEE Transactions on Industry Applications*, vol. 35, no. 5, pp. 1076–1082, 1999, doi: 10.1109/28.793368.
16. I. Takahashi and Y. Ohmori, "High-performance direct torque control of an induction motor," *IEEE Transactions on Industry Applications*, vol. 25, no. 2, pp. 257–264, 1989, doi: 10.1109/28.25540.
17. A. Bag, "Direct torque control of induction motor with fuzzy minimization torque ripple", M. Tech. Thesis, VSSUT, Burla, June 2012.
18. R.D. Lorenz, T.A. Lipo, and D.W. Novotny, "Motion control with induction motors", *Proceedings of the IEEE*, vol. 82, no. 8, pp. 1215–1240, 1994.
19. Hoang Le-Huy, "Comparison of field-oriented control and direct torque control for induction motor drives", in *Conference Record of 1999 IEEE Industry Applications Conference, Thirty-Forth IAS Annual Meeting* (Cat. No.99CH36370), vol. 2, pp. 1245–1252, 1999, doi: 10.1109/IAS.1999.801662.
20. Ranjan K. Behera and Shyama P. Das, "High performance induction motor drive: A dither injection technique", in *International Conference on Energy, Automation and Signal*, 2011, pp. 1–6, 2011, doi: 10.1109/ICEAS.2011.6147102.
21. R. Toufouti, S. Meziane, and H. Benalla, "Direct torque control for induction motor using intelligent techniques", *Journal of Theoretical and Applied Information Technology*, 3, 2007.

12 Body Wearable Antennas and Integration of Internet of Things in Vehicular Wireless Communication Systems

Arnab De, KM Vijaylaxmi, Dinesh Yadav, Soufian Lakrit, Raed M. Shubair, Bappadittya Roy, Anup Kumar Bhattacharjee

CONTENTS

12.1 INTRODUCTION

Internet of Things (IoT) is a system in which billions of physical devices all over the world are connected to the Internet and acquire and transmit data without the need for human-to-human or human-to-computer interaction. IoT is used in medical and healthcare facilities, transportation, smart homes, manufacturing, agriculture, and automation, among other places, to assist people in quick decisions in real time [1]. According to a Cisco survey, between 2003 and 2020, there was a surge in the number of physical devices connected to the Internet, ranging from 500 million to 50 billion [2]. As a result of the low data transmission rate specified by IoT systems, bandwidth requirements are lowered, resulting in ultra-narrow band (UNB) modulations [3]. Because of these characteristics, antennas for IoT applications should be miniaturised and have a narrower bandwidth. Compact antennas make it easier to integrate IoT devices, improving the antenna's quality factor, which is inversely proportional to the antenna's bandwidth [4]. Cost-effective devices and sensors are being developed for their ability to autonomously create, share, and process data in order to carry out a given task [5,6]. Because of the small bands required for IoT systems, interference effects are minimised; however, attention should be given to the antenna's decreased efficiency

DOI: 10.1201/9781003217398-12

as a result of miniaturisation [7]. In this era of information technology, a vehicle is more than just a mode of transportation of not only people and products but also information [8]. As a result, vehicles are expected to connect to an increasing number of gadgets, such as smartphones, satellites [9], base stations [10], and even other vehicles [11], [12] are examples. Dedicated short-range communication (DSRC) has lately emerged as among the most essential technologies for the development of communications-based automobiles in intelligent transportation systems (ITSs). The U.S. Department of Transportation (DOT) has stated that it would begin taking necessary footsteps to permit vehicle-to-vehicle (V2V) and vehicle-to-infrastructure (V2I) communications between light vehicles and commercial automobiles that are currently on the road for the purposes of vehicle safety [13]. Dedicated short-range communication (DSRC) is a typical technique for secure and fast communication [14]. DSRC utilizes 75 MHz bands at 5.9 GHz [5.850–5.925 GHz]. High data speeds are provided via LTE for a variety of purposes, including internet connectivity. Vehicle-to-everything (V2X), which is based primarily on IEEE 802.11p, shall permit vehicles to interact with one another as well as with road infrastructure, hence enhancing traffic safety and efficiency [15–18]. IEEE 802.11p in Europe serves as the foundation in support of the ITS-G5 standard, formed by the European Telecommunications Standard Institute (ETSI), and has a bandwidth allotment of 30 MHz centred at 5.9 GHz (5875 -5905 MHz) [19].

Because of its compact size, lightweight design, and ease of installation, the microstrip patch antenna is ideal for this communication [20–25]. For the design of wearable antennas, microstrip antennas are chosen over other varieties. However, designing a body-centric antenna is more difficult than designing a normal low-profile microstrip antenna. This is due to the technique of embedding into the garment material or skin while remaining lightweight, cost-effective, flexible, and with optimized impedance and radiation properties [26–30]. In the literature, many forms of wearable antennas have been presented [31–36]. Varkiani et al. [37] investigated a grounded CPW supplied antenna with two distinct substrates: one cotton ($\varepsilon_r = 1.65$) and another non-woven layer ($\varepsilon_r = 1.15$) with thicknesses of 1.0 mm and 5.0 mm, respectively. Abbasi et al. [38] built an EBG-backed semi-flexible monopole antenna for use in the ISM 2.45 GHz band, and Ferreira et al. [39] evaluated the effect of bending a wearable textile at the same frequency. Sundarsingh et al. [40] developed a textile antenna with rectangular and circular vertical slits for GSM-900 and GSM-1800 applications using a Jeans substrate. The electrical properties of a fully flexible 5.80 GHz e-textile antenna were studied by Ahmed et al. [41]. Many studies on DSRC antennas have lately been presented. An elevated monopole antenna accompanied by directors [42] and a nonuniform antenna array [43] were presented to implement the DSRC applications. In addition, for systems such as LTE, GPS, and DSRC systems, a multiple frequency band antenna is installed on the vehicle's roof, as in the study of Ghafari et al. [44]. Similarly, for automotive DSRC applications, a conical antenna that is small and low-profile is developed by Liou et al. [45]. A comprehensive analysis of the growth of technology allowing IoT connection and applications, as well as a study of the transformation and development of IoT-enabled smart systems for vehicles, is presented in the studies of Rahim et al., Sharma and Kaushik, and Krishnan et al. [46–48].

A simple, compact wearable antenna using Jeans material as a substrate is proposed in this chapter. Wi-MAX (5.5 GHz), WLAN (5.2/5.8 GHz), 5.8 GHz Wi-Fi (5.725–5.825 GHz), standard IEEE 802.11p DSRC band, and intelligent transportation systems (ITS) are all supported by the antenna. The goal of the project is to connect devices across many frequency bands, resulting in an integrated IoT network. The antenna fabrication is straightforward, and the parameters are thoroughly examined in the following sections. The antenna is simulated using the Zeland IE3D EM modelling platform, and the results are compared to those measured.

12.2 ANTENNA DESIGN METHODOLOGY

The complete antenna design steps are depicted in Figure 12.1, where 1(a) is the reference symmetric coplanar waveguide (CPW) fed rectangular monopole antenna (RMA) of dimensions $18.75 \times 15.00 \times$

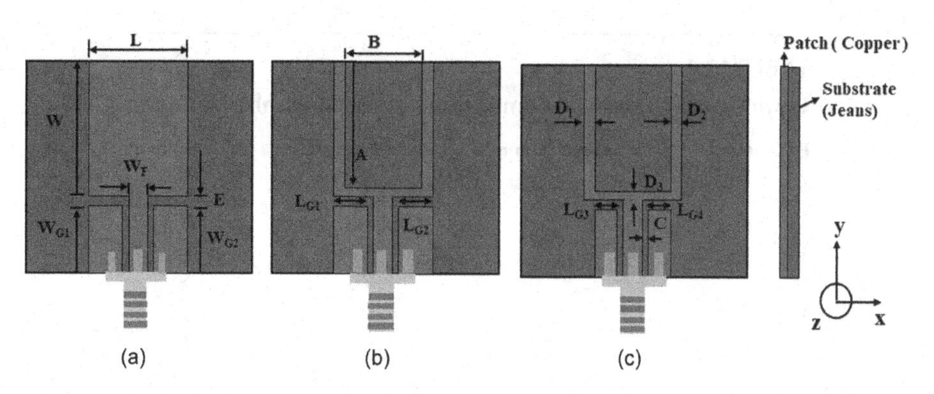

FIGURE 12.1 (a) Reference body wearable antenna (Antenna 1); (b) Tuning fork-shaped antenna (or Antenna 2); and (c) Front view of the proposed tuning fork-shaped antenna with modified ground plane (Antenna 3)

1.00 mm^3 and noted as Antenna 1. The wearable antenna consists of two layers, with the top layer consisting of copper (Cu) as the radiating patch pasted on a Jeans substrate ($\varepsilon r = 1.78$) of thickness (h) = 1.00 mm. The input impedance of the antenna is matched to 50 Ω with the help of microstrip line feed of width (W_F) = 3.00 mm. The symmetric CPW ground plane is of dimensions $W_{G1} \times L_{G1}$ mm^2 and $W_{G2} \times L_{G2}$ mm^2. In the next step, a tuning fork-shaped antenna (Antenna 2) is created by cutting a rectangular slot of dimensions $A \times B$ mm^2 in the patch and depicted in Figure 12.1(b). The two arms of the fork or the U-shaped structure have widths of D_1 and D_2. Lastly, the length of the ground plane is modified to L_{G3} and L_{G4} for better return loss response and to tune the antenna to our desired frequency band, as shown in Figure 12.1(c), and denoted as Antenna 3, which is our proposed antenna. Improvement of return loss and bandwidth can be achieved by defecting the ground structure or defecting ground structures (DGS). The overall dimensions of the fabricated antenna are $0.311\ \lambda_0 \times 0.249\ \lambda_0 \times 0.016\ \lambda_0$, where λ_0 is the free space wavelength with the lowest resonant frequency of 4.98 GHz. Preventive measures are taken to diminish the air gap between the dual layers by pasting the copper foil to the Jeans material with the help of an adhesive. The parameters along with dimensions are summarized in Table 12.1.

The lowest resonant frequency f_l can be calculated from the perimeter of the patch (antenna 3) $P = 2(2A + D_1 + D_2 + D_3) + 4(D_1 + D_2) = 90$ mm as shown in Equation (12.1)

$$f_l \approx \frac{2c}{P \times \sqrt{\varepsilon_r}} \tag{12.1}$$

where c is the velocity of light and ε_r the effective permittivity of the Jeans material.

The highest resonant frequency f_u is calculated using Equation (12.2),

$$f_u \approx \frac{4c}{\left[P + 2\left(WG_1 + LG_3\right) + 2\left(WG_2 + LG_4\right) + W_F + E\right]\sqrt{\varepsilon_r}} \tag{12.2}$$

where all the symbols have their usual meanings.

Figure 12.2 depicts a wide picture of V2V, V2I, and V2X communications. Wireless data communications between vehicles are what V2V technology is all about. This communication's main purpose is to reduce accidents by allowing cars in motion to share information about their location and speed via an IoT network. If a vehicle is intended to carry out safety interventions, the driver may get a caution signal in case of the possibility of an accident, or it may take preventive steps on its own, such as emergency braking, depending on the evolution of the technology. Unlike the V2V communication paradigm, which permits solely vehicle-to-vehicle contact, the V2I allows cars on the way to communicate with the transportation system. Traffic signals, RFID readers, lane markings, cameras,

TABLE 12.1
Optimized Parametric Dimensions of the Wearable Antenna

Parameters	Value (in mm)	Parameters	Value (in mm)
W	18.75	L_{G1}	6.50
L	15.00	L_{G2}	6.50
W_F	3.00	L_{G3}	4.50
W_{G1}	9.00	L_{G4}	4.50
W_{G2}	9.00	A	17.25
$D1$	1.50	B	12.00
$D2$	1.50	C	0.10
$D3$	1.50	E	1.00

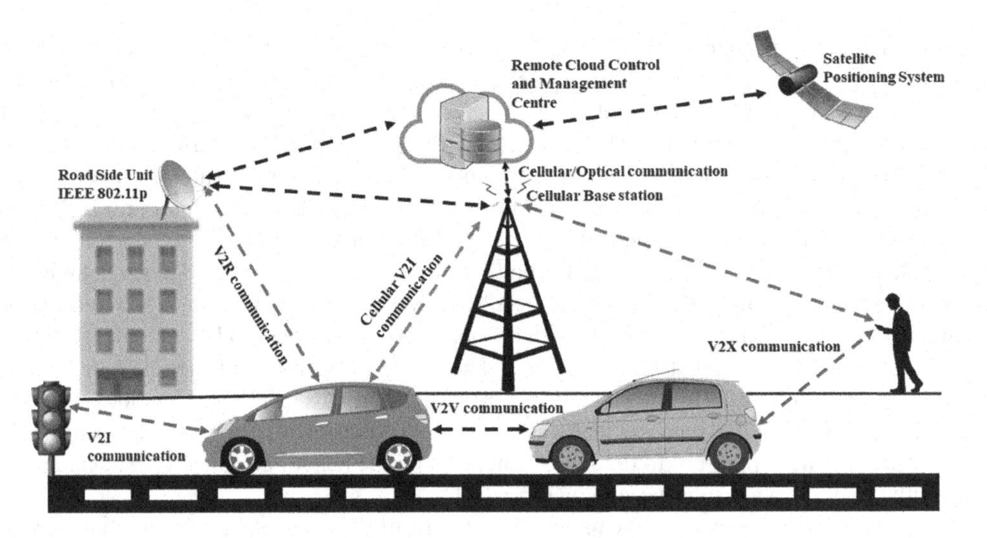

FIGURE 12.2 IoT framework for V2V, V2I, and V2X communications.

street lighting, signs, and parking metres are among these components [49]. Communications through V2I are often bidirectional, wireless, and use DSRC frequencies to transport data, similar to V2V [50]. The above-mentioned models of communication V2I and V2V are rounded out by the V2X, that is, a generalisation. Vehicle-to-pedestrian (V2P) [51], vehicle-to-roadside (V2R) [52], vehicle-to-device (V2D) [53], and vehicle-to-grid (V2G) [54] are examples of more specialised types of communication that include data flow from a vehicle to any entity that can impact it, or vice versa. According to a report on the global situation of road safety [55], over 1.25 million people die each year as a result of road accidents around the world. Pedestrians, cyclists, and motorcyclists made for about half of the victims, dubbed Vulnerable Road Users (VRU). RFID technology was originally enabled as a requisite communication tool by IoT [56]. The addition of GPS [57], Bluetooth [58], and Wi-Fi [59] to the automobile communication system advanced it even further. Since roughly 2011, the automobile industry has recognised the value of Internet of Things (IoT) technology for remotely monitoring vehicle failures and mitigating a variety of associated difficulties [60].

12.3 RESULTS AND DISCUSSION

Figure 12.3 portrays the S-parameters response for stages of development of the proposed wearable antenna.

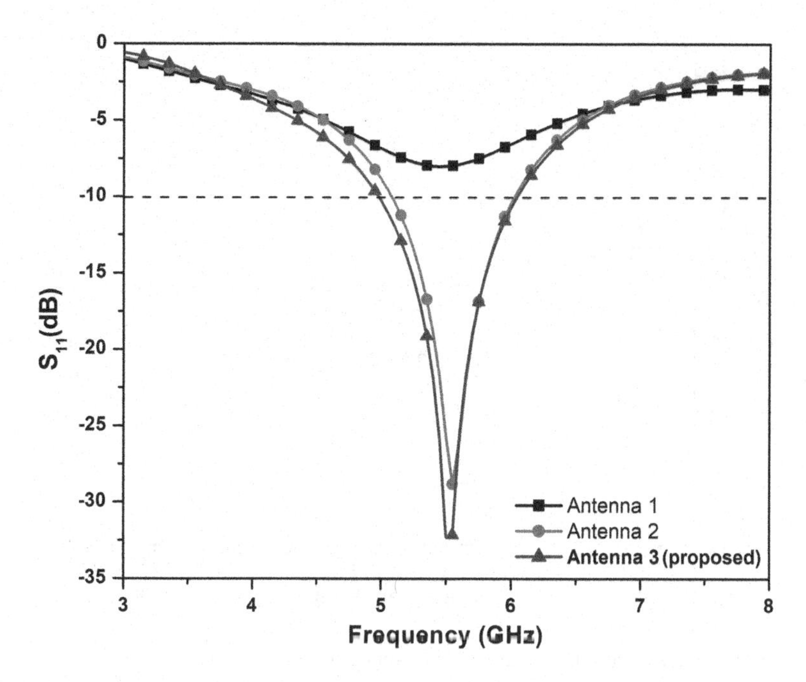

FIGURE 12.3 Variation of return losses for various design steps of the proposed antenna.

TABLE 12.2
Details of All Antennas up to Antenna 3

Type of Antennas	Resonant Frequency Bands (GHz)	Impedance Bandwidth (GHz)	Fractional Bandwidth (%)	|S11| (dB)	Peak Gain (dBi)
Antenna 1	–	–	–	–	–
Antenna 2	(5.08–6.02)	0.94	16.94	25.75	3.45
Antenna 3	(4.98–6.04)	1.06	19.24	32.24	3.50

The impedance bandwidth and Fractional Bandwidth (FBW) enhancement of 120 MHz and 2.3% are observed between Antenna 2 and our proposed antenna (Antenna 3). Return loss is improved by 6.5 dB and gain by 0.5dBi with the narrower ground plane modifications in Antenna 3 than in Antenna 2 (Table 12.2). Measured and simulated antenna gain and performance can be clearly seen in Figure 12.4, and the values are listed in Table 12.3, which shows greater gain and efficiency values for resonating frequencies of 5.20 and 5.50 GHz, other than the other frequency points.

The surface current distribution pattern at resonating frequencies of 5.20 GHz and 5.50 GHz is illustrated in Figure 12.5(b) and (c), respectively, to better comprehend the antenna's wideband performance. The current intensity is higher at 5.50 GHz (Figure 12.5(c)) and lower at 5.20 GHz, as seen in Figure 12.5(b). At 5.50 GHz, the surface current is consistently distributed in the dual arms of the fork and throughout the radiating patch area and the ground plane, resulting in a higher gain than at 5.20 GHz. The current distribution at non-resonating frequency bands of 3.00 GHz and 7.45 GHz is portrayed in Figure 12.5(a) and (d), respectively, where discontinuity in the surface electrical currents can be seen in both patch and ground plane. So the current directions are nonuniform here. The suggested design has almost omni-directional far-field patterns, as seen in Figure 12.6. The picture depicts the observed co-polar and cross-polar radiation patterns in the *y*–*z* and *x*–*z* planes at resonating frequencies of 5.20 GHz and 5.50 GHz, as well as non-resonating frequencies of 3.00 GHz and 7.45 GHz. Figure 12.7 illustrates the real and imaginary portions of the

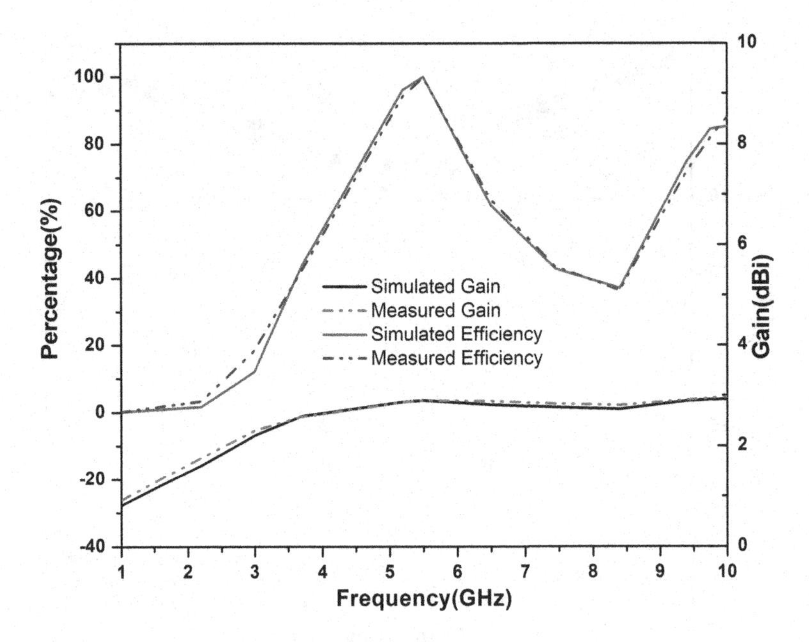

FIGURE 12.4 Measured and simulated gain and antenna efficiency of Antenna 3.

TABLE 12.3
Comparison of Simulated and Measured Gain and Antenna Efficiency Values for Antenna 2

Resonating Frequency (GHz)	Gain (dBi)		Antenna Efficiency (%)	
	Simulated	Measured	Simulated	Measured
3.00	−6.91	−5.40	12.15	18.44
5.20	3.09	3.02	96.05	94.07
5.50	3.50	3.48	99.94	99.73
7.45	1.46	2.50	42.76	43.32

input impedance with respect to frequency. The real part of the corresponding impedance is near 50 ohms at the centre frequency of 5.50 GHz, while the imaginary component is closer to 0.

12.4 PARAMETRIC ANALYSIS

The length and width of the arms of the tuning fork have a significant impact on an antenna's frequency response characteristics. In this part, a parametric study of the proposed wideband antenna was done to gain a better understanding of its behaviour.

12.4.1 Variation in the Widths of Two Arms of the Fork (*D*1 and *D*2)

When the widths of the symmetric arms of the fork *D*1 and *D*2 are increased from 1.50 mm, it is observed that the resonating frequency shifts rightwards from 5.50 GHz with degradation in return loss characteristics. When *D*1 = *D*2 is decreased from 1.50 mm, the upper-frequency level shifts rightward drastically, as seen in Figure 12.8. Simulations are carried out for various values of *D*2, keeping *D*1 fixed at 1.50 mm, and the results of return loss are shown in Figure 12.9. It is seen that

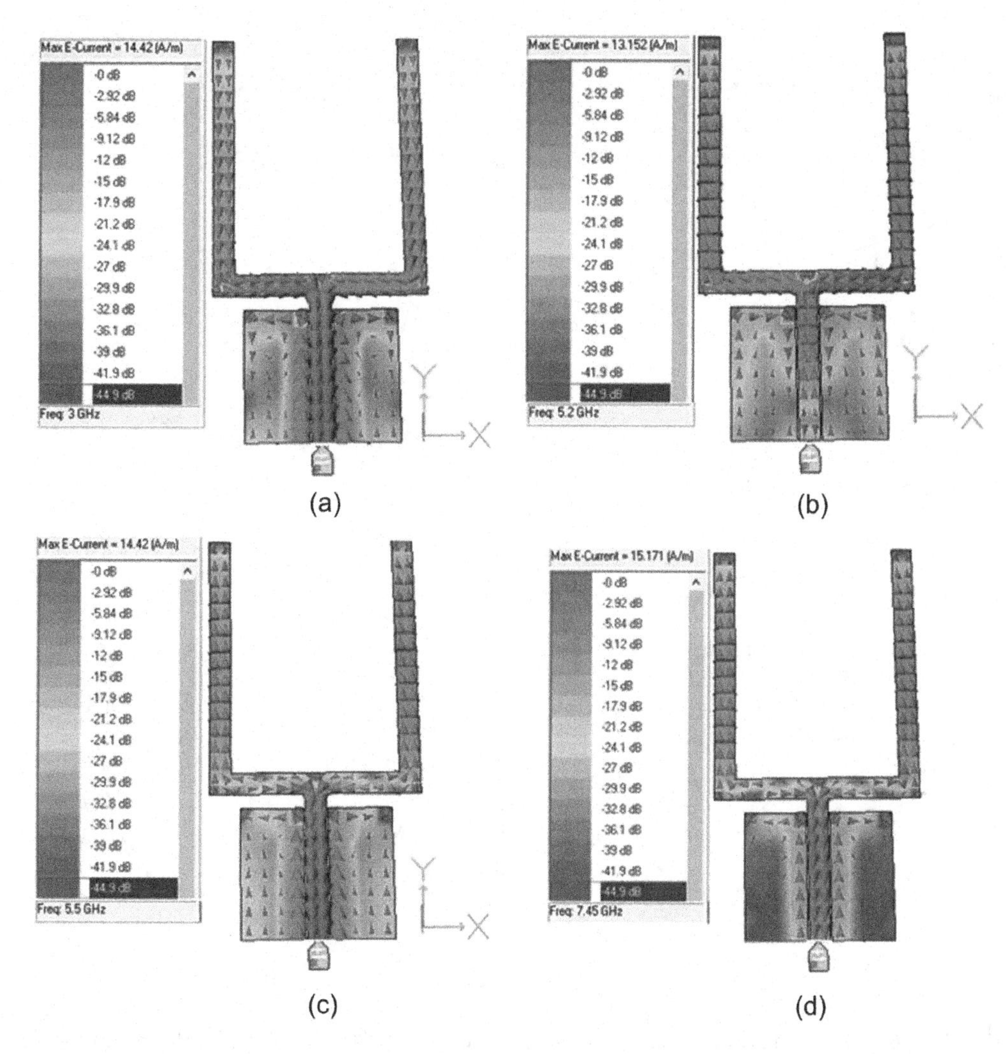

FIGURE 12.5 Surface current distribution of Antenna 3 at (a) 3.00 GHz, (b) 5.20 GHz, (c) 5.50 GHz, and (d) 7.45 GHz.

change of D2 has minimal effect on the lower frequency band, whereas an adverse effect on the higher frequency band is observed.

As both the arms of the fork are symmetric, so similar return loss characteristics can be viewed in the case of Figure 12.10, where change in D1 (keeping D2 fixed at 1.50mm) leads to a significant change in the upper resonant frequency band.

12.4.2 Effect of Using Varied Types of Substrates

The substrate material is one of the most important factors to consider when designing a body-centric wearable antenna. There are various substrate materials with varied permittivities and characteristics that are suited for specific designs and applications, such as Jeans, Nylon, Woven fibreglass fabric, and Goch. However, because it is robust (tear-resistant), durable, simple to care for, and cost-effective, this design focuses on Denim Jeans fabric as the substrate material. The S-parameter response for Jeans, Goch, Woven Fibreglass, Nylon 66, and standard FR-4 epoxy with dielectric constants of 1.78, 1.32, 2.20, 3.4, and 4.4 is shown in Figure 12.11.

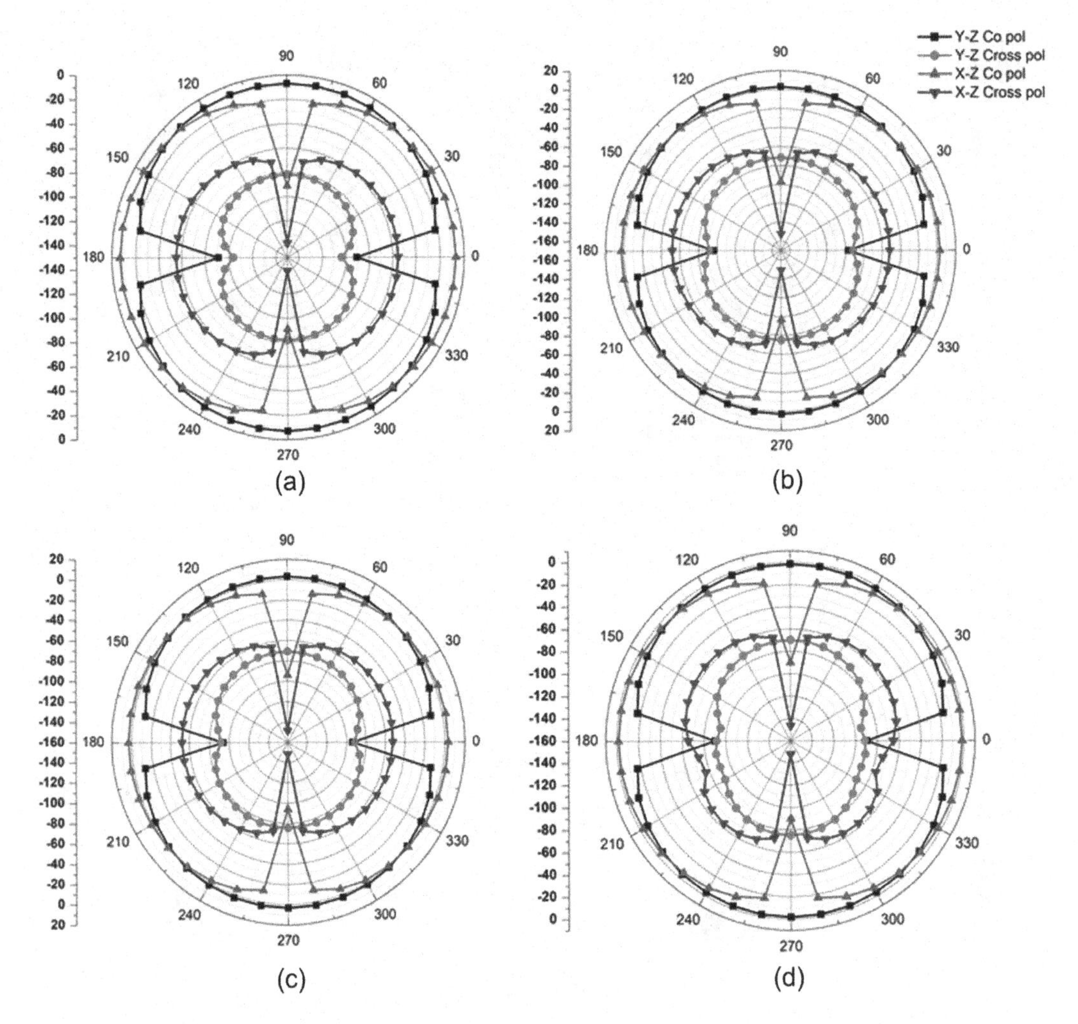

FIGURE 12.6 Measured 2D radiation pattern at (a) 3.00 GHz, (b) 5.20 GHz, (c) 5.50 GHz and (d) 7.45 GHz.

12.4.3 Effect of the Thickness of the Substrate Material

In the case of body-worn textile antennas, the thickness of the substrate material must also be chosen with care and attention for flexibility. If the thickness of the antenna is not taken into consideration, bending and mounting the antenna on a hard structure may result in a considerable loss of antenna performance. As illustrated in Figure 12.12, the thickness (*h*) is adjusted to 1.00 mm using a screw gauge, which is not excessively thick for bending issues while still providing the best S-parameter performance.

12.4.4 Variation of the Length of the Dual Arms of the Fork

The symmetric arms of the fork play a significant role in the return loss response. The length of the arms "A" is taken as 17.25 mm in the proposed design. If a reduction in the dimensions of A is performed, it is observed from Figure 12.13 that there is a right shift in the resonant frequency, which purely justifies, as we know that with an increase in resonant frequency, the length of the antenna decreases.

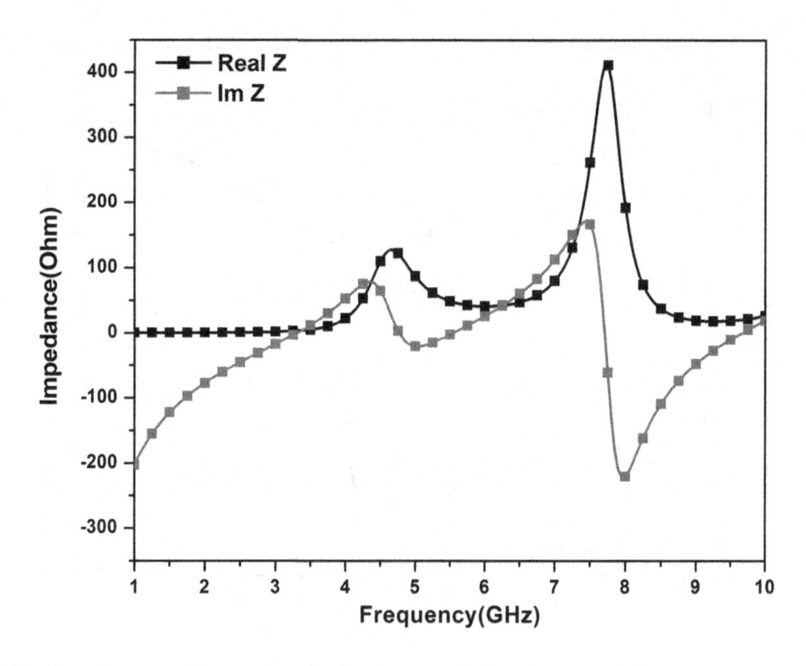

FIGURE 12.7 Impedance vs. Frequency plot for Antenna 3.

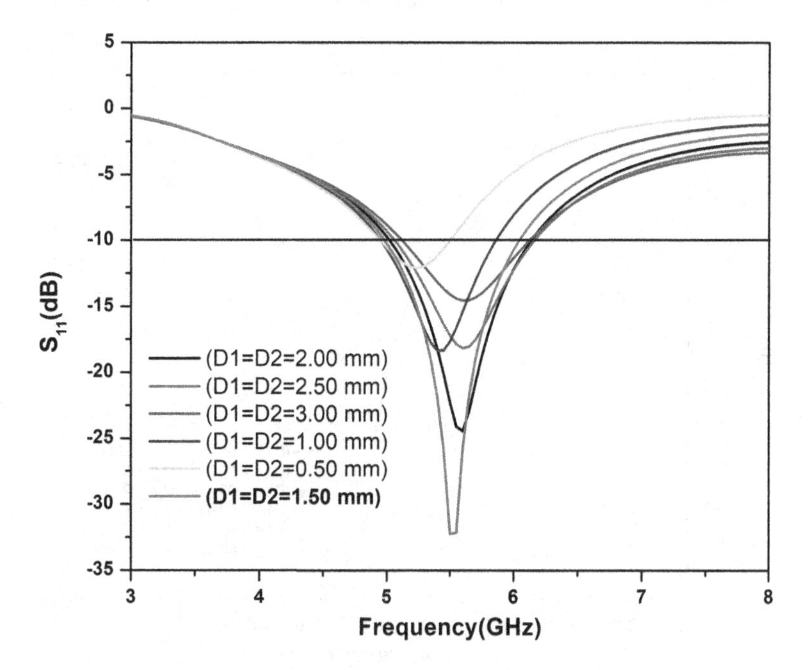

FIGURE 12.8 S-parameters response for varied values of D1 and D2.

12.4.5 Variation of Width of the Base Connecting the Two Arms of the Fork

D3 is the width of the bridge connecting the two arms of the U- shaped structure (Figure 12.1). It is observed that when D3 is fixed at 1.50 mm, we get the optimized S-parameter response as in Figure 12.14. If D3 is increased or decreased, there is a shift in the resonant frequency band and a change in the bandwidth.

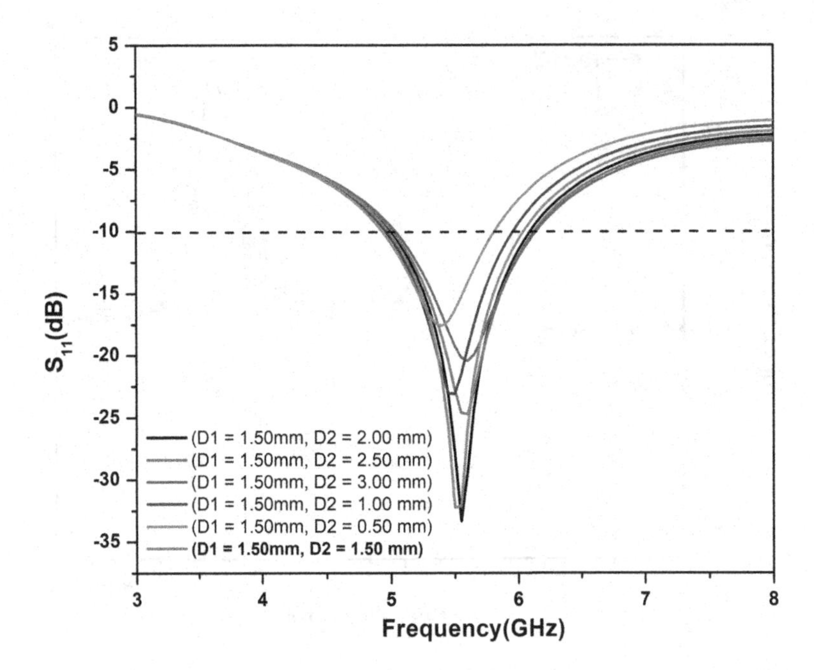

FIGURE 12.9 S-parameters vs. frequency plot by changing values of D2 (keeping Dl =1.50 mm).

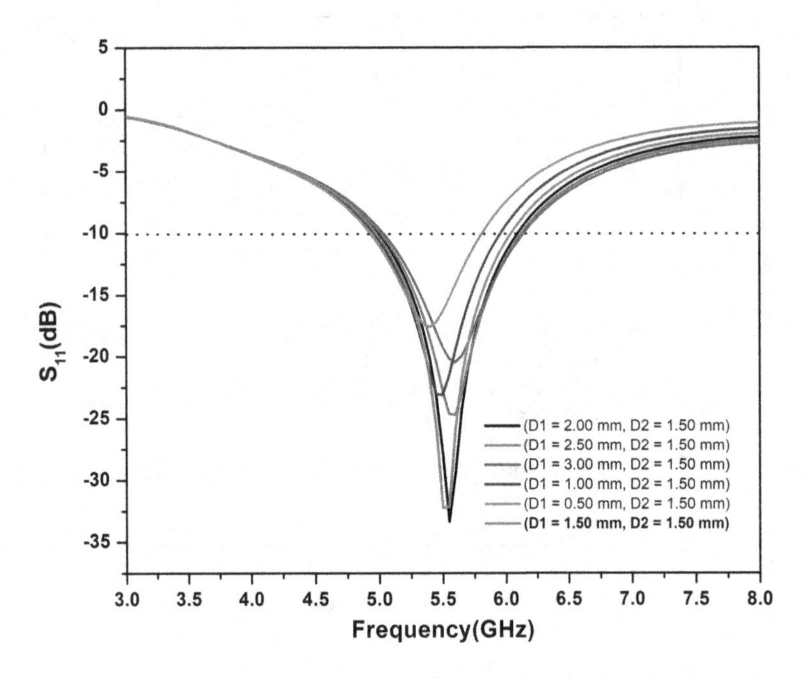

FIGURE 12.10 S11 vs. frequency curve for varied values of Dl (keeping D2 fixed at 1.50 mm).

12.4.6 Variation of Distance of the Patch from the Ground Plane

The distance of the radiating patch from the ground plane is denoted as *E* (as seen in Figure 12.1). It is an important parameter for variation of the return loss coefficient. The value of *E* is optimised and fixed to 1.00 mm to get the best return loss response at the desired frequency band, as portrayed in Figure 12.15.

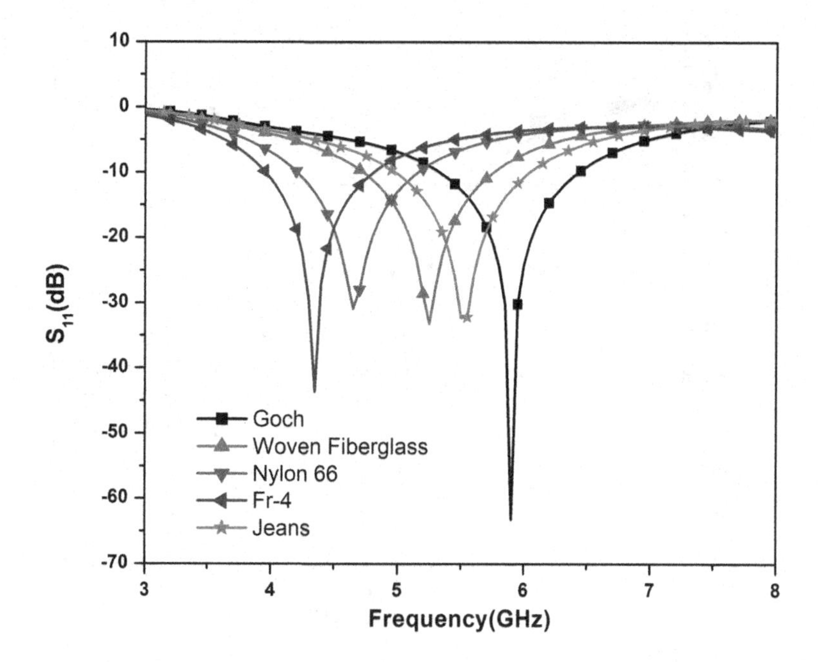

FIGURE 12.11 Comparison of S-parameters for various substrates.

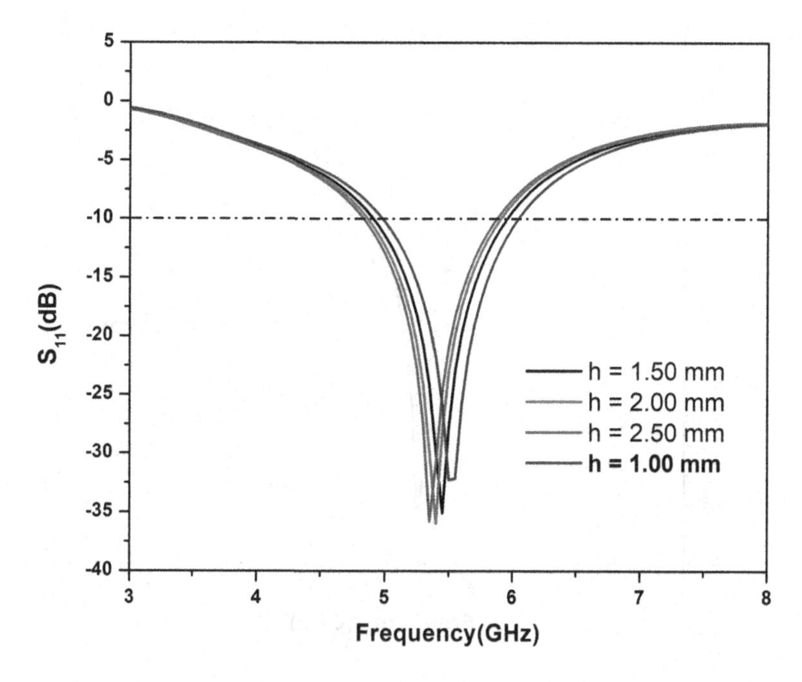

FIGURE 12.12 Comparison of return loss for variation in the thickness of the Jeans material(h).

12.5 FABRICATION AND MEASUREMENT

12.5.1 Test of Wearable Antenna at Several Positions of Human Body

The antenna is tested on the chest, thigh, and wrist, as illustrated in Figure 12.16(a, b, c) and the vector network analyser (VNA) was connected to the antenna that was being tested. The respective reflection coefficients are measured and shown in Figure 12.17, which clearly shows

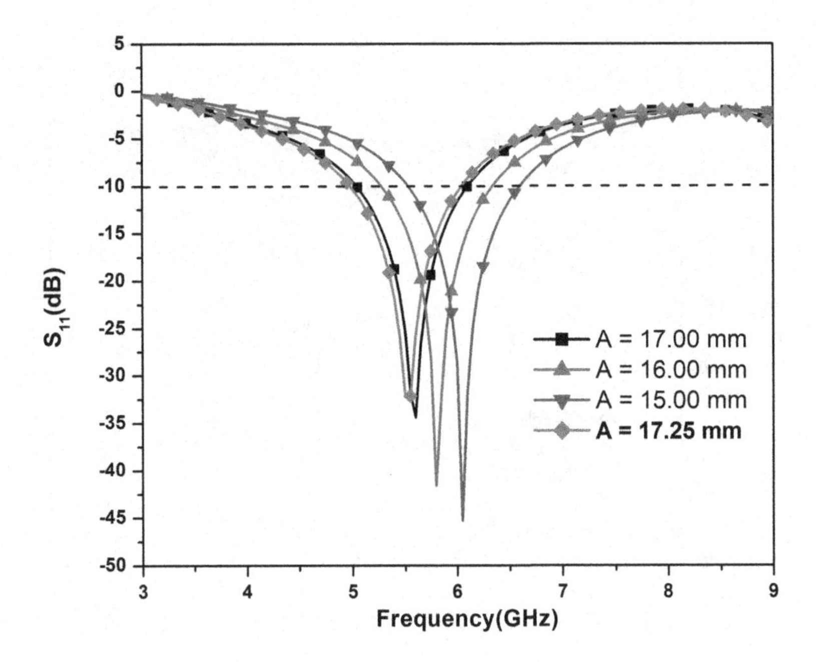

FIGURE 12.13 Variation of S-parameters for change in A.

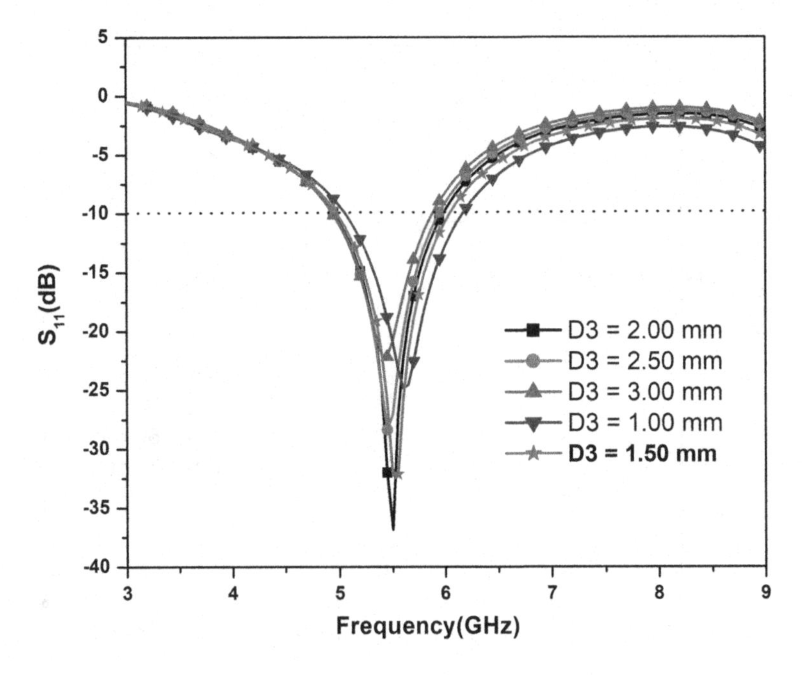

FIGURE 12.14 S-Parameter vs. frequency plot for different values of D3–

the effect of body location on antenna responses. However, all of the measured graphs show a consistent S_{11}.

12.5.2 Test of Wearable Antenna for Crumpling Conditions

As illustrated in Figure 12.18(a, bb, various crumpling effects have been applied to the antenna. Crumpling effects can degrade the performance of the antenna in terms of return loss and gain

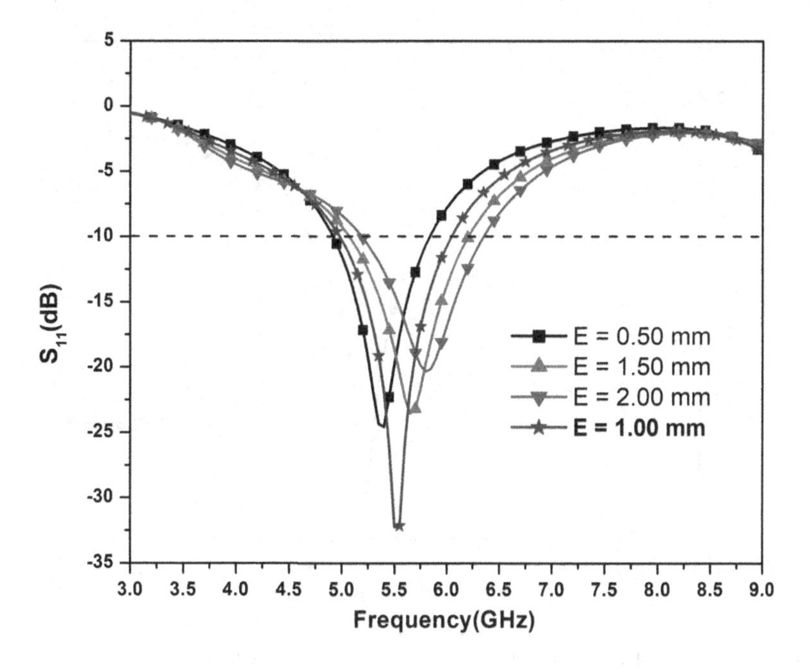

FIGURE 12.15 Return loss vs. frequency plot for different values of E.

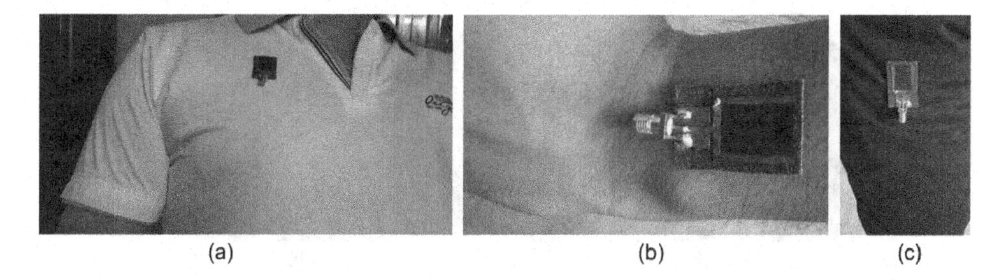

FIGURE 12.16 Fabricated antenna under test at different locations of human body (a) Chest, (b) Wrist, and (c) Thigh.

due to its deformation. As the effect of crumpling grows, it is evident from Figure 12.19 that the observed findings indicate a little right shift in the frequency band.

12.5.3 Test of Wearable Antenna for Bending Conditions

In body wearable networks, bending and structural deformation of the antenna is a typical occurrence. The bending radius of the antenna along the *y*-axis is defined by the parameter *Ry*. The upper band frequency shifts to the right when the radius *Ry* is raised from 5 mm to 20 mm, as shown in Figure 12.20.

The horizontal deformation of the antenna is defined by *Rx* (*x*-axis). When *Rx* is increased from 2.50 mm to 10.00 mm, there is a left shift in the frequency band, as shown in Figure 12.21.

Figure 12.22 depicts the fabricated wearable Jeans textile antenna. The SMA connection is designed for consistent contact to excite the antenna, minimising attenuation and reflections. Its interior dimensions are 0.25 × 0.17 inches. The antenna responses are measured using a Rohde and Schwartz Vector Network Analyser (ZVA-40). Before measuring, the VNA is calibrated to decrease or eliminate systematic errors produced by the VNA's flaws. The simulated response in Figure 12.23 validates the observed S_{11} of the manufactured textile antenna throughout a frequency band centred

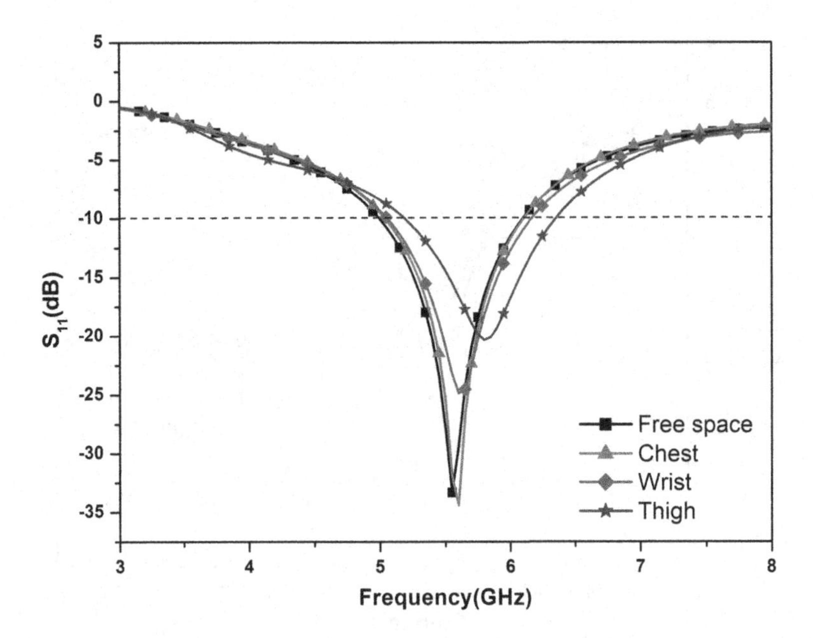

FIGURE 12.17 Measured reflection coefficients of the textile antenna at various points on the human body.

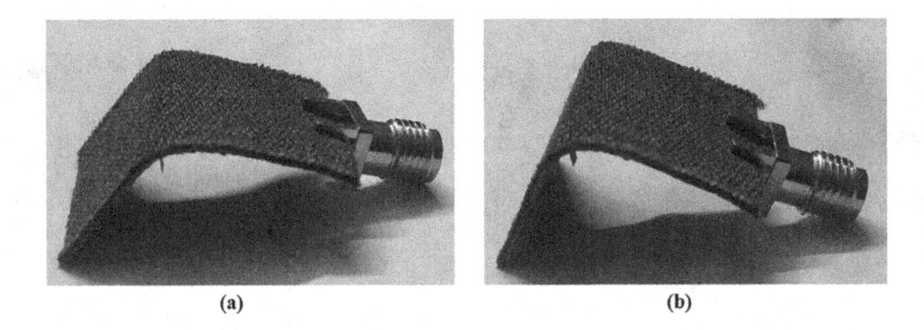

FIGURE 12.18 (a) Slight crumple (b) Severe crumple of the Jeans fabric.

at 5.50 GHz. The suggested antenna exhibits size miniaturization, gain, and bandwidth properties when compared to the most recently documented designs intended for wearable applications shown in Table 12.4.

12.6 CONCLUSION

For DSRC applications, a compact wearable antenna with dimensions of $0.311\lambda_0 \times 0.249\lambda_0 \times 0.016\lambda_0$ mm^3 was created to operate in the Wi-MAX (5.5 GHz), WLAN (5.2 GHz), 5.8G Wi-Fi, and IEEE 802.11p bands. The printed monopole design is simple, very easy to fabricate and can be mounted anywhere because of its less thickness and bending and deformation capability of the Jeans substrate. The fabricated textile antenna using Jeans substrate can be produced in large numbers than a single laboratory prototype because of its low maintenance cost, high reliability, economic purpose and good performance in terms of return loss, gain, and radiation parameters. The Jeans substrate is very durable and doesn't require regular or heavy washing like other fabrics (e.g. Cotton). It's thought to be a potential antenna for use in vehicle communication systems such as V2V, V2I, and V2X.

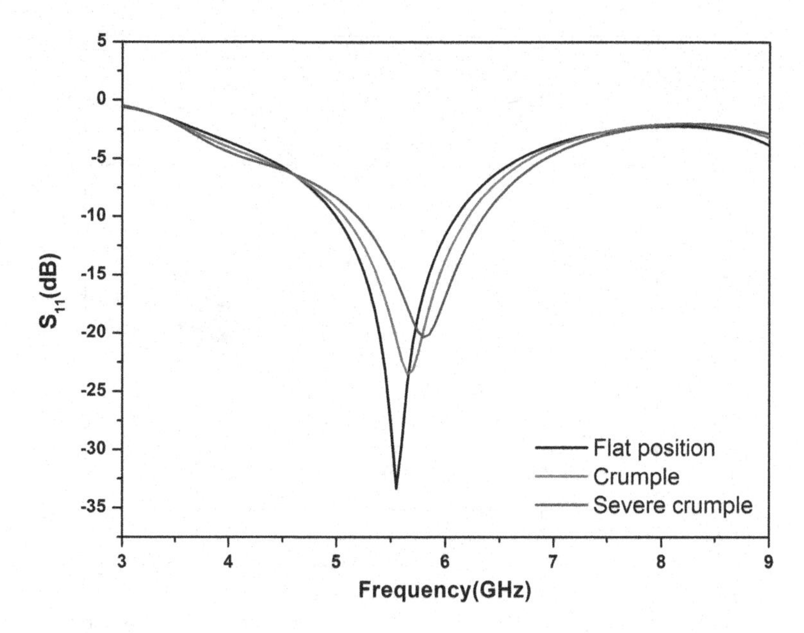

FIGURE 12.19 Reflection coefficient characteristics of the textile antenna at different crumpling circumstances.

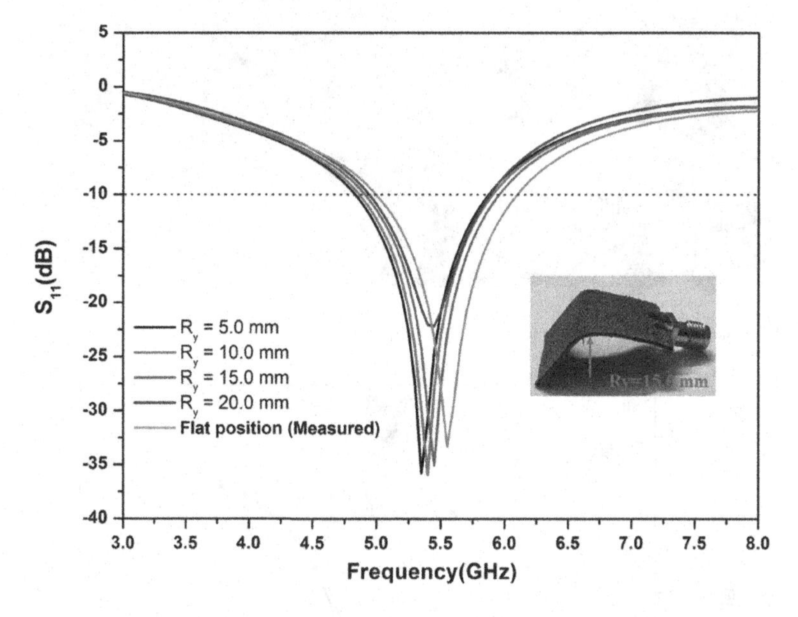

FIGURE 12.20 Measured reflection coefficient for various values of *Ry* (Inset photograph of the antenna deformed in the *y*-axis).

The ultimate goal of launching IoT technology inside this automotive sector is to provide a better level of vehicular comfort by utilising cutting-edge vehicular communications, as well as to enhance the journey with negligible travel interruptions and unpredicted incidents via smart computer-aided processing. This technology is expected to play a critical role in boosting the automotive sector's economic growth.

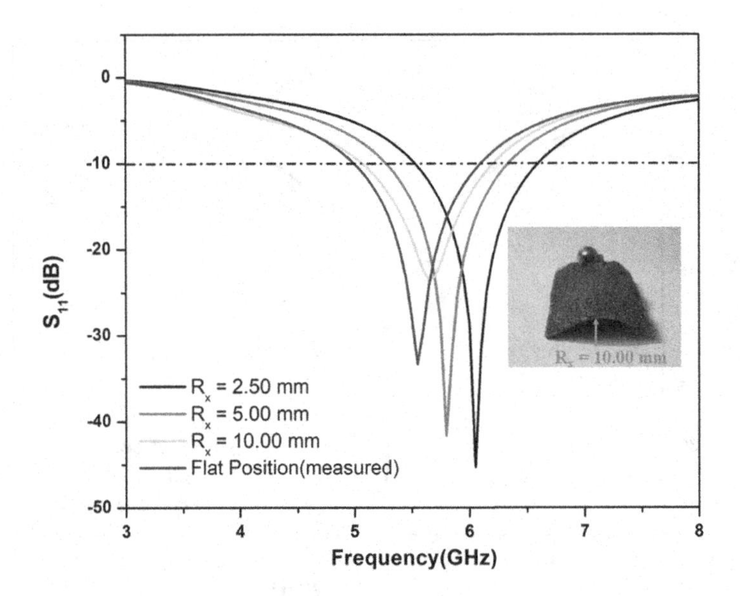

FIGURE 12.21 Measured reflection coefficient for different values of *Rx* (Inset photograph of the deformed antenna along *x*-axis).

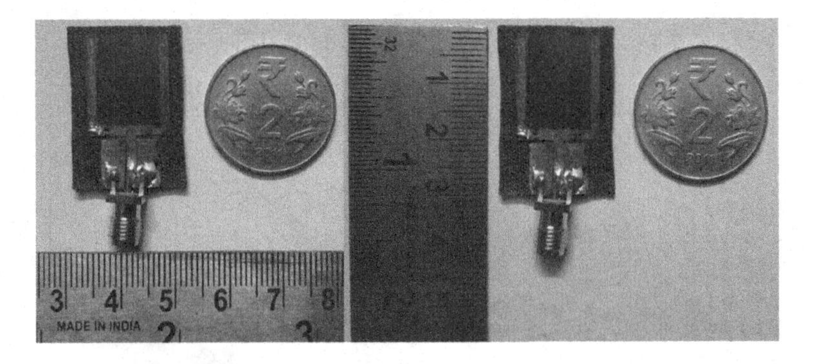

FIGURE 12.22 Photograph of the fabricated textile antenna.

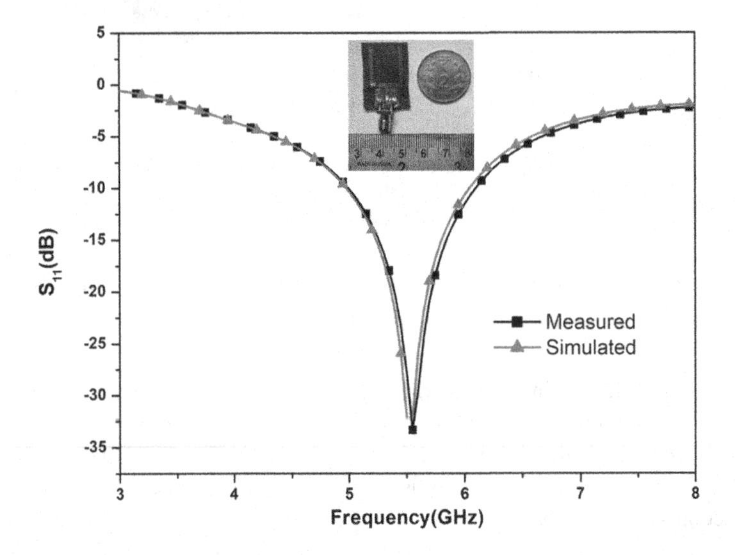

FIGURE 12.23 S-parameter curve of the antenna (measured vs. simulated).

TABLE 12.4
Contrast of the Proposed Antenna to the Current Antennas

Ref	Dimensions (in Terms of Free Space Wavelength λ_0)	Resonating Frequency (GHz)	Substrate Used	Impedance Bandwidth (GHz)	FBW (%)	Peak Gain (dBi)	Applicable Band
[28]	$0.61\lambda_0 \times 0.61\ \lambda_0 \times 0.03\ \lambda_0$	2.28–2.64	Wool ($\varepsilon_r = 1.2$)	0.36	14.63	7.3	ISM 2.4 GHz
[34]	$1.00\ \lambda_0 \times 0.84\ \lambda_0 \times 0.004\ \lambda_0$	3.5–10.6	Flexible Rogers RT/ Duroid 5880 ($\varepsilon_r = 1.67$)	7.1	100.71	4.89	UWB and WBAN
[36]	$0.70\ \lambda_0 \times 0.56\ \lambda_0 \times 0.01\ \lambda_0$	3.0–10.95	Denim ($\varepsilon_r = 1.67$)	7.95	113.98	3.57	UWB and WBAN
[37]	$0.45\ \lambda_0 \times 0.43\ \lambda_0 \times 0.007\ \lambda_0$	2.2–2.52, 3.4–3.68, 5.6–6.2, 6.5–7.0	Cotton ($\varepsilon_r = 1.65$)	0.32, 0.28, 0.60, 0.50	13.56, 7.91, 10.17, 7.41	NA	WLAN and MBAN
[38]	$0.54\ \lambda_0 \times 0.30\ \lambda_0 \times 0.012\ \lambda_0$	2.40–2.52	Semi-flexible Rogers RT/Duroid 5880	0.12	4.80	6.88	ISM 2.45 GHz
[40]	$0.36\ \lambda_0 \times 0.36\ \lambda_0 \times 0.003\lambda_0$	0.9, 1.8	Jeans ($\varepsilon_r = 1.70$)	NA	NA	1.66, 0.76 (Calculated)	GSM 900/1800
Prop	$\mathbf{0.311\lambda_0 \times 0.249\ \lambda_0 \times 0.016\ \lambda_0}$	**4.98–6.04**	**Jeans ($\varepsilon_r = 1.78$)**	**1.06**	**19.24**	**3.50**	**WI-MAX (5.5 GHz), WLAN (5.2 GHz), 5.8 GHz Wi-Fi (5.725 – 5.825 GHz), IEEE 802.11p DSRC**

REFERENCES

1. Al-Fuqaha, Ala, Mohsen Guizani, Mehdi Mohammadi, Mohammed Aledhari, and Moussa Ayyash. "Internet of things: A survey on enabling technologies, protocols, and applications." *IEEE Communications Surveys & Tutorials* 17, no. 4 (2015): 2347–2376.
2. Evans, Dave. "The internet of things: How the next evolution of the internet is changing everything." *CISCO White Paper* 1, no. 2011 (2011): 1–11.
3. Zhang, Shikai. "Spectrum analyses of UNB modulation formats." In *2013 3rd International Conference on Consumer Electronics, Communications and Networks*, pp. 594–597. IEEE, 2013.
4. Lizzi, Leonardo, and Fabien Ferrero. "Use of ultra-narrow band miniature antennas for internet-of-things applications." *Electronics Letters* 51, no. 24 (2015): 1964–1966.
5. Cetinkaya, Oktay, and Ozgur B. Akan. "Electric-field energy harvesting from lighting elements for battery-less internet of things." *IEEE Access* 5 (2017): 7423–7434.
6. Davoli, Luca, Laura Belli, Antonio Cilfone, and Gianluigi Ferrari. "From micro to macro IoT: Challenges and solutions in the integration of IEEE 802.15. 4/802.11 and sub-GHz technologies." *IEEE Internet of Things Journal* 5, no. 2 (2017): 784–793.
7. Del Barrio, S. Caporal, Pevand Bahramzy, Simon Svendsen, Ole Jagielski, and GertFrølund Pedersen. "Thermal loss in high-Q antennas." *Electronics Letters* 50, no. 13 (2014): 917–919.
8. Papadimitratos, Panos, Arnaud De La Fortelle, Knut Evenssen, Roberto Brignolo, and Stefano Cosenza. "Vehicular communication systems: Enabling technologies, applications, and future outlook on intelligent transportation." *IEEE Communications Magazine* 47, no. 11 (2009): 84–95.
9. Densmore, Arthur C., and Vahraz Jamnejad. "A satellite-tracking K-and K/sub a/-band mobile vehicle antenna system." *IEEE Transactions on Vehicular Technology* 42, no. 4 (1993): 502–513.
10. Ge, Xiaohu, Hui Cheng, Guoqiang Mao, Yang Yang, and Song Tu. "Vehicular communications for 5G cooperative small-cell networks." *IEEE Transactions on Vehicular Technology* 65, no. 10 (2016): 7882–7894.
11. He, Ruisi, Olivier Renaudin, Veli-Matti Kolmonen, Katsuyuki Haneda, Zhangdui Zhong, Bo Ai, Simon Hubert, and Claude Oestges. "Vehicle-to-vehicle radio channel characterization in crossroad scenarios." *IEEE Transactions on Vehicular Technology* 65, no. 8 (2015): 5850–5861.
12. Wong, Hang, Kwok Kan So, and Xia Gao. "Bandwidth enhancement of a monopolar patch antenna with V-shaped slot for car-to-car and WLAN communications." *IEEE Transactions on Vehicular Technology* 65, no. 3 (2015): 1130–1136.
13. Harding, John, Gregory Powell, Rebecca Yoon, Joshua Fikentscher, Charlene Doyle, Dana Sade, Mike Lukuc, Jim Simons, and Jing Wang. *Vehicle-to-Vehicle Communications: Readiness of V2V Technology for Application. No. DOT HS 812 014*. National Highway Traffic Safety Administration, 2014.
14. Jiang, Daniel, Vikas Taliwal, Andreas Meier, Wieland Holfelder, and Ralf Herrtwich. "Design of 5.9 GHz DSRC-based vehicular safety communication." *IEEE Wireless Communications* 13, no. 5 (2006): 36–43.
15. Han, Chong, Mehrdad Dianati, Rahim Tafazolli, Ralf Kernchen, and Xuemin Shen. "Analytical study of the IEEE 802.11 p MAC sublayer in vehicular networks." *IEEE Transactions on Intelligent Transportation Systems* 13, no. 2 (2012): 873–886.
16. Bazzi, Alessandro, Claudia Campolo, Barbara M. Masini, Antonella Molinaro, Alberto Zanella, and Antoine O. Berthet. "Enhancing cooperative driving in IEEE 802.11 vehicular networks through full-duplex radios." *IEEE Transactions on Wireless Communications* 17, no. 4 (2018): 2402–2416.
17. Noor-A-Rahim, Md, GG Md Nawaz Ali, Hieu Nguyen, and Yong Liang Guan. "Performance analysis of IEEE 802.11 p safety message broadcast with and without relaying at road intersection." *IEEE Access* 6 (2018): 23786–23799.
18. He, Jianhua, Zuoyin Tang, Zhong Fan, and Jie Zhang. "Enhanced collision avoidance for distributed LTE vehicle to vehicle broadcast communications." *IEEE Communications Letters* 22, no. 3 (2018): 630–633.
19. Strom, Erik G. "On medium access and physical layer standards for cooperative intelligent transport systems in Europe." *Proceedings of the IEEE* 99, no. 7 (2011): 1183–1188.
20. Huang, Chih-Yu, and En-Zo Yu. "A slot-monopole antenna for dual-band WLAN applications." *IEEE Antennas and Wireless Propagation Letters* 10 (2011): 500–502.
21. Patel, Rikikumar, and Trushit K. Upadhyaya. "Compact planar dual band antenna for WLAN application." *Progress In Electromagnetics Research Letters* 70 (2017): 89–97.
22. De, Arnab, Bappadittya Roy, and Anup Kumar Bhattacharjee. "Dual-notched monopole antenna using DGS for WLAN and Wi-MAX applications." *Journal of Circuits, Systems and Computers* 28, no. 11 (2019): 1950189.

23. Gautam, Anil K., Aditi Bisht, and Binod Kr Kanaujia. "A wideband antenna with defected ground plane for WLAN/WiMAX applications." *AEU-International Journal of Electronics and Communications* 70, no. 3 (2016): 354–358.
24. De, Arnab, Bappadittya Roy, Ankan Bhattacharya, G. V. Bharat, and Anup K. Bhattacharjee. "Compact UWB monopole antenna with WLAN and X-band satellite filtering characteristics." In *2020 International Conference on Computation, Automation and Knowledge Management (ICCAKM)*, pp. 344–347. IEEE, 2020.
25. Singh, Hari Shankar, Rahul Upadhyay, and Raed M. Shubair. "Performances study of compact printed diversity antenna in the presence of user's body for LTE mobile phone applications." *International Journal of RF and Microwave Computer-Aided Engineering* 30, no. 5 (2020): e21743.
26. Chahat, Nacer, Maxim Zhadobov, Ronan Sauleau, and Koichi Ito. "A compact UWB antenna for on-body applications." *IEEE Transactions on Antennas and Propagation* 59, no. 4 (2011): 1123–1131.
27. Ivšić, Branimir, Juraj Bartolić, Davor Bonefačić, Anja Skrivervik, and Jovanche Trajkovikj. "Design and analysis of planar UHF wearable antenna." In *2012 6th European Conference on Antennas and Propagation (EUCAP)*, pp. 1–4. IEEE, 2012.
28. Gao, Guo-Ping, Bin Hu, Shao-Fei Wang, and Chen Yang. "Wearable circular ring slot antenna with EBG structure for wireless body area network." *IEEE Antennas and Wireless Propagation Letters* 17, no. 3 (2018): 434–437.
29. Alharbi, S., R. Shubair, and A. Kiourti, "Flexible antennas for wearable applications: Recent advances and design challenges." In *Proceedings of 12th European Conference on Antennas and Propagation (EuCAP 2018)*, London, UK, April 9–14, pp. 1–2, 2018.
30. Shubair, Raed M., Amna M. AlShamsi, Kinda Khalaf, and Asimina Kiourti. "Novel miniature wearable microstrip antennas for ISM-band biomedical telemetry." In *2015 Loughborough Antennas & Propagation Conference (LAPC)*, pp. 1–4. IEEE, 2015.
31. Sankaralingam, S., and Bhaskar Gupta. "Effects of bending on impedance and radiation characteristics of rectangular wearable antenna utilizing smart clothes." *Microwave and Optical Technology Letters* 54, no. 6 (2012): 1508–1511.
32. Roy, Bappadittya, A. K. Bhattarchya, and S. K. Choudhury. "Characterization of textile substrate to design a textile antenna." In *2013 International Conference on Microwave and Photonics (ICMAP)*, pp. 1–5. IEEE, 2013.
33. Yan, Sen, and G. A. E. Vandenbosch. "Wearable antenna with tripolarisation diversity for WBAN communications." *Electronics Letters* 52, no. 7 (2016): 500–502.
34. Shafique, Kinza, Bilal A. Khawaja, Munir A. Tarar, Bilal M. Khan, Muhammad Mustaqim, and Ali Raza. "A wearable ultra-wideband antenna for wireless body area networks." *Microwave and Optical Technology Letters* 58, no. 7 (2016): 1710–1715.
35. Grilo, Marcus, Murilo Hiroaki Seko, and Fatima Salete Correra. "Wearable textile patch antenna fed by proximity coupling with increased bandwidth." *Microwave and Optical Technology Letters* 58, no. 8 (2016): 1906–1912.
36. Mustaqim, Muhammad, Bilal A. Khawaja, Hassan T. Chattha, Kinza Shafique, Muhammad J. Zafar, and Mohsin Jamil. "Ultra-wideband antenna for wearable Internet of Things devices and wireless body area network applications." *International Journal of Numerical Modelling: Electronic Networks, Devices and Fields* 32, no. 6 (2019): e2590.
37. Hosseini Varkiani, Seyed Mohsen, and Majid Afsahi. "Grounded CPW multi-band wearable antenna for MBAN and WLAN applications." *Microwave and Optical Technology Letters* 60, no. 3 (2018): 561–568.
38. Abbasi, Muhammad Ali Babar, Symeon Simos Nikolaou, Marco A. Antoniades, Marija Nikolić Stevanović, and Photos Vryonides. "Compact EBG-backed planar monopole for BAN wearable applications." *IEEE Transactions on Antennas and Propagation* 65, no. 2 (2016): 453–463.
39. Ferreira, David, Pedro Pires, Ruben Rodrigues, and Rafael FS Caldeirinha. "Wearable textile antennas: Examining the effect of bending on their performance." *IEEE Antennas and Propagation Magazine* 59, no. 3 (2017): 54–59.
40. Sundarsingh, Esther Florence, Sangeetha Velan, Malathi Kanagasabai, Aswathy K. Sarma, Chinnambeti Raviteja, and M. Gulam Nabi Alsath. "Polygon-shaped slotted dual-band antenna for wearable applications." *IEEE Antennas and Wireless Propagation Letters* 13 (2014): 611–614.
41. Ahmed, M. I., M. F. Ahmed, and A. A. Shaalan. "Investigation of electrical properties of fully wearable antenna for ISM applications." In *2018 22nd International Microwave and Radar Conference (MIKON)*, pp. 155–158. IEEE, 2018.

42. Aloi, Daniel N., Manuel Possa, Adham Barghouti, Jeff Tlusty, and Mohammad S. Sharawi. "Printed DSRC antennas for enhanced gain coverage towards front and rear of vehicle for automotive applications." In *2014 IEEE-APS Topical Conference on Antennas and Propagation in Wireless Communications (APWC)*, pp. 349–352. IEEE, 2014.
43. Varum, Tiago, João N. Matos, Ricardo Abreu, and Pedro Pinho. "Non-uniform microstrip antenna array for Rx DSRC communications." In *2014 IEEE Antennas and Propagation Society International Symposium (APSURSI)*, pp. 1071–1072. IEEE, 2014.
44. Ghafari, Elias, Andreas Fuchs, Diana Eblenkamp, and Daniel N. Aloi. "A vehicular rooftop, shark-fin, multiband antenna for the GPS/LTE/cellular/DSRC systems." In *2014 IEEE-APS Topical Conference on Antennas and Propagation in Wireless Communications (APWC)*, pp. 237–240. IEEE, 2014.
45. Liou, Chong-Yi, Shau-Gang Mao, Tsun-Chieh Chiang, and Chia-Tai Tsai. "Compact and low-profile conical antenna for automotive DSRC application." In *2016 IEEE International Symposium on Antennas and Propagation (APSURSI)*, pp. 117–118. IEEE, 2016.
46. Rahim, Md Abdur, Md Arafatur Rahman, Md Mustafizur Rahman, A. Taufiq Asyhari, Md Zakirul Alam Bhuiyan, and D. Ramasamy. "Evolution of IoT-enabled connectivity and applications in automotive industry: A review." *Vehicular Communications* 27 (2021): 100285.
47. Sharma, Surbhi, and Baijnath Kaushik. "A survey on internet of vehicles: Applications, security issues & solutions." *Vehicular Communications* 20 (2019): 100182.
48. Krishnan, G. Vidhya, M. Valan Rajkumar, and D. Umakirthika. "Role of internet of things in smart passenger cars." *International Journal of Engineering And Computer Science (IJECS)* 6, no. 5 (2017): 21410–21417.
49. Jurgen, Ronald. *V2V/V2I Communications for Improved Road Safety and Efficiency.* SAE, 2012.
50. Rahman, Kazi Atiqur, and Kemal E. Tepe. "Towards a cross-layer based MAC for smooth V2V and V2I communications for safety applications in DSRC/WAVE based systems." In *2014 IEEE Intelligent Vehicles Symposium Proceedings*, pp. 969–973. IEEE, 2014.
51. Tahmasbi-Sarvestani, Amin, Hossein Nourkhiz Mahjoub, Yaser P. Fallah, Ehsan Moradi-Pari, and Oubada Abuchaar. "Implementation and evaluation of a cooperative vehicle-to-pedestrian safety application." *IEEE Intelligent Transportation Systems Magazine* 9, no. 4 (2017): 62–75.
52. Wu, Celimuge, Tsutomu Yoshinaga, Yusheng Ji, and Yan Zhang. "Computational intelligence inspired data delivery for vehicle-to-roadside communications." *IEEE Transactions on Vehicular Technology* 67, no. 12 (2018): 12038–12048.
53. Jomaa, Diala, Siril Yella, and Mark Dougherty. "A comparative study between vehicle activated signs and speed indicator devices." *Transportation Research Procedia* 22 (2017): 115–123.
54. Endo, Masayuki, and Kenji Tanaka. "Evaluation of storage capacity of electric vehicles for vehicle to grid considering driver's perspective." In *2018 IEEE International Conference on Environment and Electrical Engineering and 2018 IEEE Industrial and Commercial Power Systems Europe (EEEIC/I&CPS Europe)*, pp. 1–5. IEEE, 2018.
55. World Health Organization. *Global Status Report on Road Safety 2015.* World Health Organization, 2015.
56. Jia, Xiaolin, Quanyuan Feng, Taihua Fan, and Quanshui Lei. "RFID technology and its applications in Internet of Things (IoT)." In *2012 2nd International Conference on Consumer Electronics, Communications and Networks (CECNet)*, pp. 1282–1285. IEEE, 2012.
57. Farrell D. O', R. Veldman, K. Schofield, *Vehicle Global Positioning System.* 1999, https://patentimages.storage.googleapis.com/53/1d/3d/1375f7ff9b4c89/US8355853.pdf.
58. Nusser, Rene, and Rodolfo Mann Pelz. "Bluetooth-based wireless connectivity in an automotive environment." In *Vehicular Technology Conference Fall 2000. IEEE VTS Fall VTC2000. 52nd Vehicular Technology Conference (Cat. No. 00CH37152)*, vol. 4, pp. 1935–1942. IEEE, 2000.
59. Oesterling, Christopher. "Method and system for implementing a vehicle WiFi Access point gateway." *U.S. Patent Application 10/809,083*, filed September 29, 2005.
60. Zhu, Xiaochun, and Yachen Zhang. "An IOT based car-bus for the 4WIDIS EV." In *2011 International Conference on Electrical and Control Engineering*, pp. 3343–3345. IEEE, 2011.

13 A Review on Wearable Antenna Design for IoT and 5G Applications

Debarati Ghosh, Ankan Bhattacharya, Arnab Nandi and Ujjal Chakraborty

CONTENTS

DOI: 10.1201/9781003217398-13

13.1 INTRODUCTION

Communication is a very crucial part of the advancement of technology. So far, the communication technology is concerned with rapid growth in demand of coverage area, channel capacity and different application-based domains, technologies are tending in smart mode. Antenna is an integral part of communication technology that could be wireless or wearable. With advancement of recent gadgets, communication is approaching to wireless-wearable form. For the requirement of a more effective and compatible communication range, body-centric wireless communication evolved in the form of off-body, on-body or in-body conditions. On-body communication includes transmitting or receiving through an antenna housed on the body by using wearable devices. Whereas in an in-body system, one implantable sensor antenna is placed inside the body. The present research trend is a wearable antenna for 5G (in the frequency range of sub-6 GHz and 24.25 GHz & above), Internet of things (IoT), telemedicine application and others. IoT refers to the network of physical objects "things" cascaded with different sensors, software and other compatible technologies with the aim of connecting and exchanging data with other devices. IoT frequency bands use 4.33GHz, 915 MHz and 2.4GHz to 5GHz. It is preferable to have a compact, flexible, low-cost wearable antenna design. A microstrip patch antenna is one of them which can meet those demands. Basically, a wearable antenna is a textile-based antenna. Textile material could be silk, wool, denim, felt etc. In this chapter, application-oriented textile-based wearable antenna design, analysis aspects and fabrication methods have been discussed.

13.2 TYPES OF WEARABLE ANTENNA

Wearable antennas are a major segment of every wearable 5G, and IoT applications. Different types of printed antennas are considered to be wearable antennas, including microstrip antenna, printed dipole, printed loop, monopole and planar inverted-F antennas (PIFAs).

13.2.1 MICROSTRIP PATCH ANTENNA

The radiating metal strip (Patch) is placed on the substrate. Being a two-dimensional structure, the patch antennas have a simple constructional feature with inherent design and manufacturing flexibility. They have additional advantageous features like conformation characteristics suitable to planar and non-planar surfaces, ability to allow linear and circular polarization etc. Furthermore, they are adaptable to modern printed circuit fabrication technology.

13.2.2 MONOPOLE ANTENNA

A monopole antenna is a straight rod-shaped conductor mounted on a physical ground plane. Monopole antennas are suitable in compact area due to their smaller size. Light weight, ease of fabrication, low production cost, and low-profile configuration drive designing wearable antenna and also offer flexibility for making smart antenna by integrating into garments.

13.2.3 PRINTED DIPOLE ANTENNA

Some special features of Dipole Antenna e.g. polarization purity, ease of fabrication, wide frequency range, printed dual arms on two sides of a dielectric-loaded substrate, substantially large bandwidth coverage etc. have attracted antenna manufacturers.

13.2.4 PRINTED LOOP ANTENNA

A circular or square or any other closed geometric form is the basic shape of printed loop antennas with single or multiple loops. In transmission and reception, large and small loop antennas are used but small loop antennas are preferred in reception. Though these antennas are fairly popular in the military and other areas, the poor efficiency overshadows their advantages to some extent.

13.2.5 PIFA

As the name suggests, PIFA has an inverted F like look. It finds many applications in the portable smart device segment. Compact size, fair specific absorption rate (SAR) value, dual-band functionality of this antenna have made it ideal for wearable forms.

13.3 MATERIAL USED IN WEARABLE ANTENNA

Wearable antennas are designed with two components namely conductive-material and flexible substrate. With respect to the applicability criteria, material choice is an integral part of designing an antenna as proper material provides requisite protection to EM radiation and ability to withstand various mechanical deformations. Apart from these, properly selected materials may neutralize non-friendly environmental incidents like a rainy storm, snowfall etc.

13.3.1 Conductive Material

Conductive materials are classified into two groups: rigid and flexible. Copper, silver and aluminium are considered suitable rigid conductors [1]. Flexible graphite film, carbon nanotube (CNT), fluorinated graphene are found to be some effective flexible conductive materials. Since polymer composites like popular flexible conductive materials used are textile, ink, liquid, graphene (FG), graphite (FGF), carbon nanotube (CNT) etc. Right at this moment, we should recall that polymer composites like PDMS-coated silica nanoparticles [2,3] and polymer yarns [4] provide suitable stretchability and flexibility and minimize loss, which qualify them as right flexible materials appropriate for wearable applications. Recent researches have highlighted the high-tensile strength, fabrication viability and hydrophobic properties of some polymer-based materials impregnated with conductive nanoparticles of gold, copper and silver having good potential for different applications [5].

There are some salient properties conductive materials must have for their use in the construction of wearable antennas. :-

- High degree of conductivity
- Ability of stretching, bending and irregular folding without losing mechanical properties
- Inertness to the environmental factors (which causes deterioration of constructional material)
- Compatible tensile strength (to withstand mechanical stress)
- Features for textile integration (for ease of sewing)

13.3.2 Substrate

Substrate material provides mechanical support to the conductive element of the antenna for improvement in radiation characteristics. This mechanically supportive nature is needed in a wearability feature. Depending on the properties of conductive material for designing a wearable antenna, different types of flexible substrates are used. Materials of low permittivity with low loss tangent have been reported to have enhanced the performance of wearable antennas. Many natural fibres have been investigated for their suitability in wearable antennas [6,7]. Other low cost and easily accessible substrate materials are reported to be effective in their use in wearable antennas [8]. The use of special grade hyper-elastic and transparent polymers like SOLARIS and ECOFLEX are gaining high demand, as they ensure an effectively strong bond between the textile and substrate. It is to note that ECOFLEX, the ultra-soft material, has unique conformational characteristics which make it suitable for fixing on human skin directly. A variety of polymer substrates are used for the construction of liquid metal (e.g. Galistan) antenna in its wearable application.

13.4 SELECTION CRITERIA OF SUBSTRATE FOR WEARABLE ANTENNA

Suitable substrates for any application are characterized by dielectric constant. It is worth recalling the expression of the dielectric constant $\epsilon=\epsilon_0\epsilon_r$, the vacuum permittivity,$\epsilon_0=8.854\times10^{-12}$.

F/m or ϵ_r is the relative permittivity [9]. Textile materials (as substrate) to be used in the antenna design, the role of their dielectric properties (e.g. dielectric constant and loss tangent) are very important in deciding the antenna performance [10]. In general, the dielectric properties depend on the frequency, environment temperature, surface roughness [11] and also purity and homogeneity of the concerned material; the moisture content is the influencing factor of dielectric constant. Dielectric constant is a function of the temperature. Increase in temperature results in increase in the dielectric constant. This is due to the increased mobility of polar molecules that permit them to align more easily with the electric field. The dielectric constant value is sensitive to efficiency and high gain of an antenna. A low dielectric constant provides better impedance bandwidth of the antenna due to a reduction in surface wave losses, which influences wave propagation within the substrates. As far as the antenna substrate is concerned, the dielectric constant bears great importance during its selection.

13.4.1 Thickness of Substrate

Textiles being a compressible material the thickness of this substrate is a challengeable issue in wearable technology. Since the antenna is integrated onto clothes or attached to the human body, with pressure caused by the diverse movements of the human body, the thickness of the substrate is changed. So, the thickness of the substrate plays an important role in antenna performance. As a ready reference, the thickness "h" of the substrate is calculated as $0.003\lambda\leq h\leq0.005\lambda$, with being the λ guided wavelength. The value of "h" has a bearing on the Q-factor of radiation.

$$Q\propto 1/h \qquad \left[\text{For thin substrates}\right]$$

So with an increase in the height of the substrate, the Q-factor drops. Predictably using a thicker substrate larger antenna bandwidth (BW) (to note Q= 1/BW) may be achieved [12]. This is because of the fact that with an increase in the aperture between the patch and the ground planes of the antenna, the Q-factor decreases.

13.5 DESIGN PROCEDURE

To initiate the design process, based on various properties like electrical conductivity (for conductive materials) and permittivity and loss tangent (for dielectric materials) first comes the selection of the materials to be associated with the design of flexible and wearable antennas. Antenna (radiating element) and feeding structures are then used in the next stage utilizing the gathered data, followed by simulation and optimization at the penultimate stage. The design is then given physical form with the help of a suitable fabrication technique. For picking up a suitable fabrication technique, the developer has to consider the characteristics of material and must go through the critical study of antenna topology.

The designed fabricated antenna of a wearable category has to go through different phases of performance tests, which will reveal its performance characteristics like radiation patterns, S-parameters, specific absorption rate (SAR), efficiency etc. But all these are not sufficient proof of compatibility of the designed antenna in wearable applications. For this additional qualitative test must be conducted. A few important tests worth mentioning are the durability test, bending effect

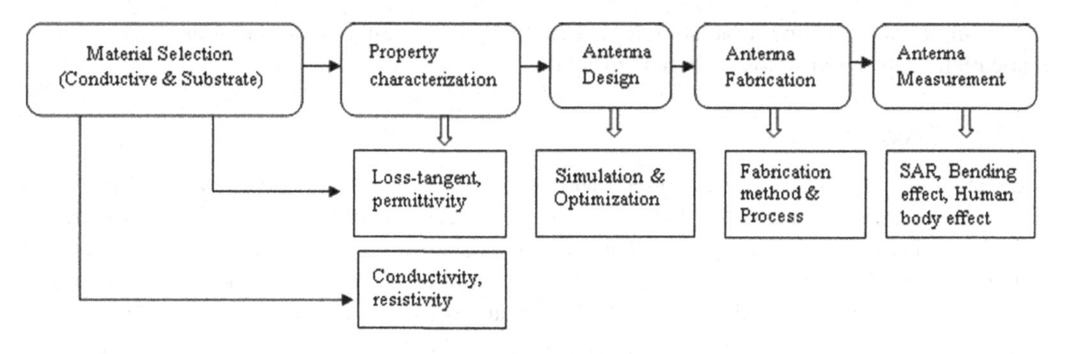

FIGURE 13.1 Design steps.

test, robustness test, humidity test, and thermal test. The secondary tests project the technical and application-oriented viability of the designed antenna in a more profound manner. Design steps are shown in Figure 13.1.

13.6 DESIGN OF WEARABLE ANTENNA (FOR IOT APPLICATION)

13.6.1 Design 1

A partial ground plane-based hexagonal-shaped patch antenna operating on 2.6 GHz and 5.2 GHz bands has been proposed in the study of Kumar and Mathur [13]. The ground plane under reference is rectangular shape. To enhance the bandwidth, slot has been created in the partial ground plane. The proposed elliptical patch is having six segments. Structural flexibility has been reported by the authors using substrates ethylene-vinyl acetate and Felt. Felt material with loss tangent 0.044 is positioned above the partial ground plane. Another substrate, EVA foam, is stacked on Felt substrate acrylic. In this design, microstrip feed line is used. The proposed antenna is applicable in the IoT domain. The antenna offers reflection coefficient of −13 dB at 2.6 GHz and −11 dB at 5.2 GHz. 160 MHz bandwidth is reported at first resonance (2.6 GHz) and 75 MHz at second resonance (5.2 GHz). The measured SAR value is 1.33 mW/gm for 1 gm of human tissue, which is fairly acceptable for wearable applications. CST software has been used for the simulation of this designed wearable antenna.

13.6.2 Design 2

In [14], a 60 GHz compact and flexible mm-Wave wearable antenna is proposed. The designed antenna has two U-shaped slotted radiating patches with a rectangular loop. A flexible printed circuit board has been incorporated to maintain ideal mechanical properties for wearable devices. Microstrip feedline is used in this design. This simulation of a designed antenna in CST software projects bandwidth in the range of 8.4 GHz with a 9.6 dBi gain, which is useful for IoT applications.

13.6.3 Design 3

Semi-circular antenna with a half-mode substrate-integrated waveguide (HMSIW) has been reported in the study of Banerjee et al. [15]. The operating frequency of the designed antenna is 5.8 GHz, which is an IoT compatible frequency band. Substrate-integrated waveguide offers high efficiency with minimum dimension. The paper mentions jeans as chosen substrate. The three-layered SIW structure consists of the dielectric substrate jeans sandwiched between the conductive ground plane and the semi-circular patch. It uses rows of inter-connecting cylindrical via of 1 mm diameter at the edges of the semi-circular patch. The antenna is designed and simulated in HFSS software. Coaxial feeding is employed in this design. The distance between the *Via* centres is kept at 1.5 mm to have minimum radiation loss. This SIW structure-based design offers cost-effective fabrication, –18 dB return loss with 6.02 dBi gain.

13.6.4 Design 4

A double C-shaped meta-material unit-cell with polypropylene substrate (non-woven category geo-textile) material is designed in the study of Selvan [16]. Meta-material is an artificial material developed by realizing physical properties that are non-existent in natural material [17]. Availability of the polypropylene sheets of desirable thickness light weight etc. are the additional advantages offered by this substrate. In this design, double negative ($\varepsilon < 0$ and $\mu < 0$)or left –handed medium is used. Polypropylene substrate is a copper patch, and the radiating element uses a thickness of 0.035 mm. The designed antenna offers bandwidth of 9.8–10.6 GHz and 4.8–6.1 GHz. IoT frequency band suitably falls under this category. Meta-material-based antenna provides size reduction of the antenna with improved antenna performance.

13.6.5 Design 5

In the study of Biswas and Chakraborty [18], Jeans substrate-based Multiple Input Multiple Output (MIMO) category antenna is presented with two copper patches of rectangular shape. When a single "I"-shaped stub is used, the frequency band of the proposed antenna ranges from 1.85 to 5.87 GHz with poor port isolation. To deal with this problem, two series of interconnected etched "I"-shaped stubs are incorporated on the ground surface, which showed improved port isolation. The antenna is designed and simulated in HFSS software. Bandwidth enhancement and reduced interference are important in mobile communication for better performance. The introduction of two "I"-shaped stubs, as mentioned earlier, has improved those parameters, as demonstrated by their wide frequency range (1830–8000 MHz) performance with port-to-port isolation at a high value. The design adopts a microstrip filtering mechanism to simulate the stop band filtering effect. This antenna is useful for IoT applications. Figures 13.2 and 13.3 show the picture of the MIMO antennas.

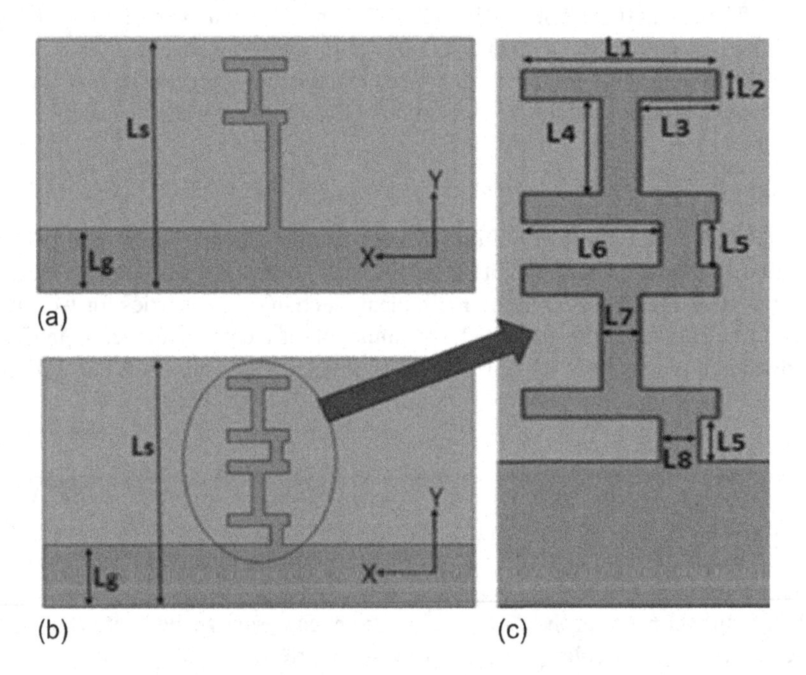

FIGURE 13.2 MIMO antenna bottom layer showing (a) single "I" stubs, (b) double "I" stub and (c) configuration of the double "I" stub (Source: [18], Copyright (2019) Wiley).

13.6.6 Design 6

A wearable antenna (dual wideband) with on/off body communications features and made of metamaterial is designed in the study of Roy and Chakraborty [19] on the jeans substrate with 50-ohm microstrip feed line. The design is simulated and analysed with different substrate heights using HFSS software. The paper reports that higher the value of substrate-height, better the performance is. The antenna (with the highest substrate height) introduces 2.4–2.48 GHz and 5.15–5.85 GHz frequency range suitable for WLAN and IoT applications. Bending analysis for the effect of bandwidth change on the designed antenna performance is reported in chest, arm and leg positions. It is observed that the chest position provides a better result. The designed antenna provides an omnidirectional pattern. Figures 13.4–13.6 show the picture of the proposed antennas.

13.7 DESIGN OF WEARABLE ANTENNA (FOR 5G APPLICATIONS)

13.7.1 Design 1

In the study of Sharma et al. [20], the designed antenna patch consists of a circular ring section with a cut diamond. The operating frequency is 28 GHz. The fabric jeans material is used as substrate. The antenna patch is made of thin-film copper foil. The design is done in FEKO software. The parametric analysis is done based on microstrip line width, length of the transmission line, and smaller circle radius. It is seen that with an increase in the value of the circular radius, a shift in resonant

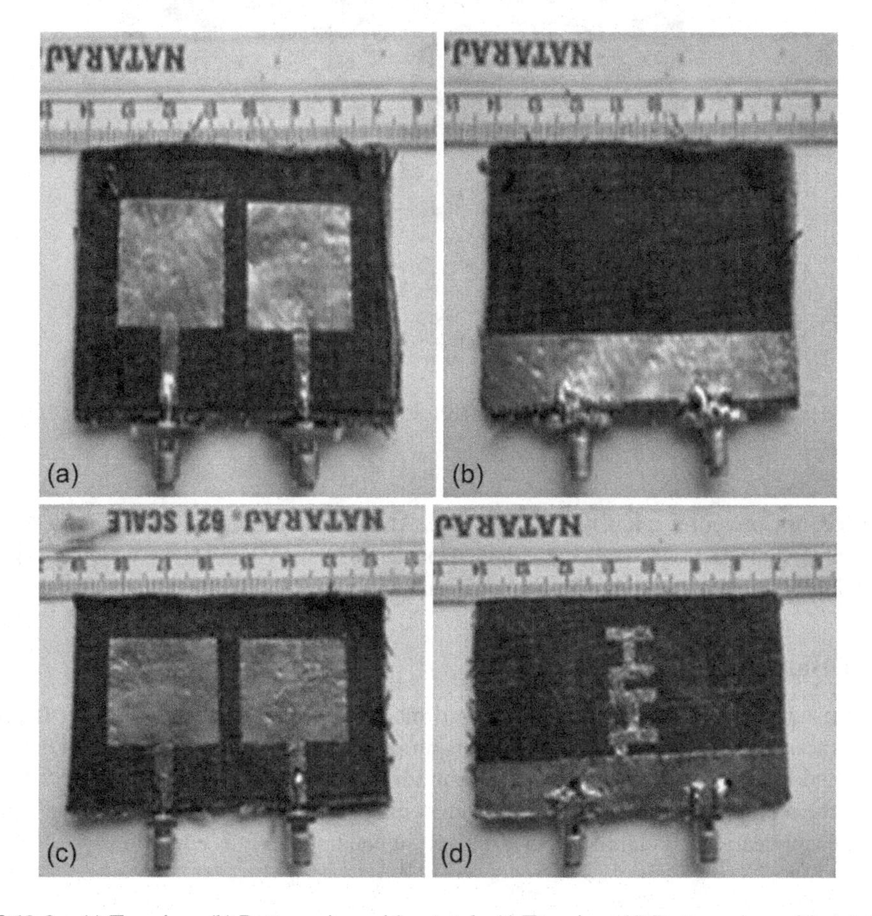

FIGURE 13.3 (a) Top view; (b) Bottom view without stub; (c) Top view; (d) Bottom view with a stub of fabricated MIMO antenna (Source: [18], Copyright (2019) Wiley).

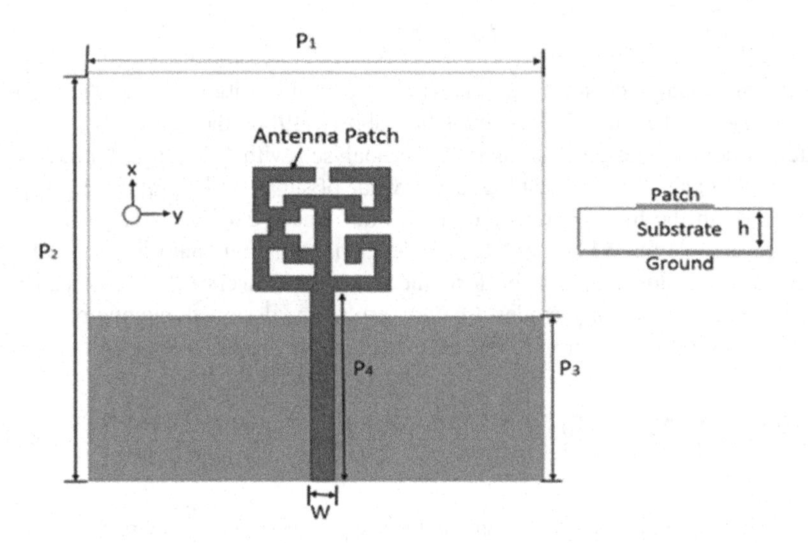

FIGURE 13.4 Geometry of the wearable Antenna (Source: [19], Copyright (2019) Springer).

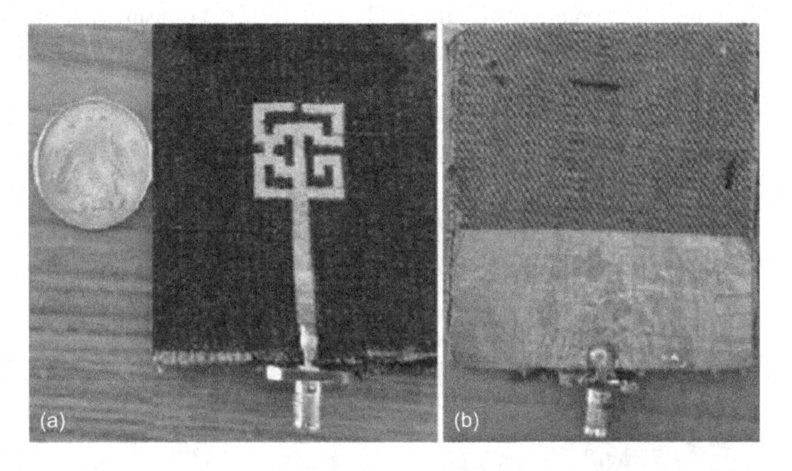

FIGURE 13.5 (a) Top and (b) Bottom view of fabricated prototype of antenna (Source: [19], Copyright (2019) Springer)

frequency occurs, providing a low return loss value. At optimum radius, return loss is 59.61 dB. The designed antenna offers a wide frequency range from 21.18 GHz to 36.59 GHz, which covers the 5G frequency band. One advantage of this design is that it requires less space.

13.7.2 Design 2

Polyethylene terephthalate (PET) substrate-based modified microstrip patch antenna is proposed with a thickness of 0.125 mm for 5G applications in [21]. Its novel fabrication method uses an ink-jet printer and highly effective conductive ink in admixture with silver nanoparticles. The paper referred to use a co-planar waveguide for good matching. This antenna offers a suitable bandwidth range for 5G applications. It claims to perform well in bending analysis conditions.

13.7.3 Design 3

Inset-Fed square patch antennas with an operating frequency of 3.5 GHz for sub-6GHz 5G applications and rectangular patch antennas with an operating frequency of 28 GHz for 5G-millimetre

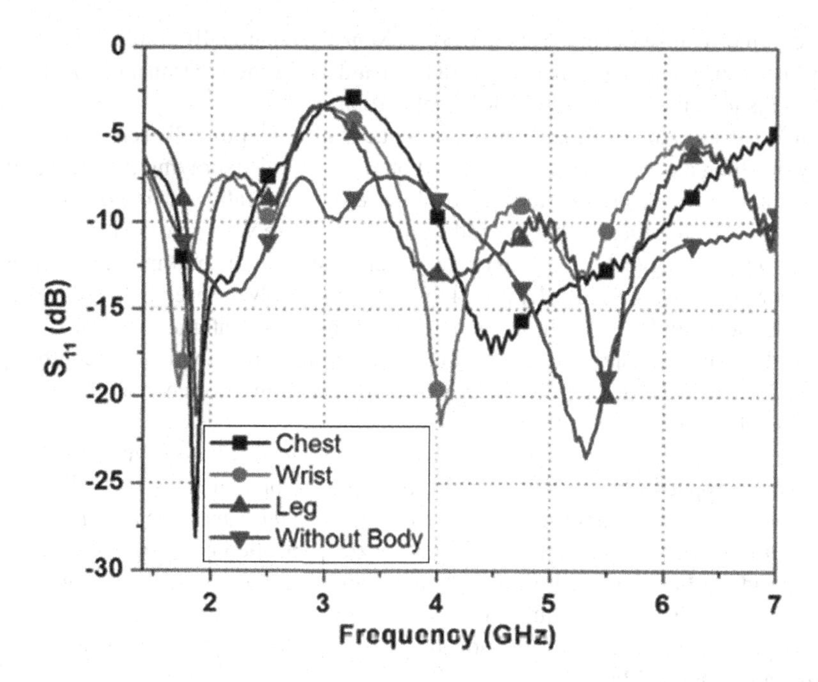

FIGURE 13.6 Comparative graphical representation of measured S_{11} (dB) parameters of on-body and off-body positions (Source: [19], Copyright (2019) Springer)

wave applications are presented in the article by Vivek et al. [22]. For wearability features, polycarbonate is considered as substrate. It is observed by parametric analysis that the inset feed length and dimension of a patch antenna affect antenna performance in the form of mismatch in impedance and variation in return loss. This is observed by the researchers in the designed antennas. The designed antenna offers BW of 41.2 MHz (3.4458 to 3.487 GHz) and 1.49 GHz (27.604 to 29.094 GHz) for square patch and rectangular patch which are applicable to 5G applications with good gain. For mobile communication, information on the effect of radiation on the human body is required, for which SAR analysis is necessary, which is missing in the referred paper.

13.7.4 Design 4

Dual-band rectangular patch antenna with six U-slot loaded on the patch structure is proposed in the study of Ahmed and Ahmed [23]. Flexible material "ULTRALAM® 3850HT" is used as a substrate having a thickness of 0.05 mm. The patch and the ground planes are rectangular and etched on the opposite sides of the substrate. This design claims to achieve effective impedance matching. The design is simulated in HFSS and CST software. The simulation result shows that the S_{11} value of −13.996 dB is obtained at 37.95–38.39 GHz and −19.27 dB is obtained at 59.49–60.15 GHz which covers the 5G frequency band. This antenna is integrated into a smartwatch as a wearable device.

13.8 WEARABLE ANTENNA FABRICATION METHOD

A number of techniques are available for the fabrication of wearable flexible antennas in commercial and research and development fields. The fabrication method is based on the choice of materials like substrates and conductive materials [24]. This method ensures the speed, accuracy, durability and wearability of the antenna.

Some fabrication methods are discussed below.

1. **Conductive Spray Technique:** In this technique, conductive materials like copper (in admixture with a gas) and other suitable materials can be sprayed on surfaces like fabric to create a thin, lightweight and flexible antenna. Some special conductive materials have

been reported by researchers. For example MXenes, a chemically stable, hard conductive material which can be made in a very thin form and well suited to transmit and direct radio waves. This technique is useful for IoT applications.

2. **Screen Printing:** Antenna fabrication technique is also adopting 3D screen printing technology in which a printed pattern is created on the screen by spraying ink on the specified exposed area of the desired pattern [25], followed by evaporative drying of a used solvent. Though apart from others polyester and stainless steel are very commonly used materials in 3D screen printing technology, in recent developments in the making of wearable antennas, researchers have successfully tested the potential of silver-based ink on *Aramid* fabric. This technology finds its use in manufacturing transparent antennas and RFIDs. Despite several advantageous aspects of this technology, it suffers from inadequate control over the deposited ink thickness. This technology also suffers from poor control of the associated resolution of the deposited patterns.
3. **Inkjet Printing:** This is another 3D printing technology where highly conductive ink laced with nanoparticles is used to achieve high-resolution antenna [24]. Variations in the procedure under this technology include *Continuous Inkjet* and *Drop-on-Demand print.* The *Drop-on-Demand print* technique uses nozzle-controlled pressurized ink pulses.
4. **Sewing and Embroidering:** It is an easy fabrication technique used by sewing or embroidering machine. It doesn't require adhesive. So this fabrication technique doesn't affect antenna performance. This fabrication method is preferable for wearable antennas for clothing applications [24].

13.9 WEARABLE ANTENNA MEASUREMENT

For wearability purposes, some validation parameters through measurements are considered with respect to environmental conditions and comfortability. For that, apart from basic measurements, SAR, robustness, durability, bending and crumpling effects tests are performed. Antenna radiation effect on the human body is characterized by SAR (Specific absorption rate) value. Taking the average over a small volume of 1 or 10 gm of human tissue, SAR is measured. In the United States, for a given wireless system, the mandatory SAR value is <1.6 W/Kg averaging on 1 gm tissue; and in Europe, SAR is restricted at ≤ 2.0 mW/gm or less based on 10 gm tissue average [24].

Bending or crumpling is one of the most sensitive properties for wearable applications. Since the antenna is integrated on a wearable surface, a slight change of movement of the human body affects the performance of an antenna. So it is better to simulate the antenna under different bending conditions. It is important to characterize the resonant frequency and return loss under different bending conditions. To check distortion or degradation of antennas, radiation patterns and directivity tests are performed. Durability and robustness tests are also conducted under different bending conditions for ensuring the non-existence of wrinkles or permanent folds which may have impact on the performance of the fabricated antenna.

13.10 ANTENNA-BASED IoT APPLICATIONS

There are various dual/multi-band antennas integrated into IoT devices. These devices also accommodate flexible/wearable antennas. It is worthy of mentioning that the antennas to be used in IoT devices must be compatible with respect to the antenna's bandwidth. Different fields like avionics, education, and medical use a variety of IoT technologies. Some of them are LoRa, Bluetooth, Wi-Fi, medical body area networks (MBAN), wireless avionics intra-communications (WAIC) etc. working in the frequency range 433 MHz–5.9GHz, all inclusive. IoT application has compatibility with planar inverted-F antenna design. Radio frequency identification (RFID)-based antennas are also becoming popular in IoT applications because of their special features which enable a device to share its unique digital code across a wireless network and to capture its physical positioning status globally as well.

13.11 CONCLUSION

This chapter describes various developmental aspects of different types of wearable antennas, their application and fabrication methods. In the era of wearable wireless technology, a new trend is taking a different way for improving antenna performance along with minimizing the manufacturing cost for affordability. Material life-time enhancement is also considered by considering washability, humidity and thermal test on wearable antenna substrates along with bending, crumpling and SAR measurement. To miniaturize the design and for cost-effectiveness, many researchers are using the SIW–based, Electromagnetic Band Gap (EBG) structure-based and meta-material surface-based antenna. Depending on application, proper selection of conductive material, substrate and modern fabrication techniques cumulatively make the wearable antenna purposeful for different IoT-based applications. Because of the miniaturization, the fields of application of wearable antennas are expanding very fast. Thus, the possibility of growth of wearable antennas is exponential.

REFERENCES

1. S. M. Ali, C. Sovuthy, M. A. Imran, S. Socheatra, Q. H. Abbasi, and Z. Z. Abidin, "Recent advances of wearable antennas in materials, fabrication methods, designs, and their applications: State-of-the-art," *Micromachines*, vol. 11, no. 10, p. 888, 2020.
2. E. J. Park, J. K. Sim, M.-G. Jeong, H. O. Seo, and Y. D. Kim, "Transparent and superhydrophobic films prepared with polydimethylsiloxane-coated silica nanoparticles," *RSC Adv.*, vol. 3, no. 31, pp. 12571–12576, 2013.
3. C.-P. Lin, C.-H. Chang, Y.-T. Cheng, and C. F. Jou, "Development of a flexible SU-8/PDMS-based antenna," *IEEE Antennas Wirel. Propag. Lett.*, vol. 10, pp. 1108–1111, 2011.
4. X. Liao et al., "High strength in combination with high toughness in robust and sustainable polymeric materials," *Science*, vol. 366, no. 6471, pp. 1376–1379, 2019.
5. K. N. Paracha, S. K. Abdul Rahim, P. J. Soh, and M. Khalily, "Wearable antennas: A review of materials, structures, and innovative features for autonomous communication and sensing," *IEEE Access*, vol. 7, pp. 56694–56712, 2019, doi: 10.1109/ACCESS.2019.2909146.
6. S. B. Roshni, M. P. Jayakrishnan, P. Mohanan, and K. P. Surendran, "Design and fabrication of an E-shaped wearable textile antenna on PVB-coated hydrophobic polyester fabric," *Smart Mater. Struct.*, vol. 26, no. 10, p. 105011, 2017.
7. Y. Kim, H. Kim, and H.-J. Yoo, "Electrical characterization of screen-printed circuits on the fabric," *IEEE Trans. Adv. Packag.*, vol. 33, no. 1, pp. 196–205, 2009.
8. V. Lakafosis, A. Rida, R. Vyas, L. Yang, S. Nikolaou, and M. M. Tentzeris, "Progress towards the first wireless sensor networks consisting of inkjet-printed, paper-based RFID-enabled sensor tags," *Proc. IEEE*, vol. 98, no. 9, pp. 1601–1609, 2010.
9. S. Sankaralingam and B. Gupta, "Determination of dielectric constant of fabric materials and their use as substrates for design and development of antennas for wearable applications," *IEEE Trans. Instrum. Meas.*, vol. 59, no. 12, pp. 3122–3130, 2010.
10. M. I. Ahmed, M. F. Ahmed, and A. H. A. Shaalan, "Novel electro-textile patch antenna on jeans substrate for wearable applications," *Prog. Electromagn. Res. C*, vol. 83, pp. 255–265, 2018.
11. R. Salvado, C. Loss, R. Gonçalves, and P. Pinho, "Textile materials for the design of wearable antennas: A survey," *Sensors*, vol. 12, no. 11, pp. 15841–15857, 2012.
12. G. Kaur, A. Kaur, and A. Kaur, "Wearable antennas for on-body communication systems," *Int. J. Eng. Sci. Adv. Technol.*, vol. 4, no. 6, pp. 568–575, 2014.
13. D. Kumar and D. Mathur, "Dual band wearable antenna for IoT applications," *Int. J. Innov. Technol. Explor. Eng.*, vol. 9, no. 1, pp. 1515–1518, 2019, doi: 10.35940/ijitee.A4344.119119.
14. M. Ur-Rehman et al., "A wearable antenna for mmWave IoT applications," in *2018 IEEE International Symposium on Antennas and Propagation & USNC/URSI National Radio Science Meeting*, 2018, pp. 1211–1212.

15. S. Banerjee, A. Singh, S. Dey, S. Chattopadhyay, S. Mukherjee, and S. Saha, "SIW based body wearable antenna for IoT applications," in *2019 International Conference on Opto-Electronics and Applied Optics (Optronix)*, 2019, pp. 1–4.
16. P. T. Selvan, B. G. Priya, T. Dhivya, and T. Keerthana, "A novel double C-shaped compact wearable substrate antenna using metamaterial for dualband applications," *International Journal Of Engineering Research & Technology (Ijert) Iconnect – 2017* vol. 5, no. 13, 2017.
17. W. J. Krzysztofik and T. N. Cao, "Metamaterials in application to improve antenna parameters," *Metamaterials and Metasurfaces*, vol. 12, no. 2, pp. 63–85, 2018.
18. A. K. Biswas and U. Chakraborty, "A compact wide band textile MIMO antenna with very low mutual coupling for wearable applications," *Int. J. RF Microw. Comput. Eng.*, vol. 29, no. 8, p. e21769, 2019.
19. S. Roy and U. Chakraborty, "Metamaterial based dual wideband wearable antenna for wireless applications," *Wirel. Pers. Commun.*, vol. 106, no. 3, pp. 1117–1133, 2019.
20. D. Sharma, S. K. Dubey, and V. N. Ojha, "Wearable antenna for millimeter wave 5G communications," in *2018 IEEE Indian Conference on Antennas and Propogation (InCAP)*, 2018, pp. 1–4.
21. M. Tighezza, S. K. A. Rahim, and M. T. Islam, "Flexible wideband antenna for 5G applications," *Microw. Opt. Technol. Lett.*, vol. 60, no. 1, pp. 38–44, 2018.
22. Narukurthi Vivek, Sandeep Kumar B, DrK. Shambavi, "Design of wearable antennas for 5G," vol. 12, no. 5, pp. 148–156, 2021, doi: 10.34218/IJEET.12.5.2021.014.
23. M. I. Ahmed and M. F. Ahmed, "A wearable flexible antenna integrated on a smart watch for 5G applications," *J. Physics: Conference Series*, vol. 1447, no. 1, p. 12005, 2020.
24. Y. Li, Z. Zhang, Z. Feng, and H. R. Khaleel, "Fabrication and measurement techniques of wearable and flexible antennas," *Cult. Tour*, vol. 1, pp. 7–23, 2014.
25. M. A. Monne, X. Lan, and M. Y. Chen, "Material selection and fabrication processes for flexible conformal antennas," *Int. J. Antennas Propag.*, vol. 2018, pp. 1–15, 2018. https://doi.org/10.1155/2018/9815631.

14 Investigation of Interface Trap Charges and Temperature on RF Performance with Noise Analysis for IoT Application of a Heterojunction Tunnel FET

Debika Das and Ujjal Chakraborty

CONTENTS

14.1 INTRODUCTION

In the recent past, the CMOS technology has been unceasingly scaled down in order to shrink the device dimensions to the extent of a nanometre regime to enhance the overall performance and preserve the integrity of revolutionary Moore's law [1]. Conversely, this trend of miniaturization in CMOS technology leads to fundamental physical restrictions owing to the existence of numerous detrimental effects including high subthreshold swing (SS), high OFF current (I_{OFF}), rapid rise in power dissipation along with different short-channel effects (SCEs) [2]. Further, decreasing supply-voltage (V_{DD}) while maintaining low I_{OFF} is found to be critical for limiting energy consumption and enhancing the battery lifespan of a device. In MOSFETs, the thermal constraint of SS forbids threshold voltage (V_T) reduction which restricts optimum device performance at low values of V_{DD}. Further, the computation duration and communication technologies are experiencing tremendous issues with CMOS-based technology for further reduction in power dissipation [3], [4]. It forbids the incorporation of functionality and areas in which IoT devices are well operated by batteries. An inbuilt feature of quantum tunnelling is inherent in the unconventional device Tunnel FET (TFET) that ensures better performance at low V_{DD} as well as it is devoid of the thermal tail present in MOSFETs [5]. The gate modulated interband TFETs comprising a Zener tunnel junction at the source region appear to be a perfect alternative for the microelectronics industry [6], [7], [8].

DOI: 10.1201/9781003217398-14

TFETs are basically a gated structure of p-i-n diode that employs the mechanism of Zener tunnelling at the reverse-bias junction to provoke band to band tunnelling (BTBT). This phenomenon of BTBT in TFETs aids in providing low I_{OFF} and steeper SS, which is much lower than the kT/q limit, and thereby, TFET becomes an attractive device for low-power applications as demanded International Technology Roadmap for Semiconductors (ITRS) roadmap and beyond CMOS technology. Besides, the constraint of fabrication complexity in FET architectures is also overcome. This facilitates superior Internet of Things (IoT) sensing and signal processing units in TFET-based memory elements and circuits [9].

Despite providing low I_{OFF} and steeper SS, TFETs face the challenging issues of comparatively low ON current (I_{ON}) and ambipolar behaviour, which may restrict a device's behaviour in digital circuits [10, 11]. The tunnelling current in TFET is found to be a complex function which depends on the effective mass of the carrier, steepness of tunnelling barrier and energy-gap of material [12, 13]. Various improvements in TFET performance have been obtained by different engineering aspects, including structure, material and work function, which are accessible from published literature. Commonly, double gate TFET [14], low k spacers [15], vertical TFET [7], nanowire TFET [16], symmetric TFET [17], germanium TFET [18] etc. are investigated to achieve superior performance of a TFET device.

However, recent works reported in published literature emphasize primarily the analyses of general characteristics of various novel geometries of TFETs under ideal conditions of the device [19, 20]. It appears that slight consideration is paid towards the reliability of a TFET design. As the trend of rigorous scaling is in practice, the complete analyses of a device's performance for low-power applications stay inadequate unless the impact of interface traps is considered. This existence of trap charges arises from the stress and various process-induced harm that occurs during the process of fabrication [21, 22]. The unconventional technique of carrier transport in TFET makes its behaviour critical under the influence of interface traps. The reliability is found to be a more prominent issue in TFETs than in MOSFET [23]. The first work on degradation caused by acceptor-type interface traps on drain current in a fabricated gate all around nanowire TFET was reported by Huang et al [24].

Scaling down of devices in recent times has also brought hindrance to the thermal budget due to dopant fluctuations in the regions of high doping. Furthermore, heat dissipation drastically increases with the rise in on-chip transistors, which leads to a rise in a transistor's operating temperature. Thus, temperature dependence at different ambient temperatures of a device is also a vital matter of concern for assuring reliability of a device. Moreover, an assessment of a device's RF characteristics is of utmost importance to investigate the perspective of the device for analogue-based applications. It has been observed that the temperature sensitivity features of TFET have already been presented in previously reported works [25, 26, 27]. However, an elaborate study on temperature-dependent analogue and different RF figures of merits (FOMs) as well as influence of interface trap charge polarity and density under different ambient temperature has been seldom reported.

Additionally, to certify optimum supremacy of a device's behaviour, exploration of electrical noise is indispensable; even though this zone is less explored up to now. Recently, few works have been reported [1, 28, 29] on noise analysis and modelling of TFET; still, a widespread exposure is tremendously essential to inspect the supremacy of a device. It is owing to various high frequency noise sources, serious impediments to RF/analogue application of a device appear. Also, various defect centres and impacts of concentration and distribution of ITC have prominent adverse effects on the noise characteristics of a device.

This chapter discusses the reliability aspects and various limiting factors that can deviate the optimum performance of a TFET device. A heterojunction TFET reported in the study of Das et al. [30] has been considered for the investigation and analysis of reliability concerns of a TFET device in general. The chapter is ordered as follows: the device architecture and simulation strategy are presented in section 14.2, the operation mechanism is discussed in section 14.3, the various results and discussions are drawn in section 14.4 followed by future scope in section 14.5, and the chapter is summarized in section 14.6.

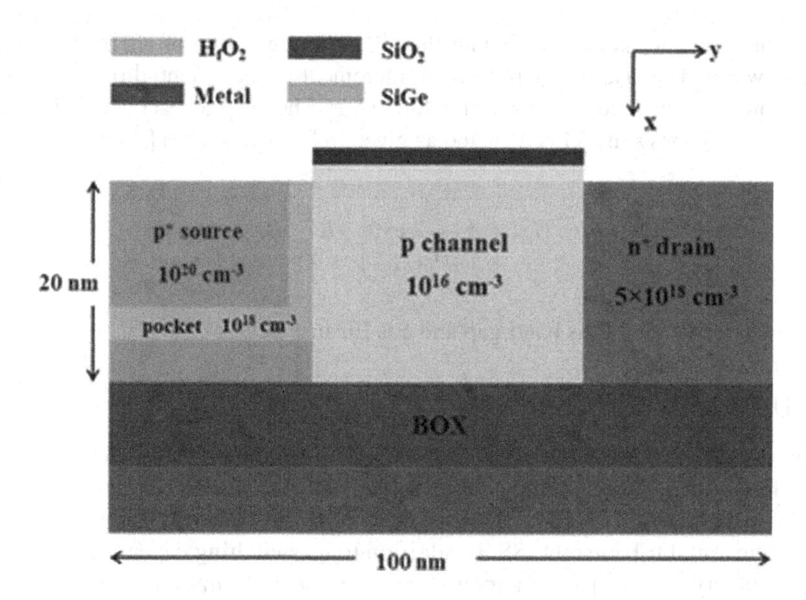

FIGURE 14.1 2-D schematic illustration of a heterojunction TFET (Source: [30], Copyright (2020) IEEE).

14.2 DEVICE ARCHITECTURE AND SIMULATION STRATEGY

A heterojunction TFET comprising silicon-silicon germanium (Si-SiGe) pocket at the source/channel junction which has been adapted from Das et al. [30] is considered for different reliability characterizations in this chapter, as shown in Figure 14.1. Heterojunction TFETs are advantageous in removing discrepancies that occur between fabricated and simulated results due to the existence of parasitic thermionic leakage current caused by parasitic components [31]. A δp^+ Si-Ge layer is infused at the source/channel junction to promote high I_{ON} with the aid of low band-gap material Ge which suppresses the energy bands more abruptly. A high-k (HfO_2) dielectric gate material is applied to deliver improved capacitive coupling. The device length is 100 nm having source and drain lengths of 20 nm and 30 nm, respectively. The length of the channel is 47 nm with a Si body of 5 nm thickness. Different doping concentrations are taken into consideration at source (1×10^{20} cm^3), drain (5×10^{18} cm^3), substrate (1×10^{18} cm^3) and channel (1×10^{16} cm^3), respectively.

The simulations are accomplished by employing Sentaurus 2D technology computer-aided design (TCAD) simulator [32]. A non-local BTBT model is enabled to control the tunnelling phenomenon more efficiently. To consider the impact of the greater doping concentration of the source as well as the drain region, Fermi–Dirac statistics is activated as a substitute for Boltzmann statistics. Further, to account temperature effects, an advanced hydrodynamic model is activated. The Shockley-Read-Hall (SRH) recombination model is used. A band gap narrowing model is activated to control the tunnelling probability of charge carriers as well as a doping-dependent mobility model is also initiated.

14.3 BASIC OPERATION MECHANISM OF TFET

MOSFET functions on the mechanism of charge variation in the channel, while, TFETs basic working phenomenon is based on the mechanism of potential variation that permits or restricts the tunnelling mechanism. When positive gate voltage (V_{GS}) is applied, the energy bands on the channel get suppressed, contracting the energy barrier that exists between source and channel. V_{GS} of TFETs is changed until the valence band (VB) at the source region and conduction band (CB) at the channel region are aligned to each other. This lets the flow of current all through the device. The BTBT is implemented by TFET for driving its current, thereby permitting the charge carriers to tunnel through a potential barrier between VB and the CB. The tunnelling of charge carriers relies on energy barrier width. The rise in V_{GS} reflects an increment in the potential of the channel, which results in a greater electric field and generation rate (G_{tun}). The G_{tun} caused by inter-band tunnelling rate as proposed by Kanes's model is depicted as given in Equation (14.1) [1].

$$G_{tun} = A\frac{|\xi^2|}{\sqrt{E_g}}\exp\left(-B\frac{E_g^{\frac{3}{2}}}{|\xi|}\right) \quad (14.1)$$

where A and B are constants, E_g is band-gap and ξ is Electric field.

14.4 RESULTS AND DISCUSSION

This section indulges in the behaviour of a TFET under the impact of different reliability issues considering trap effect, temperature sensitivity and electrical noise characteristics. The emergent structure of TFET is examined with regard to several performance parameters including ON current, OFF current, SS, in addition to its switching capacitance characteristics to discover its utility for compact low-power, greater-speed digital and memory applications, which form a fundamental fragment of portable intelligent devices to be employed in IoT applications.

14.4.1 Impact of Interface Trap Charge

The influence of interface-trap charges (ITCs) is one of the primary causes of degradation in a device's performance, reliability issues and lifetime as well. The existence of the fourth-bond in the interface having energy level between band gaps of Si due to the presence of ITCs initiate defect centres in the device [33]. ITCs can be basically divided into two categories depending upon polarity: donor type and acceptor type traps. The donor traps behave as positive ITCs in an empty state but it is pronounced as a neutral charge when it is occupied by an electron. Whereas acceptor traps behave as neutral charges in the empty state, on the other hand, they behave as negative ITCs when occupied by an electron. The donor traps lie above VB and acceptor traps lie below CB in the energy level. These ITCs in TFETs are generated from high electric fields that exist in the tunnelling junction. Besides, instability owing to hot-carriers induced stress is also responsible for the generation of ITCs [34]. The trap charges located on the surface of a Si body also vary the electric field at the source/channel junction to influence the tunnelling current and the BTBT phenomenon. To illustrate, a PNIN gate all around (GAA) TFET as referred to in [35] and its behaviour depending on the concentration of ITC and polarity is taken into consideration here. It is observed that the positive trap increases, whereas the negative trap lowers the drain current. In the case of positive ITCs, the rise in drain current (I_{DS}) is caused by enhanced effective gate bias (V_{GS}) under the influence of reduced flat band voltage (V_{FB}). On the contrary, the I_{DS} decreases as a consequence of reduced effective V_{GS} due to high V_{FB} as obtained and presented in [35]. The presence of ITCs varies the behaviour of electric fields at the tunnelling junction [35]. This rise (drop) in the electric field is caused by the decrease (increase) in V_{FB} under the impact of donor (acceptor) type traps which is related as given by Equation (14.2) [35].

$$\Delta V_{FB} - \frac{qN_f}{C_{ox}} \quad (14.2)$$

where q is the electric charge, N_f is the ITC density and C_{ox} is the gate-oxide capacitance. The degradation due to the donor trap is more pronounced at the subthreshold regime than at the super-threshold regime. It is also observed that severe degradation in I_{OFF} is obtained with a rise in donor charge density [35]).

Moreover, the traps can be classified into two more types based on their distribution, uniform and Gaussian traps. The Gaussian trap influence is expected to be further severe than its counterpart, the uniform trap, which is evident from Figure 14.2 (referred from the work of Das and Chakraborty [29]). This can be attributed to better similarities of Gaussian distribution with experimental results [36]. Also, fluctuation in charge carriers caused by Gaussian traps lessens the surface potential to yield behaviour degradation [29]. Such behaviours are also expected to occur in the device considered in this chapter when it is under influence of the interface trap.

14.4.2 Impact of Temperature Sensitivity

Present literature exposes that TFETs yield low-temperature sensitivity characteristics in comparison to conventional MOSFET. This can be owed to the unconventional phenomenon of the BTBT conduction mechanism in contrast to conventional thermionic transport in MOSFETs. Therefore, TFETs offer resistance against temperature sensitivity characteristics [37]. The activation of an advanced hydrodynamic model is essential to take account of the impact ionization that occurs at high temperatures. It has been seen that there is a rising trend in I_{ON} and I_{OFF} with the increase in temperature, as seen in Figure 14.3 (referred from [37]); however, the effect is more dominant in leakage current. This behaviour can be explained as given by Equation (14.3) [38].

$$I_{ds} = A\frac{|E|^2}{E_g^{\frac{1}{2}}}\exp\left(-\frac{BE_g^{\frac{3}{2}}}{|E|}\right) \tag{14.3}$$

where E_g is band-gap, E is electric-field, A and B are parameters that rely on material with default values. The semiconductor band-gap that relies on temperature follows the below relation, given by Equation (14.4) [38].

$$E_g(T) = E_g(300) - \frac{\alpha T^2}{1+\beta} \tag{14.4}$$

where $\alpha = 4.73 \times 10^{-4}$ eV/K, $\beta = 636$ K and E_g (300) = 1.08 eV for silicon.

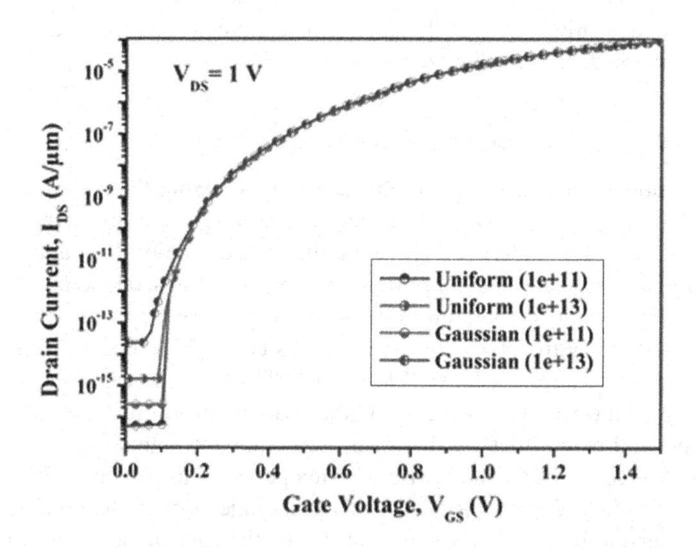

FIGURE 14.2 Transfer characteristic considering the effect of uniform and Gaussian traps (Source: [29], Copyright (2020) Wiley).

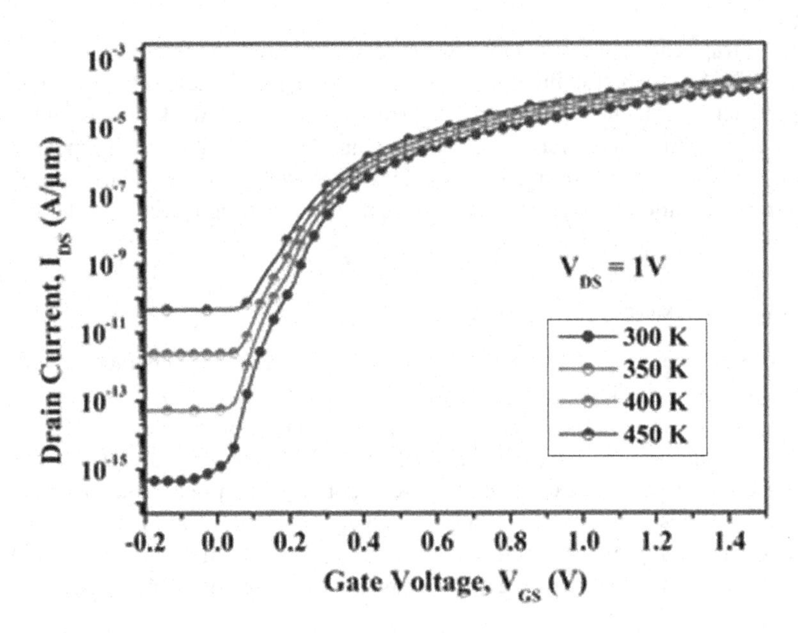

FIGURE 14.3 Impact of temperature variation on transfer characteristics (Source: [39], Copyright (2020) Wiley).

Thus, Equations (14.3) and (14.4) reflect the rising behaviour of I_{DS} owing to band-gap reduction with the rise in temperature. But, there is a noticeable effect of temperature on I_{OFF} than on I_{ON}. This difference in temperature dependence characteristics on I_{ON} and I_{OFF} is due to different mechanisms that are influencing both the states. The I_{ON} relies on the BTBT phenomenon which is controlled by the width of the tunnelling barrier. The tunnelling barrier width, on the other hand, is a weak function of temperature. Hence, I_{ON} has better immunity over temperature fluctuations. Besides, high governance of temperature on I_{OFF} is because of the control of Shockley Read Hall (SRH) at low electric fields, which is highly affected by temperature [37]. There is also a generation of a large number of charge carriers at rising temperatures owing to the reverse bias junction in TFET [38, 39]. Furthermore, when the influence of traps with different polarities is considered, the temperature sensitivity characteristics do not alter, irrespective of whether it is a positive or a negative trap, although the effect of a positive trap is still detected to be more pronounced [35]. Such behaviour is expected to appear in the device considered in this chapter too.

14.4.3 RF/Analogue Behaviour Characterization

The RF characterization is an utmost requirement for investigating the calibre of a device in the analogue circuit domain. Even in any modern communication system, the minimum distortion in signals should be preserved to understand the suitability of a device for RF / analogue based applications, maintaining high speed. The amplification capability transconductance (g_{m}) of a device escalates with an increase in temperature, owing to the positive temperature coefficient of I_{DS}. This trend is reflected in Figure 14.4 (referred from Das et al. [37]). The g_m helps to attain better switching speed and offers improved cut off frequency. The parasitic capacitances accompanying a device play a significant part in shaping its AC behaviour. These are responsible for generating paths between input and output that are liable for oscillation and signal distortion in circuits. The total gate capacitance (C_{gg}) is observed to rise with temperature, as shown in Figure 14.5 (referred from Das et al. [37]). These capacitances occur from the injection of charge carriers from drain. At high V_{GS}, an inversion-layer is created that increases the capacitance due to reduction of the drain potential barrier. At high temperatures, the energy barrier is contracted to enhance the carrier

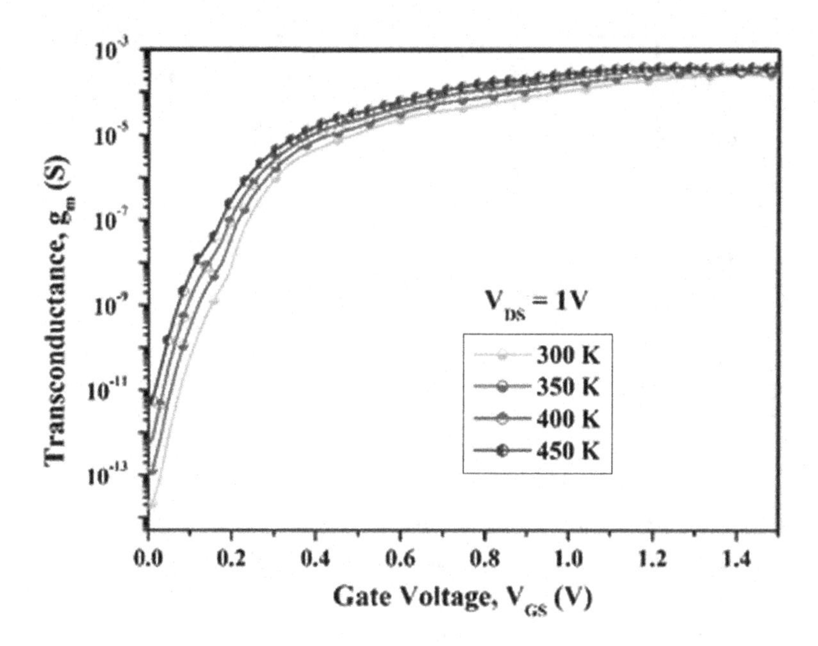

FIGURE 14.4 Effect of temperature variation on transconductance (Source: [39], Copyright (2020) Wiley).

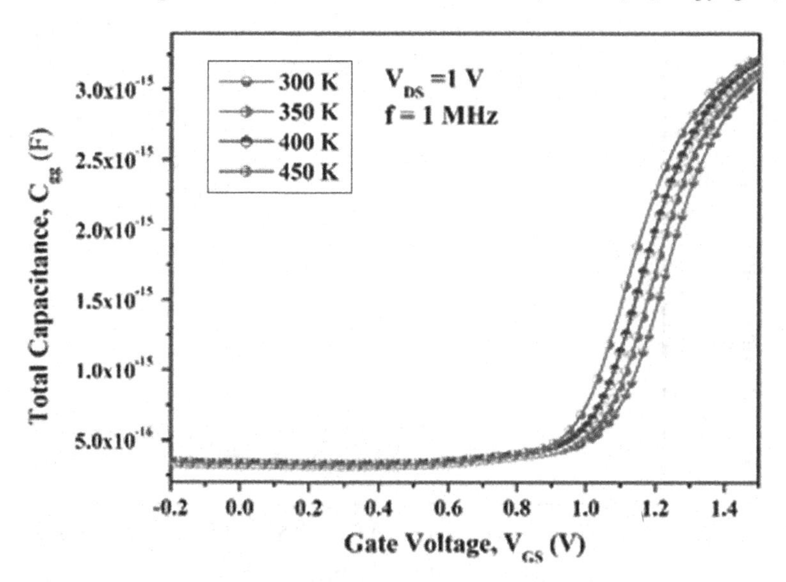

FIGURE 14.5 Effect of temperature variation on total capacitance (Source: [39], Copyright (2020) Wiley).

concentration at the surface. Further, this rise in temperature yields a thermal generation of carriers in the Si body that is responsible for generation of electron-hole pairs. This growth of channel carrier concentration at high temperatures plays a major part in parasitic capacitance composition [40]. Likewise, cut-off frequency (f_t) (which is established as a particular frequency where current gain drops to 0 dB) also reflects an inclining trend with a rise in temperature as seen in Figure 14.6 (referred from Das et al. [37]) due to its directly proportional relationship with g_m as expressed by Equation (14.5) [38].

$$f_t = \frac{g_m}{2\pi\left(C_{gg}\right)} \tag{14.5}$$

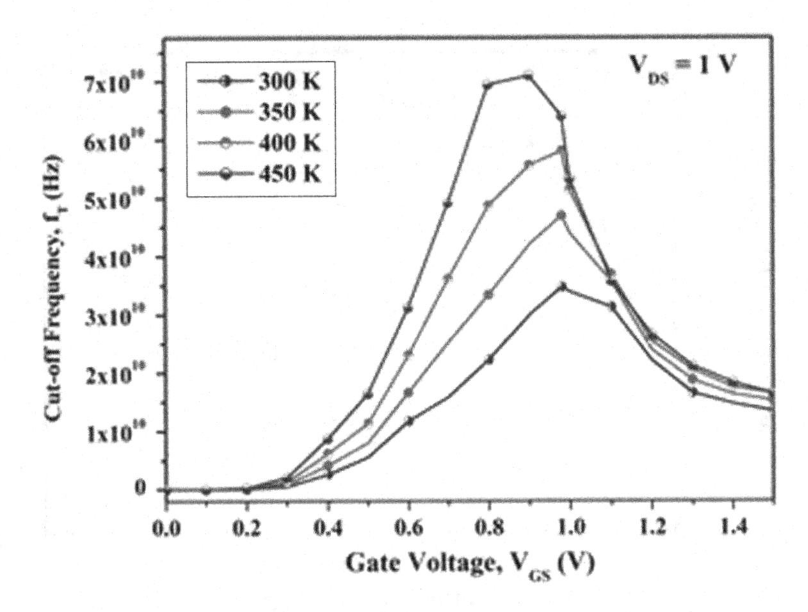

FIGURE 14.6 Effect of temperature variation on f_t (Source: [39], Copyright (2020) Wiley).

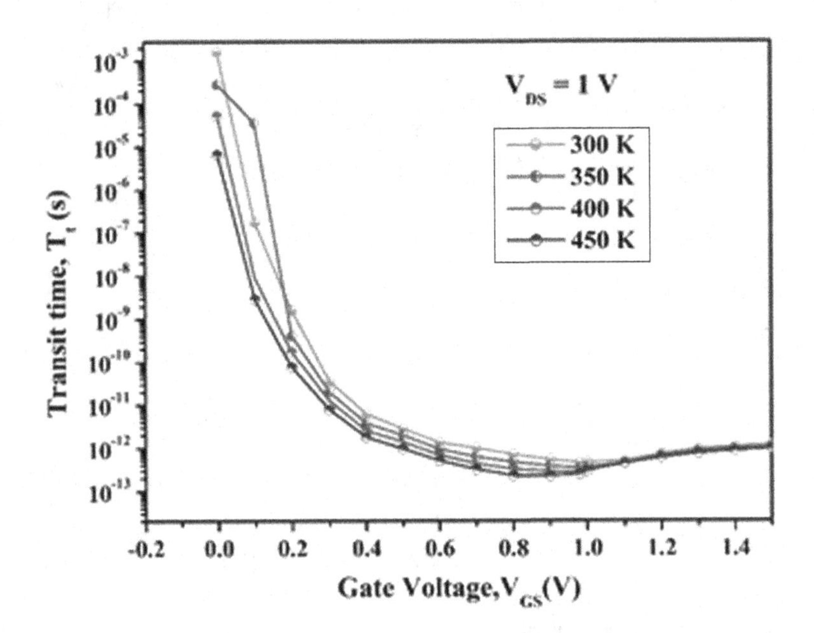

FIGURE 14.7 Effect of temperature variation on T_t (Source: [39], Copyright (2020) Wiley).

It has also been observed that the inclining trend of f_t with augmentation in temperature is still prevalent in presence of traps [35]. Although, the effect of the donor trap is witnessed to be more dominant than the acceptor trap [22]. Similarly, the transit time (T_t) as expressed by Equation (14.6), [37] and shown in Figure 14.7 (referred from [37]) is basically an important parameter for high-speed applications, which follows a declining trend with a rise in temperature.

$$T_t = \frac{1}{20\pi f_t} \tag{14.6}$$

As well as, T_t is detected to drop at high V_{GS} that can be attributed to higher inversion-charge density causing a narrower tunnelling path. Accordingly, carriers have to traverse smaller paths to facilitate reduced T_t.

14.4.4 Impact of Electrical Noise

TFETs have emerged as a replacement of the traditional MOSFETs, but to guarantee optimum performance and reliability of a device electrical noise analysis is a serious matter of concern. However, the noise aspect of TFET is underexplored when compared to other electrical parameters. The noise characteristics can be explained by considering the effect of voltage noise spectral density ($S_{vg}ee$) and current noise spectral density (S_{ID}). The random telegraph noise (RTN), flicker noise and generation-recombination (GR) noise are low-frequency noise sources which scale reciprocally with design layout and degrade the operation of both analogue, mixed-analogue and digital circuits. On the contrary, diffusion noise is found to be dominant at high frequency and this behaviour is evident from Figure 14.8 (referred from [37]).

The GR noise in TFETs exists due to instabilities that occur in the amount of available carriers generated by BTBT in the channel. GR noise is completely dominant at low frequency caused by the carrier fluctuations throughout the channel primarily due to various SRH centres and defect centres present in the channel [41]. The S_{ID} representing GR noise is expressed as given by Equation (14.7) [1]. It can be seen that the inverse square dependence on frequency reduces its effect at high frequency.

$$S_{IG-R} = \frac{N_t \tau}{N^2 1 + \omega^2} \tag{14.7}$$

where, N_t is trap concentration, N is total carrier density, τ is time constant and ω is frequency. Contrariwise, this mentioned behaviour decreases at high frequency due to a minor chance of channel carriers being influenced by the recombination centre existing in the channel. At higher frequency, V_{GS} varies at a very fast rate to result in a fast change of diffusion rate which causes variation

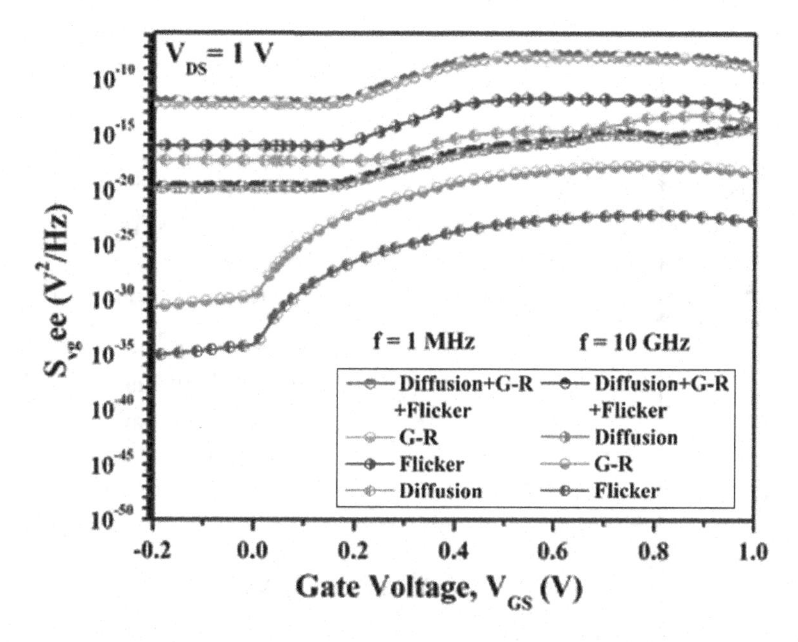

FIGURE 14.8 Impact of different components electrical noise on $S_{vg}ee$ behaviour (Source: [39], Copyright (2020) Wiley).

in the concentration of charge carriers. This results in a dominant effect of diffusion noise at high frequency which depends on the mobility fluctuation of charge carriers [40]. Diffusion noise is generated from the diffusion component of channel current.

Additionally, flicker (1/*f*) noise is deliberated as an additive outcome of a large number of GR noise formed by sub-bands impurities/defects and fluctuation in mobility that significantly deteriorates at high frequencies [1]. It is expressed as given by Equation (14.8), [1]

$$S_{\mathrm{ID}} = \left(\frac{2}{F} + \frac{B}{F^2}\right)\frac{q^2 I_{DN_t}^2 \left(E_{\mathrm{FN}}\right)}{\xi_{\mathrm{ox}}^2 W L' \alpha f^{\gamma}} \tag{14.8}$$

here F is electric-field, B is a constant, L' is the effective gate length, W is gate-width, α is an attenuation factor, ξ_{ox} is gate oxide dielectric constant, f is frequency and the exponential factor γ states how S_{ID} is reliant on frequency [28]. Typically, the spectrum of $1/f$ dependent on frequency is formed by the accumulation of a number of Lorentzian-spectra [1].

The electrical noise behaviour can also be investigated under the influence of interface traps considering both the distribution and density of trap charges. It has been observed from Figure 14.9 and Figure 14.10 (referred from work of Das and Chakraborty [29]) that there is a change in the trend of S_{ID} behaviour with respect to change in concentration of traps as well as distribution of traps. However, the Gaussian trap is found to cause further degradation compared to the uniform trap. The trend of S_{vg}ee under impact different density of trap charge and distribution is reflected in Figure 14.11 and Figure 14.12, respectively (referred from [29]) which follows an analogous trend with S_{ID}. This is owing to a directly proportional relation between both the parameters [29].

14.5 FUTURE SCOPE

Benchmarking of various emerging devices in recent times for digital applicability has exposed the TFETs compatibility for beyond-CMOS low power applications among other contemporary devices. Although there is advancement in benchmarking of TFET for digital applications, analogue designs have not received the required attention yet. Thus, utilization of TFETs for improved

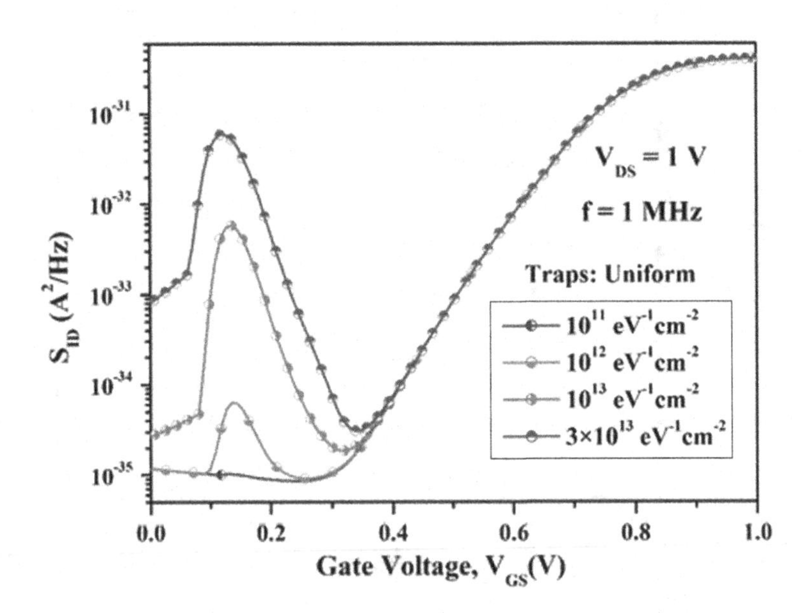

FIGURE 14.9 Impact of Uniform trap on S_{ID} behaviour for variation in trap density (Source: [29], Copyright (2020) Springer).

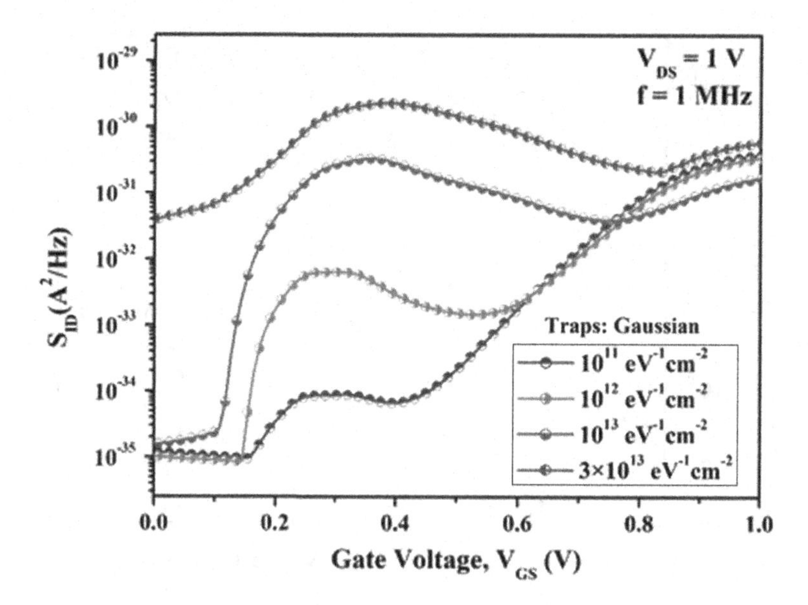

FIGURE 14.10 Impact of Gaussian trap on S_{ID} behaviour for variation in trap density. (Source: [29], Copyright (2020) Springer)

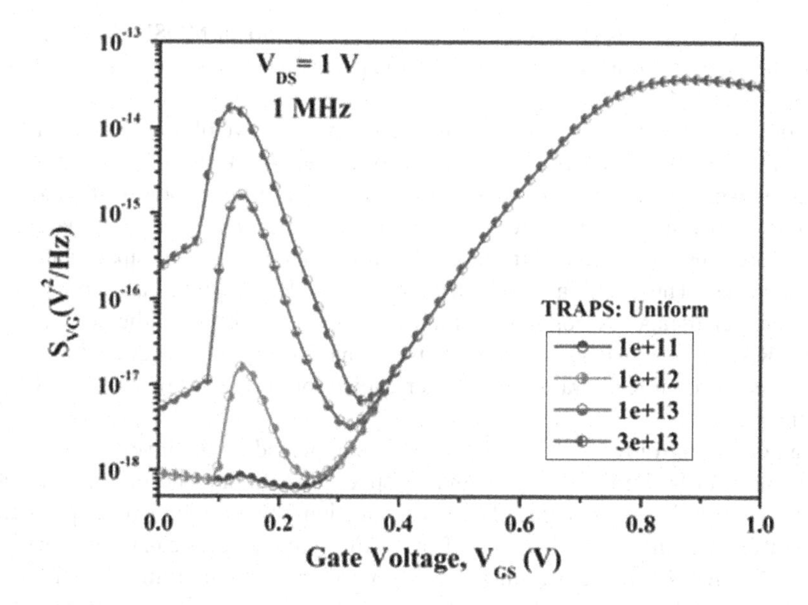

FIGURE 14.11 Impact of Uniform trap on S_{vg}ee behaviour for variation in trap density (Source: [29], Copyright (2020) Springer).

analogue circuits like operational transconductance amplifiers (OTA), low noise amplifiers etc. can be adopted as future scope by adopting proper methodologies. The design of TFET is mostly performed in Sentaurus TCAD simulator, thus for implementing analogue circuit, Verilog-A-based table models should be built by interpolation of values with quadratic-spline. These Verilog-A models generated can then be utilized for the accomplishment of spice simulations to analyse analogue characteristics. The advantages of TFET over non-scalability issues, SCE's and low leakage are due to sub-60 mV/dec SS feasibility, which acts as a major breakthrough. Thus, due to sub-60 mV/dec SS, the transconductance generation efficiency (g_m/I_D) in TFETs can be obtained to even a high

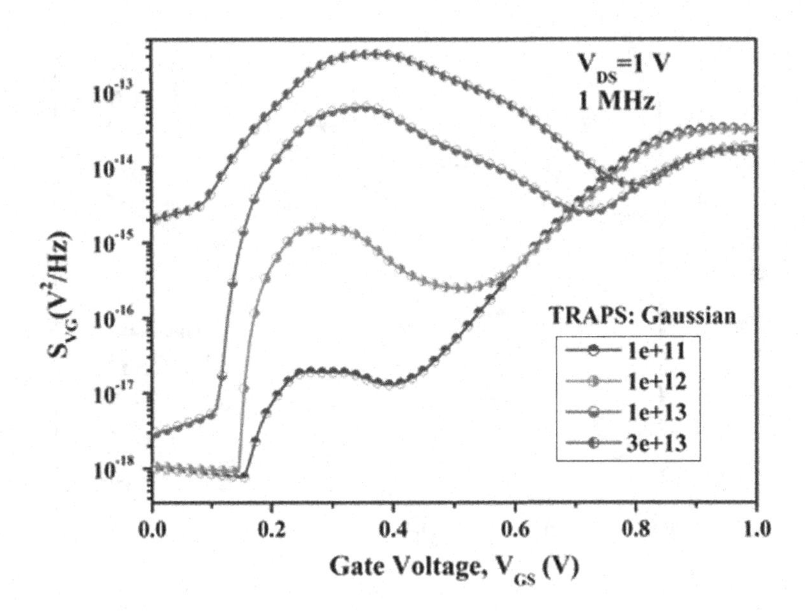

FIGURE 14.12 Impact of Gaussian trap on S_{vg}ee behaviour for variation in trap density (Source: [29], Copyright (2020) Springer).

value of 150 V^{-1}, whereas it is confined at 38.5 V^{-1} in conventional MOSFETs [42]. Additionally, TFET excels the state-of-the-art characteristic for the gain of a single stage amplifier that consumes very less chip area too [43].

Furthermore, the tremendous rise in IoTs as a future perspective of the microelectronics industry increases the demand for energy efficient sensor nodes. A variety of applications, including body sensing network (BSN), remote surveillance etc. need ultralow power and energy-efficient operation in order to sustain battery life. These IoT devices demand significantly larger embedded memories to store sensor data and instructions. However, major power dissipation occurs in these embedded memories. Thus, design of an ultra-low power SRAM (static random access memory) for IoTs is a new challenge. A popular solution for energy reduction is the subthreshold region operation of SRAM [3], [9]. Hence, the non-conventional TFET which is devoid of the SS limitation of 60mV/dec at room temperature is a better choice for design of robust SRAM for different IoT applications.

The design of an innovative TFET architecture accompanied by the investigation of its various reliability factors can be implemented in greater speed of memory and digital applications that appears as a key task for IoT systems. The heterojunction TFET architectures presented can be employed in different memory architectures. These TFET architectures can be exploited for similar 7-T, 8-T and 9-T memory architectures in addition to improvement in optimised circuit technologies which provide support for the great demand for reduced power consumable memory in handy and smart IoT applications [44]. Even the ambipolar behaviour of TFET, whereby current flow occurs in both positive and negative gate voltages is appropriate for extremely random and unclonable circuit and hence develop the hardware security [45], [46], [47]. The ambipolar delay can be announced to lessen the prospect of hardware outbreaks and raise the randomness behaviour of a circuit. Various IoT applications including sensing of risky environmental situations, wearable and compact fitness checking systems, bio medical sensors, remote surveillance, traffic watching and numerous other sensing networks involve low power and energy proficient devices in order to sustain a longer battery lifespan along with infused self-energy harvesting method. Therefore, compatible TFET structures can be employed in the application of IoT.

14.6 SUMMARY

A detailed survey of a TFET device considering the impact of various reliability issues is deliberated in this chapter. The TFETs are preferred over conventional MOSFETs due to their exceptional super steeper subthreshold swing and low leakage current. However, this dawn of TFET in the microelectronics industry is somehow affected by its low I_{ON}; hence, different investigations on structural variation and materials of TFETs are performed to obtain optimum behaviour. With the prevalent rigorous scaling down of devices, analyses of reliability factors are of utmost importance. The presence of ITCs in the vicinity of a device can have a hazardous impact on its performance. Thus, analyses on the impact of different densities and distribution of ITCs on electrical behaviour of a device have been carefully looked upon. At the same time, the ambient temperature also has adverse effects on device characteristics. Further, analysis of different RF FOMs is necessary to investigate the prospective of a device in analogue along with mixed-mode circuits. Thus, the trend of temperature sensitivity on these RF FOMs along with the impact of density and type of ITCs are inspected. The investigation of electrical noise features of TFET, which is comparatively underexplored is a serious matter of concern. Different noise components are observed to dominate at different frequency ranges. The noise characteristics also get degraded depending on the density and distribution of ITCs. The reliability issues of the device considered in this chapter are also expected to behave in a similar way as explained considering the effects in general. Further, the benchmarking of a TFET device in analogue applications such as OTAs and LNA is also discussed that can be adopted as future indulgence through appropriate methodologies. This work also indicates the suitability of TFETs for energy efficient as well as secured hardware design platforms in upcoming IoT systems.

REFERENCES

1. R. Goswami, B. Bhowmick, and S. Baishya, "Effect of scaling on noise in circular gate TFET and its application as a digital inverter," *Microelectron*, vol. 53, pp. 16–24, 2016.
2. K. Roy, S. Mukhopadhyay, and H. Mahmoodi-Meimand, "Leakage current mechanisms and leakage reduction techniques in deep submicrometer CMOS circuits," *Proceedings of IEEE*, vol. 91, no. 2, pp. 305–327, 2003.
3. S. P. Anju, S. Yadav, K. Nigam, D. Sharma, and P. N. Kondekar, "Realization of junctionless TFET-based power efficient 6T SRAM memory cell for Internet of Things applications," *Proceedings of First International Conference on Smart System, Innovations and Computing*, Smart Innovation, Systems and Technologies, vol. 79, pp. 515–523, 2018.
4. A. M. Ionescu and H. Riel, "Tunnel field-effect transistors as energy efficient electronic switches," *Nature*, vol. 479, pp. 329–337, 2011.
5. W. Y. Choi, B.-G. Park, J. D. Lee, and T.-J. K. Liu, "Tunneling field-effect transistors (TFETs) with subthreshold swing (SS) less than 60 mV/dec," *IEEE Electron Device Letters*, vol. 28, no. 8, pp. 743–745, 2007.
6. W. M. Reddick and G. A. J. Amaratunga, "Silicon surface tunnel transistor," *Applied Physics Letters*, vol. 67, no. 4, pp. 494–496, 1995.
7. K. K. Bhuwalka, S. Sedlmaier, A. K. Ludsteck, C. Toksdorf, J. Schulz, and I. Eisele, "Vertical tunnel field-effect transistor," *IEEE Transactions on Electron Devices*, vol. 51, no. 2, pp. 279–282, 2004.
8. S. Mookerjea and S. Datta, "Comparative study of Si, Ge and InAs based steep subthreshold slope tunnel transistors for 0.25 V supply voltage logic applications," in *Proceedings of 66th Device Research Conference*, pp. 47–48, June, 2008.
9. S. Ahmad, N. Alam, and M. Hasan, "Robust TFET SRAM cell for ultra-low power IoT application," in *2017 International Conference on Electron Devices and Solid-State Circuits (EDSSC)*, pp. 1–2, 2017, doi: 10.1109/EDSSC.2017.8333263
10. U. E. Avci, D. H. Morris, and I. A. Young, "Tunnel field-effect transistors: Prospects and challenges," *IEEE Journal of Electron Devices Society*, vol. 3, no. 3, pp. 88–95, 2015.
11. S. O. Koswatta, S. J. Koester, and W. Haensch, "On the possibility of obtaining MOSFET-like performance and sub-60-mV/dec swing in 1-D broken-gap tunnel transistors," *IEEE Transactions on Electron Devices*, vol. 57, no. 12, pp. 3222–3230, 2010.

12. E. O. Kane, "Theory of tunneling," *Journal of Applied Physics*, vol. 32, no. 1, pp. 83–91, 1961.
13. D. Sarkar, M. Krall, and K. Banerjee, "Electron-hole duality during the band-to-band tunneling process in graphene-nanoribbon tunnel field- effect-transistors," *Applied Physics Letters*, vol. 97, no. 26, p. 263109, 2010.
14. K. Boucart and A. M. Ionescu, "Double-gate tunnel FET With High k gate dielectric," *IEEE Transactions on Electron Devices*, vol. 54, pp. 1725–1733, 2007.
15. A. S. Verhulst, W. G. Vandenberghe, K. Maex, and G. Groeseneken, "Tunnel field-effect transistor without gate-drain overlap," *Applied Physics Letters*, vol. 91, no. 5, pp. 053102–053103, 2007.
16. Y. Lv, Q. Huang, H. Wang, S. Chang, and J. He, "A numerical study on graphene nano-ribbon heterojunction dual-material gate tunnel FET," *IEEE Electron Device Letters*, vol. 37, pp. 1354–1357, 2016.
17. H. Nam, M. H. Cho, and C. Shin, "Symmetric tunnel field-effect transistor (S-TFET)," *Current Applied Physics*, vol. 15, no. 2, pp. 71–77, 2015.
18. K. Vanlalawmpuia and B. Bhowmick, "Investigation of a Ge-source vertical TFET with delta-doped layer," *IEEE Transactions on Electron Devices*, vol. 66, pp. 4439–4445, 2019.
19. J. Appenzeller, Y.-M. Lin, J. Knoch, Z. Chen, and P. Avouris, "Comparing carbon nanotube transistors-the ideal choice: A novel tunneling device design," *IEEE Transactions on Electron Devices*, vol. 52, no. 12, pp. 2568–2576, 2005.
20. S. Kumar, E. Goel, K. Singh, B. Singh, M. Kumar, S. Jit, and A. Compact, "2-D analytical model for electrical characteristics of double-gate tunnel field-effect transistors with a SiO2/high-k stacked gate-oxide structure," *IEEE Transactions on Electron Devices*, vol. 63, no. 8, pp. 3291–3299, 2016.
21. R. Wang, Xiaobo Jiang, Tao Yu, Jiewen Fan, Jiang Chen, David Z. Pan and Ru HuangR. Wang et al., "Investigations on line-edge roughness (LER) and line-width roughness (LWR) in nanoscale CMOS technology: Part II—Experimental results and impacts on device variability," *IEEE Transaction on Electron Devices*, vol. 60, no. 11, pp. 3676–3682, 2013.
22. M. G. Pala, D. Esseni, and F. Conzatti, "Impact of interface traps on the IV curves of InAs tunnel-FETs and MOSFETs: A full quantum study," in *Proceedings of IEEE IEDM*, San Francisco, CA, pp. 1–4, December, 2012.
23. G. F. Jiao, Z.X. Chen, H. Y. Yu, X. Y. Huang, D.M. Huang, N. Singh, G. Q. Lo, D.-L. Kwong, Ming Fu Li and G. F. Jiao et al., "New degradation mechanisms and reliability performance in tunneling field effect transistors," in *Proceedings of IEEE IEDM*, pp. 1–4, December, 2009.
24. X. Y. Huang, G. F. Jiao, W. Cao, D. Huang, H. Y. Yu, Z. X. Chen, N. Singh, G. Q. Lo, D. L. Kwong and Ming Fu Li et al., "Effect of interface traps and oxide charge on drain current degradation in tunneling field-effect transistors," *IEEE Electron Device Letters*, vol. 31, no. 8, pp. 779–781, 2010.
25. M. Born, K. K. Bhuwalka, M. Schindler, U. Abilene, M. Schmidt, T. Sulima, and I. Eisele, "Tunnel FET: A CMOS device for high temperature applications," in *Proceedings of 25th International Conference on Microelectronics*, pp. 124–127, 2006.
26. T. Nirschl, P. F. Wang, W. Hansch, and D. S. Landsiedel, "The tunnelling field effect transistors (TFET): The temperature dependence, the simulation model, and its application," in *Proceedings of International Symposium of Circuits Systems*, pp. 713–716, 2004.
27. S. Migita, K. Fukuda, Y. Morita, and H. Ota, "Experimental demonstration of temperature stability of Si-tunnel FET over Si-MOSFET," in *Proceedings of Silicon Nanoelectronics Workshop*, pp. 1–2, 2012.
28. Rahul Pandey, Saurabh Mookerjea and Suman Datta, "Electrical noise in heterojunction interband tunnel FETs," *IEEE Transactions on Electron Devices*, vol. 61, pp. 552–560, 2014.
29. D. Das and U. Chakraborty, "A study on dual dielectric pocket heterojunction SOI tunnel FET performance and flicker noise analysis in presence of interface traps," *Silicon*, vol. 13, pp. 787–798 May 2020.
30. D. Das, R. Pandey, S. Baishya, and U. Chakraborty, "Impact of temperature and trap charges on heterojunction tunnel FET," in *2020 National Conference on Emerging Trends on Sustainable Technology and Engineering Applications (NCETSTEA)*, pp. 1–5, 2020, doi: 10.1109/NCETSTEA48365.2020.9119953.
31. Gilbert Hillsboro Dewey, Benjamin F. Chu-Kung, J. Boardman, Joel M. Fastenau, Jack T. Kavalieros, Roza Kotlyar, W. K. Liu, Dmitri Lubyshev, Matthew V. Metz, N. Mukherjee, P. E. Oakey, Ravi Pillarisetty, Marko Radosavljevic, Han Wui Then and Robert Chau, "Fabrication, characterization, and physics of III-V heterojunction tunneling field effect transistors (H-TFET) for steep sub-threshold swing," in *2011 International Electron Devices Meeting*, 33.6.1–33.6.4, 2011.
32. TCAD, *Sentaurus Device User's Manual*, Synopsys, Mountain View, CA; 2009.
33. J. Madan and R. Chaujar, "Interfacial charge analysis of heterogeneous gate dielectric-gate all around-tunnel FET for improved device reliability," IEEE Transactions on Device and Materials Reliability, vol. 16, no. 2, pp. 227–234, 2016.

34. Y. Qiu, R. Wang, Q. Huang, and R. Huang, "A comparative study on the impacts of interface traps on tunneling FET and MOSFET," *IEEE Transactions on Electron Devices*, vol. 61, no. 5, pp. 1284–1291, 2014.
35. J. Madan and R. Chaujar, "Numerical simulation of N^+ source pocket PIN-GAA-tunnel FET: Impact of interface trap charges and temperature," *IEEE Transactions on Electron Devices*, vol. 64, no. 4, pp. 1482–1488, 2017.
36. W. Wang, J. Hwang, Y. Xuan, and P. D. Ye, "Analysis of electron mobility in inversion-mode MOSFETs," *IEEE Transactions on Electron Devices*, vol. 58, pp. 1972–1978, 2011.
37. D. Das, S. Baishya, and U. Chakraborty, "Impact of temperature on RF characteristics and electrical noise analysis of an L-shaped gate tunnel FET with hetero-stacked source configuration," *International Journal of RF and Microwave Computer-Aided Engineering*, vol. 30, p. e22310, 2020.
38. N. Paras and S. S. Chauhan, "Temperature sensitivity analysis of vertical tunneling based dual metal gate TFET on analog/RF FOMs," *Applied Physics A*, vol. 125, no. 316, 2019. https://doi.org/10.1007/s00339-019-2621-x.
39. R. Narang, M. Saxena, R. S. Gupta, and M. Gupta, "Impact of temperature variations on the device and circuit performance of tunnel FET: A simulation study," *IEEE Transactions on Nanotechnology*, vol. 12, no. 6, pp. 951–957, 2013.
40. S. Mookerjea, D. Mohata, T. Mayer, V. Narayanan, and S. Datta, "Temperature- dependent I-V characteristics of a vertical $In_{0.53}Ga_{0.47}As$ tunnel FET," *IEEE Electron Device Letters*, vol. 31, pp. 564–566, 2010.
41. S. Y. Wu, "Theory of generation-recombination noise in MOS transistors," *Solid State Electron*, vol. 11, pp. 25–32, 1968.
42. B. Leonardo, S. Mariana, and R. S. Berardi, "TFET-based circuit design using the transconductance generation efficiency gm/Id method," *IEEE Journal of the Electron Devices Society*, vol. 3, pp. 208–216, 2015.
43. R. S. Rangel and P. G. D. Agopian, "Performance evaluation of Tunnel-FET basic amplifier circuits," in *IEEE 10th Latin American Symposium on Circuits & Systems (LASCAS)*, pp. 21–24, 2019, doi: 10.1109/LASCAS.2019.8667587.
44. H. Liu, X. Li, R. Vaddi, K. Ma, S. Datta, and V. Narayanan, "Tunnel FET RF rectifier design for energy harvesting applications," *IEEE Journal on Emerging and Selected Topics in Circuits and Systems*, vol. 4, pp. 400–411, 2014.
45. S. Taheri and J.-S. Yuan, "Security analysis of tunnel field-effect transistor for low power hardware," *International Journal of Computer Science and Information Technologies*, vol. 8, no. 2, pp. 271–275, 2017.
46. Y. Lee, D. Yoon, Y. Kim, D. Blaauw, and D. Sylvester, "Circuit and system design guidelines for ultra-low power sensor nodes," *IPSJ Transactions on System LSI Design Methodology*, vol. 6, no. 2, pp. 17–26, 2013.
47. S. L. Tripathi, "Low-power high performance tunnel FET with analysis for IoT applications," *Handbook of Research on the Internet of Things Applications in Robotics and Automation*, 2019. https://doi.org/10.4018/978-1-5225-9574-8.ch002.

15 Application and Utilization of High-Aspect-Ratio Anti-reflective Si Nanostructure-Embedded Optical Sensor for IoT Applications

Arijit Bardhan Roy, Kalluri Vinay Kumar, and Moumita Saha

CONTENTS

15.1 INTRODUCTION

Smart and sustainable growth of human technologies is the first and foremost criteria for the socio-economic development of civilization. So nurture of smart technologies with sustainable approaches will be more agreeable in the coming future. Not only that, in the upcoming time, IoT-based technologies will be able to occupy most of the industrial sectors through smartwatches, home appliances, smart lights, wearable devices, and more. Further, these types of devices may be able to offer valuable contributions to the health, defence, and farming sectors. To design an efficient and smart Internet of Things (IoT) system, a vast quantity of sensors, actuators, and other apparatus for data acquisition and handling will be needed. To develop a smart cultivation system, the measurement of solar irradiation is a very crucial parameter. Pyranometers and irradiance meters are the most popular devices to measure solar irradiance. These tools could determine irradiance with high correctness and a broad range of spectral range. These devices can be high-priced and sometimes need specific equipment before the measurement. Therefore, low cost and much effective approaches are needed to introduce the solar irradiance system in the initial stage. For this reason, efficient low-cost optical PV sensors play a very vital role in that type of system. But due to high material costs in addition to low efficiencies of different PV devices, these cannot still be introduced as a primary sensor in the IoT sector [1–3].

In this context through this study, we try to resolve the barrier with the facilitation of just a 10 μc thin silicon substrate embedded with some optimized nanostructures. In conventional methods mainly most of the industries prefer 180 μc silicon substrate with some micro texturing. But when we reduce the thickness of the substrate to cut out the material consumption of the sensor,

DOI: 10.1201/9781003217398-15

some photons may be unabsorbed by the substrate. So nano-texturing on top of the cell will be more effective in absorbing photons by thin substrate than the conventional wafer (180 μc). So through this study, we try to investigate the proper aspect ratio for nanostructured geometry embedded on top of the silicon substrate. During this learning, we have investigated mainly the optical responses from the nanostructured geometry through finite element method (FEM) simulations.

15.2 SIMULATION AND OPTIMIZATION

In this study, we primarily focused on making a nanostructured silicon geometry with the help of FEM-based software like COMSOL. During this simulation study, we mainly focused on the reflectance behaviour and electric field profile of a particular structure in the visible wavelength region. Different aspect-ratio nanostructured geometries will be simulated through a 2D simulation model with a triangular arrangement made by the same material, silicon, on top of the thin silicon substrate. To find out proper anti-reflective nanostructured geometry, we have to compare structures (having base or width (*d*) and height (*h*)) that have two types of aspect ratios (high and low). The basic simulation models are shown in Figure 15.1.

15.3 SIMULATION SETUP

The simulation setup will be done on COMSOL Multiphysics 5.4 software to estimate the electric fields and the reflection of the model, which is shown in Figure 15.2.

Two ports used to obtain the results on the light will appear on port 1, and for the meshing of electromagnetic fields in the frequency domain, port 2 will be boundary conditions at perfect electric conductor / perfect matched layer (PEC/PML). The wavelength range lies between 300 nm and 1100 nm, with a zero-degree angle of incidence in the simulation setup [4,5].

15.4 RESULTS AND ANALYSIS

The light wave coming from the sun will be irradiance on top of the sensor, and the silicon nanostructures absorb the photons, which cultivate an electron–hole pair into the substrate. The absorption of the photon into the silicon will be denoted by the electric field profile of a particular structure. The injected photon into the substrate will be distributed uniformly throughout the device. If the

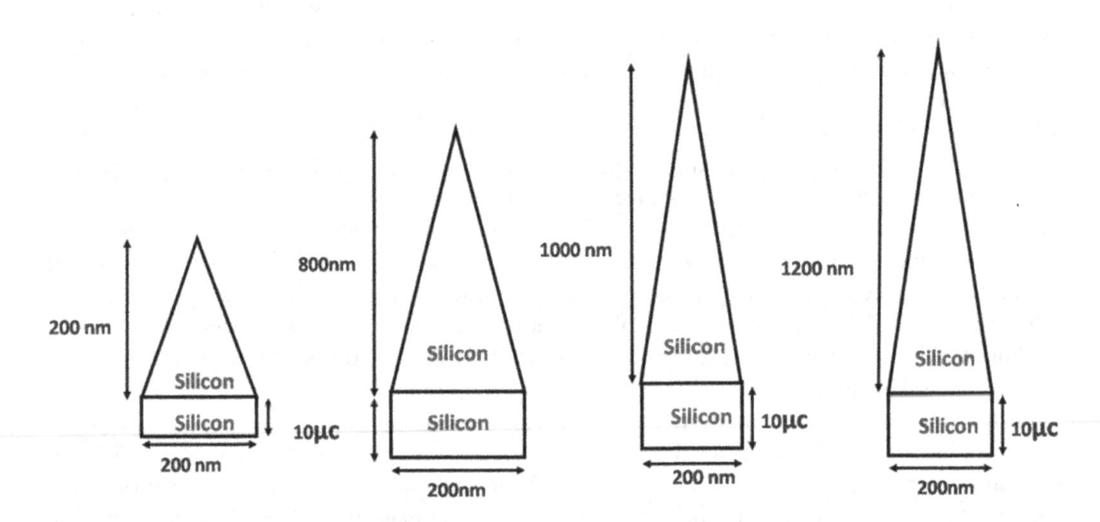

FIGURE 15.1 Graphical depiction of different aspect ratios of silicon nanostructures.

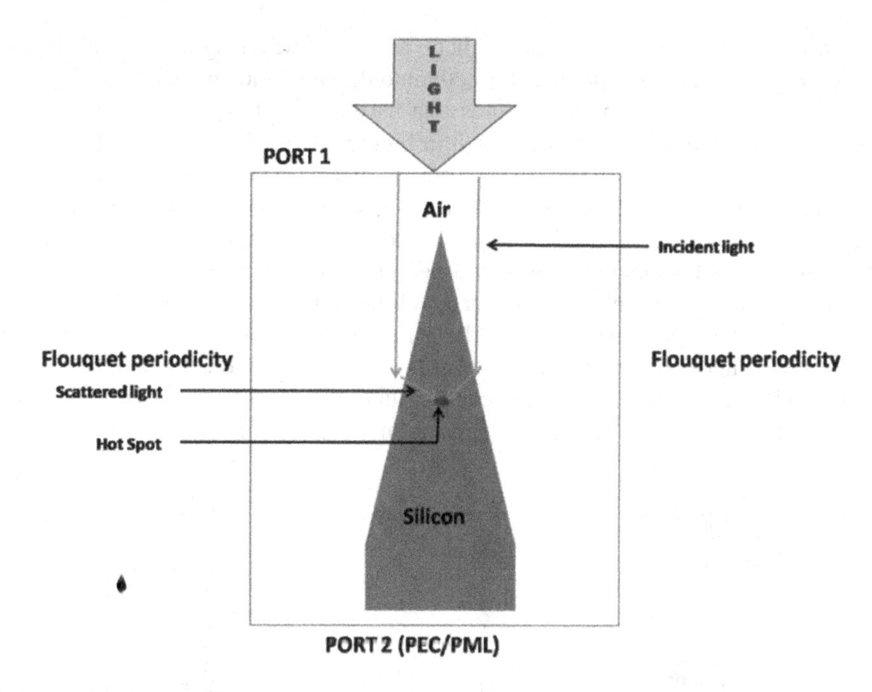

FIGURE 15.2 Simulation setup and photon generation technique.

photon density increases, it will be proportional to the short circuit current of the device, which results in enhancing the power production of the optical sensor.

To make a comparison between the two types of nanostructures (high and low), we presume aspect ratio (AR) one structure as low AR structure having a base (d) and height (h) both as 200 nm. For high-AR nanostructures, all bases were assumed as 200 nm with different heights like 800, 1000, and 1200 nm. All high- and low-AR Si nanostructures are modelled in the software of COMSOL Multiphysics 5.4 by wave optics (electromagnetic field, frequency domain model). In Figure 15.2, the lower side is indicated as the silicon substrate region and on top of the silicon layer will be the air region. The models, procedures, and further meshing will be internally inbuilt into the software.

The optical model properties of the reflection, electric field, transmission, absorption etc. will be analyzed with the support of the scattering parameters (s-parameters)[4].

$$S_{11} = \sqrt{\frac{\text{Power\_Reflected\_Port1}}{\text{Power\_Incident\_Port1}}} \tag{15.1}$$

$$S_{21} = \sqrt{\frac{\text{Power\_Delivered\_Port2}}{\text{Power\_Incident\_Port1}}} \tag{15.2}$$

$$\nabla \times E = 0 \tag{15.3}$$

where S_{11} and S_{12} are reflectance and absorption, respectively, and E=electric field.

To find out the reflection characteristics from a (~10 μc) thin silicon substrate, a PML boundary condition was connected at the back end to capture the response due to metallization. Port 1 is excited by the sun's light AM 1.5. The incident sunlight will be trapped by the geometry of the nanostructures through the air region. During the whole simulation process, we mainly prefer the 400–700 nm wavelength of light to determine the optical responses given by different types of nanostructures. The refractive incidences of silicon in various wavelengths were taken from Palik et al., and these values were incorporated perfectly into the simulation model [4, 5].

The electric field profiles of nanostructures that have different aspect ratios under the wavelength between 400 nm and 700 nm are shown in Figures 15.3, 15.4, 15.5, and 15.6. In all these figures, we have provided the electric field responses of four types of nanostructures with four different aspect ratios like 1, 4, 5, and 6. If we do investigate all the electric field figures, then we can understand that more photons will be trapped and captured by the high-aspect-ratio structures (aspect ratios 4, 5, and 6) compared to the low-aspect-ratio (aspect ratio 1) structure. Not only that, most of the hot spots (red portion) generated on top of the high-aspect-ratio nanostructures indicate maximum electron–hole pair generation onto the upper surface of the geometry where the junction of the device will be made up. Further influence of hotspots will be more dominant in high-photon-density regions (500, 600, and 700 nm wavelength). But one question that will come from the study is why are the high-aspect-ratio structures capable of trapping maximum photons compared to

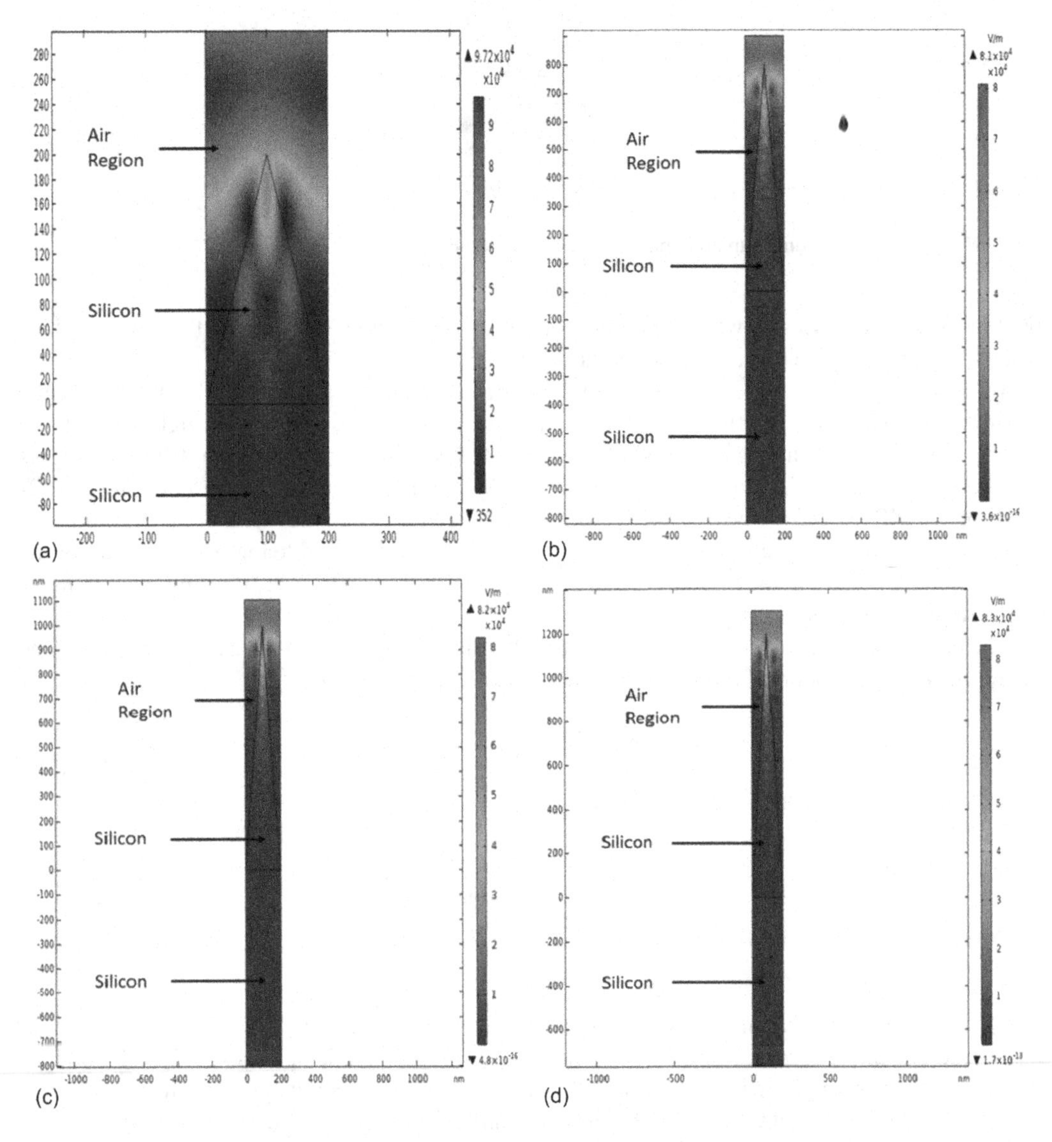

FIGURE 15.3 Electric field profile of 200 nm base with (a) 200 nm, (b) 800 nm, (c) 1000 nm, and (d) 1200 nm height silicon nanostructure in 400 nm wavelength.

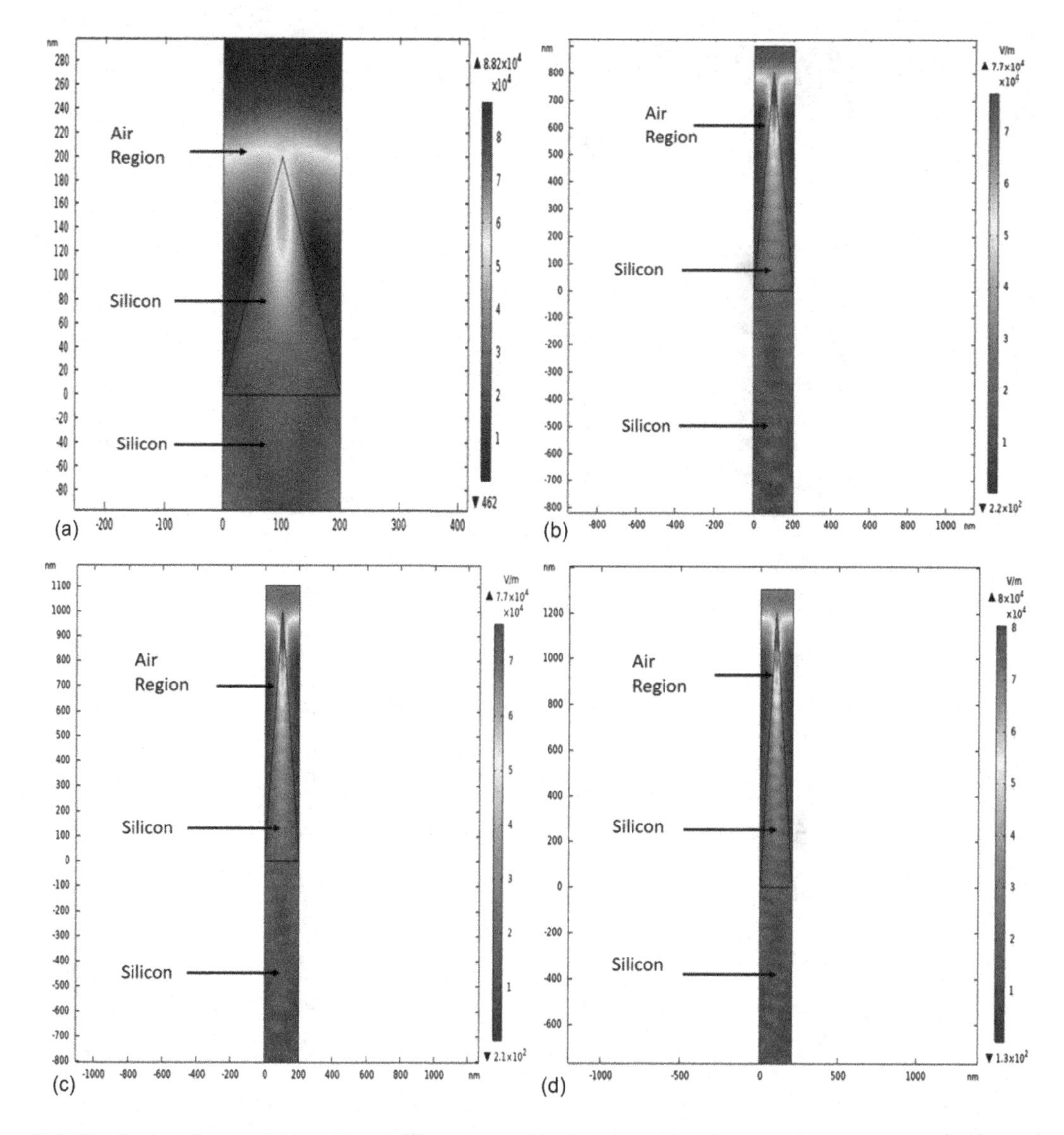

FIGURE 15.4 Electric field profile of 200 nm base with (a) 200 nm, (b) 800 nm, (c) 1000 nm, and (d) 1200 nm height silicon nanostructure in 500 nm wavelength.

low-aspect-ratio geometry? The smooth variation (low to high) of refractive indices of the structure from top to bottom will more efficiently bound the light rays that enter into the nanostructure geometry. Further due to the high-aspect-ratio nanostructures, the maximum scattering and multiple bounces of lights will occur that will generate maximum electron and hole pair into the absorber layer (silicon substrate). These incidences directly correlate with the increment of the short circuit current of the device and enhance the efficiency of the solar cells very effectively.

15.5 REFLECTANCE PROFILE

To increase the absorption of photons into the substrate, at first we have to make sure that the reflection of the substrate must be very less. Forming the surface of solar cell, the reflection must be decreased by using different types of nanostructures make to scatter the light rays into many angles. So in this study, we try to investigate the reflection characteristics of nanostructures with different

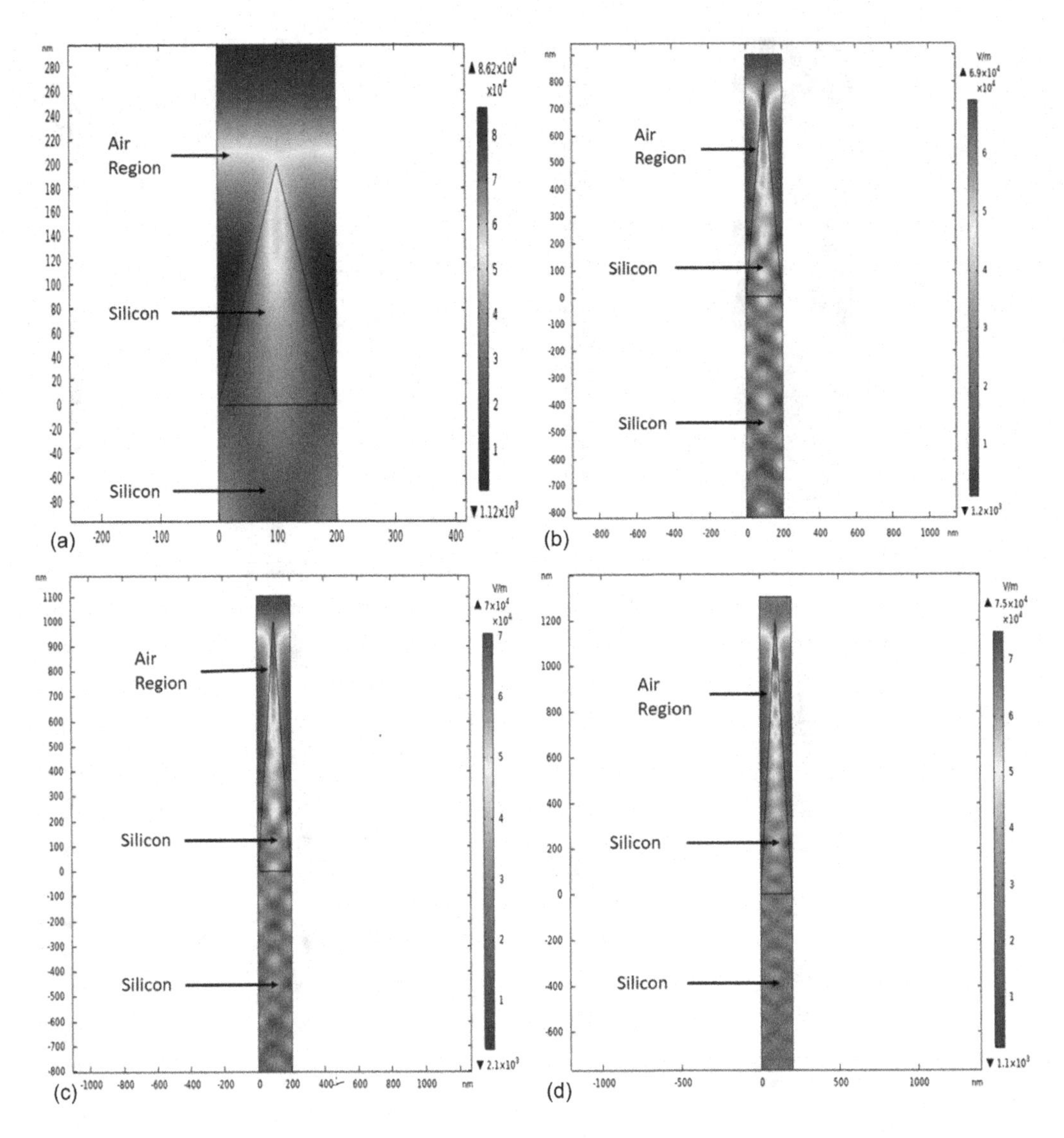

FIGURE 15.5 Electric field profile of 200 nm base with (a) 200 nm, (b) 800 nm, (c) 1000 nm, and (d) 1200 nm height silicon nanostructure in 600 nm wavelength.

aspect ratios through the optical simulation. Through this study, it was quite clear that the low-AR structure will be able to collect fewer photons than high-AR structures due to the extra height of the structure. Due to high AR, the path length of the light rays will be increased and maximum photons will be absorbed by the silicon substrate. Another point is that due to the multiple bounces of the light with the super scattering effect, the maximum photons enter into the high-AR structure. So in the high-AR structures, the reflectance loss will be less than 6% (<6%) compared to low-aspect-ratio structures during the entire wavelength range of 300–1100 nm in zero-degree incidence. On the other hand, the low-aspect-ratio structure is not able to give even less than 12% in any wavelength, which is validated by Figure 15.7.

Further, if we investigate the reflectance profile of the high-aspect-ratio nanostructures, then we can easily notice that all of the structures offered lower than 6% integrated reflectance (shown in Figure 15.8).

In conventional solar cell technology, this type of low reflectance was achieved by micro texturing with anti-reflection coating (ARC). To realize perfect anti-reflection coating, we have to

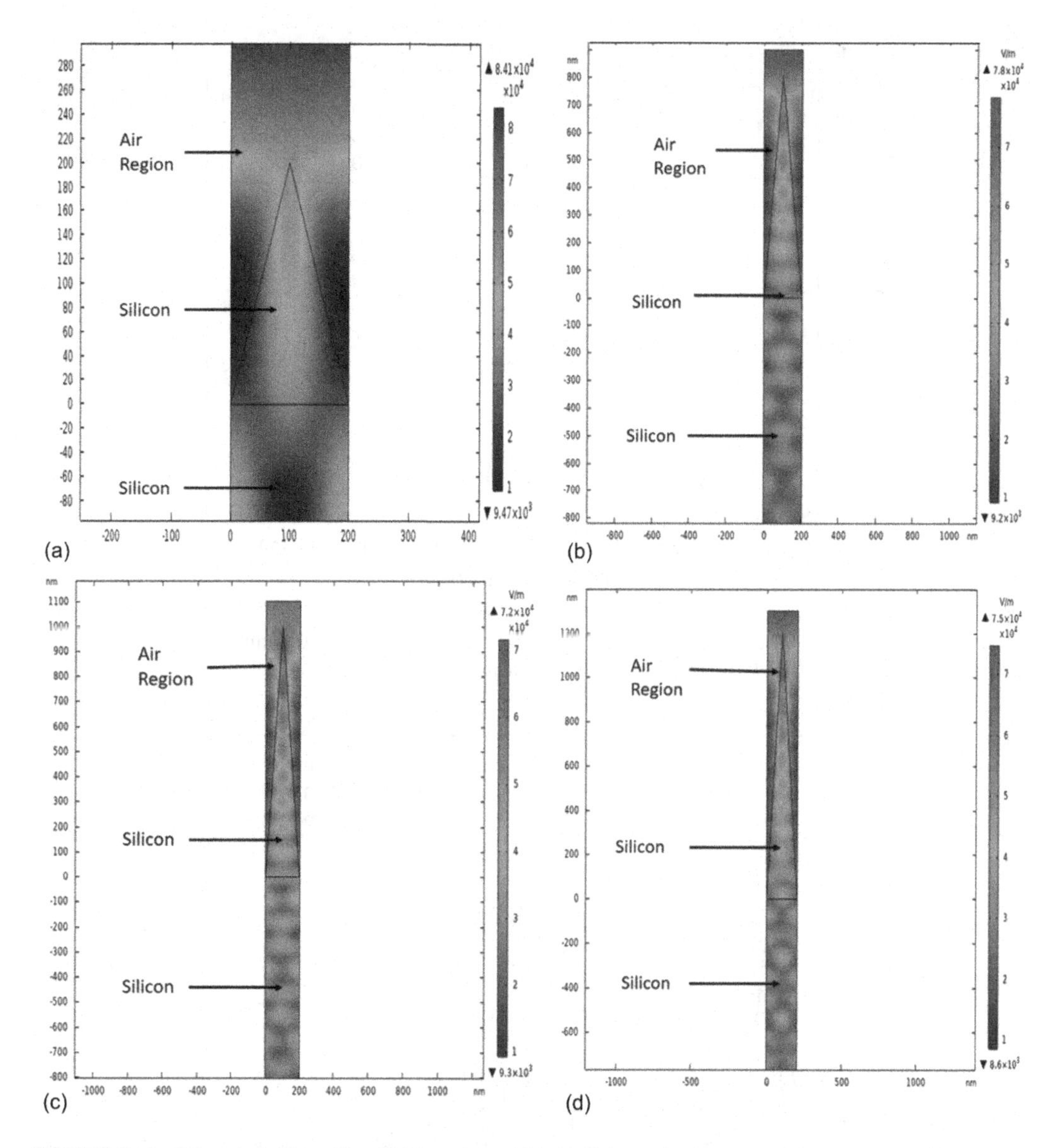

FIGURE 15.6 Electric field profile of 200 nm base with (a) 200 nm, (b) 800 nm, (c) 1000 nm, and (d) 1200 nm height silicon nanostructures in 700 nm wavelength.

incorporate some high-cost vacuum devices like PECVD and sputtering, which further increase the market price of the solar cell. By integrating the proposed high-aspect-ratio nanostructures into the fabrication process with the help of some chemical or lithography process, we can achieve the same or even more output power from the solar cell without involving any anti-reflection coating (ARC). But many increases in aspect ratios (more than 6) will immensely increase the surface area of the geometry that may raise the recombination loss of the PV sensor [6–10].

15.6 OPTICAL RESPONSE IN HIGHER ANGLE OF INCIDENCE

Capturing the incident photons from all directions is mandatory for developing an effective optical PV sensor. For this reason, utilizing the photons from a high angle of incidence (AOI) is very much vital. So investigating the reflectance profile under a high angle of incidence of light is essential in this study [11,12]. During this work, three types of higher angle incidences (30°, 45°, and 60°) were

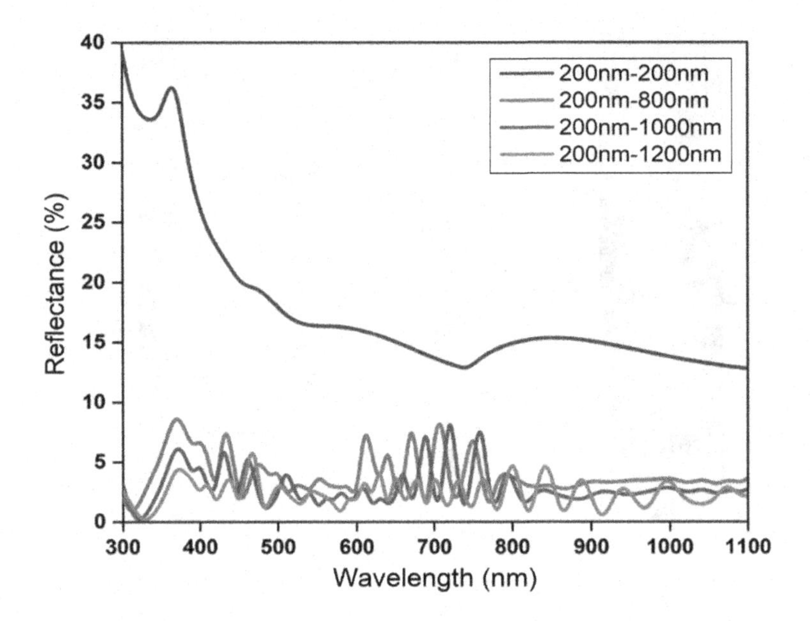

FIGURE 15.7 The reflectance profiles of high- (200 nm bases with 800 nm, 1000 nm, and 1200 nm height) and low–aspect-ratio (200 nm base with 200 nm height) nanostructures.

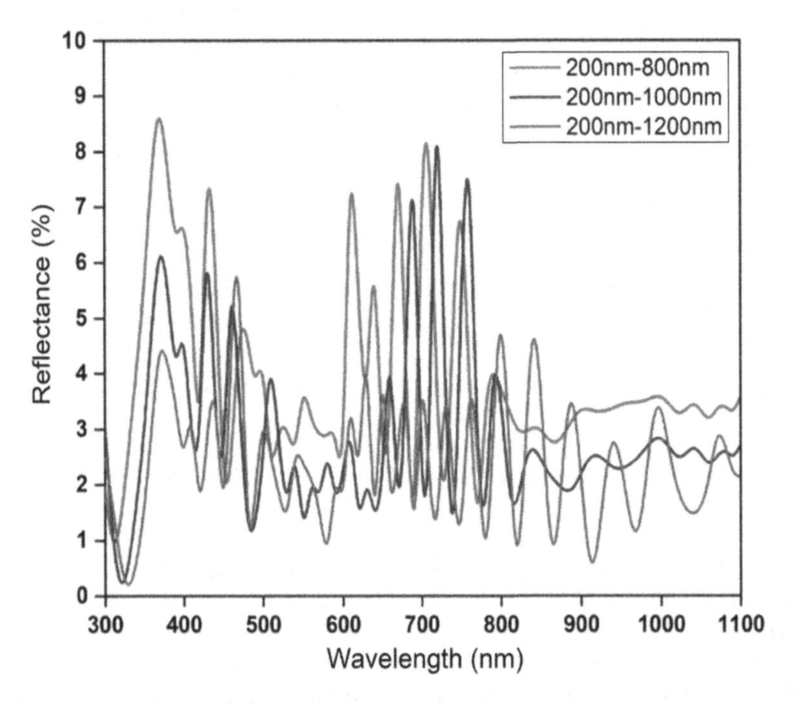

FIGURE 15.8 The reflectance profiles of 200 nm base with 800 nm, 1000 nm, and 1200 nm heights of high-aspect-ratio nanostructures.

taken for analysis. From that investigation, it was observed that high-aspect-ratio nanostructures offered more proficiency than lower-aspect-ratio structures in a higher angle of incidence of light described by Table 15.1 and Figure 15.9.

From Table 15.1, it was observed that the low-aspect-ratio nanostructured geometries from S.No 1 to 5 offered high reflectances in a higher angle of incidences compared to high-aspect-ratio

TABLE 15.1
Integrated Reflectance of Different Nanostructured Geometries in Different Angles of Incidences of Light

S.No	Morphology of Nanostructured Geometry	Integrated Reflectance			
		AOI[a] = 0°	AOI = 30°	AOI = 45°	AOI = 60°
1	200 nm base with 100 nm height	25.15	29.51	37.03	49.2
2	200 nm base with 200 nm height	16.2	20.18	26.89	39.54
3	200 nm base with 300 nm height	11.23	15.06	21.32	33.86
4	200 nm base with 400 nm height	8.35	11.45	17.12	28.8
5	200 nm base with 500 nm height	6.33	9.21	14.39	25.32
6	200 nm base with 600 nm height	5.26	7.6	12.36	23.01
7	200 nm base with 700 nm height	4.34	6.49	11.09	21.01
8	200 nm base with 800 nm height	3.88	5.74	9.62	18.76
9	200 nm base with 900 nm height	3.52	5.18	8.76	17.64
10	200 nm base with 1000 nm height	2.81	4.22	7.55	16.49

AOI[a]: angle of incidence.

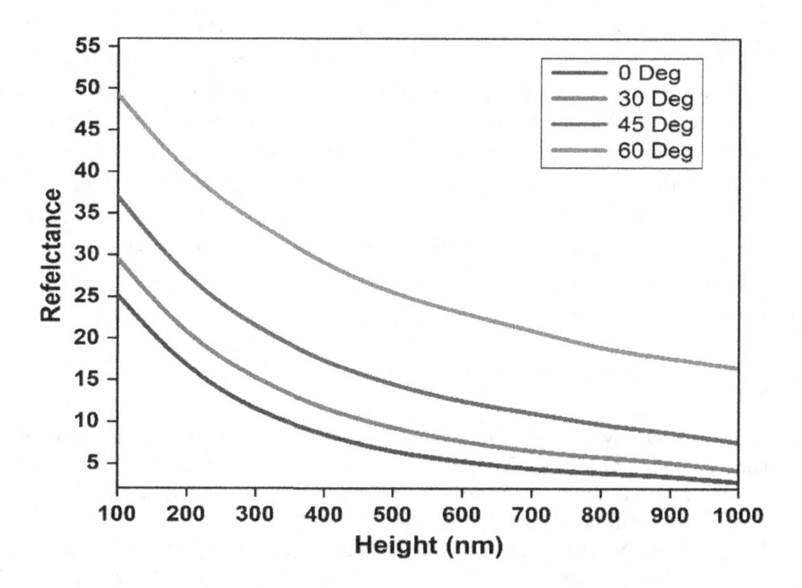

FIGURE 15.9 The reflectance profiles of 200 nm base with 100 nm to 1000 nm height of nanostructure geometries in different angles of incidence (AOI) of light.

geometries (S.No 6 to 10). But this whole work mostly focused on the smart cultivation system. So we have to develop such kind of sensor which can capture the sunlight not only in the middle of the day but also in other daytime periods. In this context, the PV sensor with high-aspect-ratio nanostructures has the potential to offer significant results compared to other structures.

To validate the optical responses in the higher angle of incidence of light, the electric field profiles of both geometries (high and low aspect ratios) have been investigated in Figure 15.10a and b. Through this investigation, it was observed that a high-aspect-ratio silicon nanostructure (with 200 nm base and 1000 nm height) was a better contender for trapping the photons than a low-aspect-ratio structure (Figure 15.10a). The hotspots (red region) generated on top of the high-aspect-ratio nanostructured geometry validated the fact that much more light is absorbed onto the surface. The

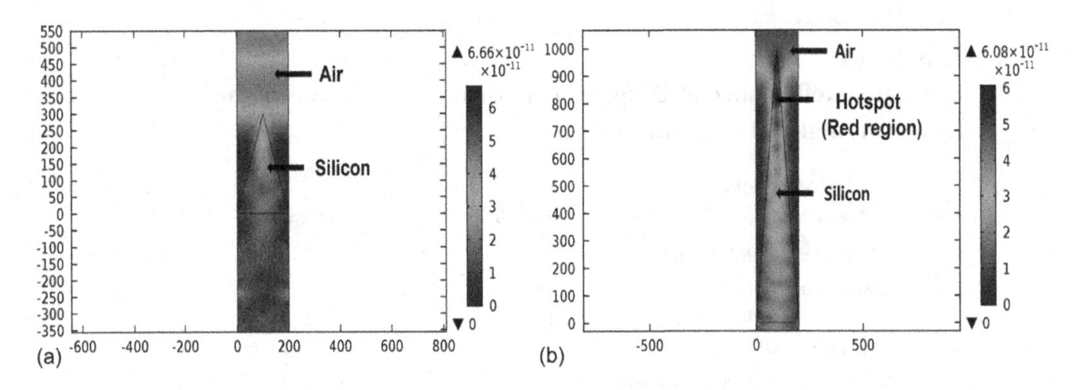

FIGURE 15.10 The electric field profiles of 200 nm base with (a)100 nm and (b)1000 nm height of nanostructure geometries in 550 nm wavelength at 45° angle of incidence (AOI).

super scattering, as well as multiple bounces of light rays, offered much more absorption of photons in high-aspect-ratio nanostructures than low-aspect-ratio structures.

15.7 CONCLUSION

At the end of this study, we proposed some high-aspect-ratio anti-reflective nanostructures for thin silicon optical PV sensors with a minimum loss of material. This study can also help validate the importance of high-aspect-ratio triangular nanostructures in optical sensor research in the future. In this study, we observed that embedding these optimized structures on top of the thin silicon substrate will accelerate the photon generation very effectively compared to the low-aspect-ratio structures. Further any dielectric nanoparticles or metamaterials on top of this structure will be able to give us a more satisfactory result. At last, the authors strongly believed that in the future, this type of study will encourage more research communities to work on other high-aspect-ratio nanostructures implemented on different materials for enhancing the efficiency of PV sensors, which also helps make a smart and eco-friendly IoT sector.

REFERENCES

1. Aleksic, S., 2019. A survey on optical technologies for IoT, smart industry, and smart infrastructures, *Journal of Sensor and Actuator*, 8, 47, p. 18.
2. Lorenzo, I., Alberto, B., Lorenzo, P., Mauro, B., Paola, P., 2017. Sensing light with LEDs: Performance evaluation for IoT applications, *Journal of Imaging*, 3, 50, p. 12.
3. Hussein, A.-T., Arabasi, S., 2018. Solar irradiance measurements using smart devices: A cost-effective technique for estimation of solar irradiance for sustainable energy systems, *Sustainability*, 10, 508, p. 11.
4. Roy, A. B., Dhar, A., Choudhuri, M., Das, S., Hossain, S. M., Kundu, A., 2016. Black silicon solar cell: Analysis optimization and evolution towards a thinner and flexible future, *Nanotechnology*, 27, 305302, p. 12.
5. Palik, E. D., 1985. *Handbook of Optical Constants of Solids*. San Diego, CA: Academic.
6. Banerjee, S., Mandal, S., Sukanta, D., Roy, A. B., Mukherjee, N., 2019. Nano-mirror embedded back reflector layer (BRL) for advanced light management in thin silicon solar cells. *Industrial & Engineering Chemistry Research*, 58, 28, pp. 12678–12686.
7. Glunz, S. W., Preu, R., Biro, D., 2012. Crystalline Silicon Solar Cells: State-of-the-Art and Future Developments, *Comprehensive Renewable Energy*, pp. 353–387. https://doi.org/10.1016/B978-0-08-087872-0.00117-7
8. Han, K. S., Shin, J. H., Yoon, W. Y., Lee, H., 2011. Enhanced performance of solar cells with antireflection layer fabricated by nano-imprint lithography, *Solar Energy Materials and Solar Cells*, 95, 1, pp. 288–291.

9. Roy, A. B., Das, S., Kundu, A., Banerjee, C., Mukherjee, N., 2017. c-Si/n-ZnO based flexible solar cells with silica nanoparticles as light trapping metamaterial, *Physical Chemistry Chemical Physics*, 19, 20, pp. 12838–12844.
10. Sharma, J., Das, G., Roy, A. B., Bose, S., Mukhopadhyay, S., 2019. Design analysis of heterojunction solar cells with aligned AZO nanorods embedded in p-type Si wafer, *Silicon*, 12, 82, pp. 305–316.
11. Roy, A. B., Kumar, K. V., Saha, M., 2021. Light management studies by using different surface texturing for thin cSi solar cells, *Applied Physics A*, 127, 129, pp. 1–12.
12. Sharma, J., Roy, A. B., Das, G., Patra, S., Barua, A. K., Mukhopadhyay, S., 2019. Application of N-doped ZnO Nanorods in Heterojunction Si Solar Cells, in R. Sharma, and D. Rawal. (eds) The Physics of Semiconductor Devices. IWPSD 2017. Springer Proceedings in Physics, vol. 215. Springer, Cham. https://doi.org/10.1007/978-3-319-97604-4_55.

16 RF and Microwave Energy Harvesting Antennas for Self-Sustainable IoT

Samik Chakraborty and Ayona Chakraborty

CONTENTS

16.1 INTRODUCTION

Wireless electrical communication in its present form was initiated by Maxwell and Hertz by the replacement of transmission lines or cables with high-frequency electromagnetic (EM) radio waves. Since Marconi's use of radio communication, its emergence from broadcast radio to the recent inundation of technology developments have made advanced antenna systems (ASS) a viable option for the development of radio frequency (RF) and microwave energy harvesting antennas, towards the use in self-sustainable Internet of Things (IoT) devices in many commercial applications.

The rise in average temperature to mitigate the global energy demand is becoming an increasingly burning issue. In this regard, nonconventional green energy harvesting becomes a big subject for exploration. Among many other ways of nonconventional energy harvesting like solar energy, vibration energy, and thermal energy, which are particularly useful for small hand-held IoT devices, microwave/RF energy harvesting is a promising competitor, because of its over-the-clock unconditional existence and compactness of the relevant device, thus establishing its superiority over the others, particularly in IoT-based applications [1]. Open source energy harvesting in its state of the art form is applied in single or combinational methods in various areas, such as mobile charging and smart building, but in areas like smart packing, microwave/RF energy is a preferred method to power the small devices. While harvesting open environmental energy, the main difference in the various kind of power sources used is the power density, as an example microwave/RF (0.01 to 0.1 mW/cm^2), different vibrations (4 to 100 mW/cm^2), photovoltaic (10 to 10 mW/cm^2) and thermal (20 mW/cm^2 to 10 mW/cm^2). Though the abundance of RF energy is widespread, densitywise, it is limited, except in areas very close to the RF sources. Hence, efficient RF power harvesting circuits, including high gain, broadband antenna, and array, must be developed to operate for the most optimal performances [1–2].

DOI: 10.1201/9781003217398-16

Some peer-reviewed papers have reported RF to DC conversion with incident powers as low as –20 dBm with adequate circuitry for the conversion. This leads us to conclude that if available surrounding RF energy in the concerned areas is around –20 dBm, then it may be potentially harvested. In Figure 16.1(a), power levels better than the –20 dBm spectrum level are achieved and hence the probability of RF energy harvesting is high. Again in Figure 16.1(b), spectrum level below –20 dBm has been observed and the signal strength increases as the distance from the RF source, i.e., the mobile base station (BTS), decreases [3].

Table 16.1 shows the calculation of estimated received power level, assuming normalized transmitter with 0 dBi and receiver antenna system gain with ideal condition free space EM signal propagation loss (FSPL), it is obvious that FM radio transmitter has the highest electric field intensity producing the highest electric potential for RF energy harvesting [4].

It is also observed [5] that power from RF to DC is roughly the integral over the spectrum of digital TV band and is significantly higher than the narrow band mobile cellular RF energy harvesting cases.

$$P_{\mathrm{DC(DTV)}} = \alpha \int_{470}^{770} \delta P_{\mathrm{DC}}\left(f\right) df \tag{16.1}$$

Here, the power attenuation factor is α in the specified signal spectrum of 470–770 MHz frequency.

In case of RF power harvesting using an antenna with receiver systems (rectenna), the incident angle $S\left(\theta, \varphi, f, t\right)$ can vary over the frequency band with respect to time. $A_{\mathrm{eff}}\left(\theta, \varphi, f\right)$ is the effective aperture of the receiving antenna, which is a dependent variable of frequencies and polarizations of the revived spectrum and different incidence angles. Therefore, at any instant of time average, received RF power over a range of frequencies can be expressed as

$$P_{\mathrm{RF}} = \frac{1}{f_{\mathrm{high}} - f_{\mathrm{low}}} \int_{f_{\mathrm{low}}}^{f_{\mathrm{high}}} \int_{0}^{4\text{À}} S\left(\theta, \varphi, f, t\right) A_{\mathrm{eff}}\left(\theta, \varphi, f\right) d\text{©} df \tag{16.2}$$

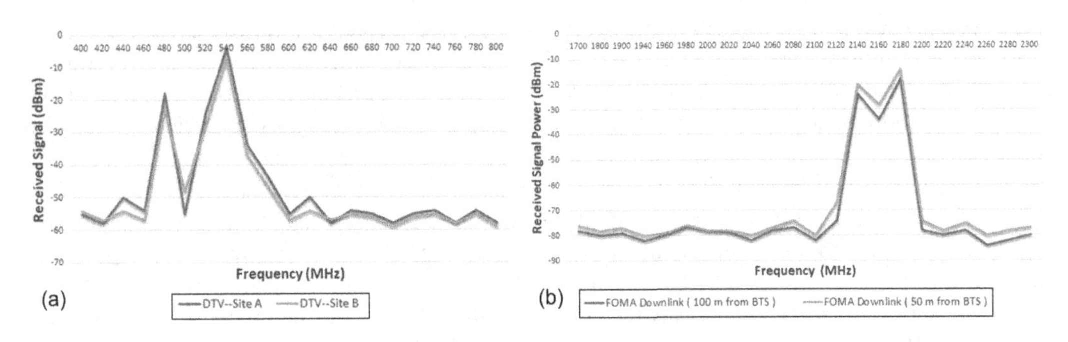

FIGURE 16.1 (a) Measured signal spectrum; (b) measured GSM cellular signal spectrum.

TABLE 16.1
RF Energy Sources, Measured Data

Source	V/m	dBm
FM transmitter radio	0.15 to 3	
City-based analogue TV	0.3 to 2	
Satellite-based digital TV	0.2 to 2.4	–40 to 0.0
City-based cellular network		–65 to 0.0
Small-range Wi-Fi network		Nearly –30

Thus, converted DC power for a particular frequency will be

$$P_{DC}(f_i) = P_{RF}(f_i, t).\eta(P_{RF}(f_i, t), \rho, Z_{DC}) \tag{16.3}$$

Here, the conversion efficiency is a variable of impedance mismatch ($\rho(P_{RF}, f)$) between the rectifier circuit, antennas, and load impedance. Here reflection coefficient is non-linear in nature and is a function of input power and incident frequency.

16.2 DESIGN OF RF ENERGY HARVEST SYSTEM

The block diagram shown in Figure 16.2 antennas chosen are microstrip or dielectric in nature due to their easy manufacturing process, low cost and easy incorporation with matching circuits. In the case of microwave/RF energy, the harvesting system target is to achieve maximum available RF power; for that purpose some useful low power harvesting circuits and antennas (including an array of antennas) are described in the following sections.

16.2.1 Antenna Design Requirements

An antenna is a basic element for transmitting and receiving electromagnetic (RF/microwave) waves, as well as it can convert an EM wave to an electrical signal and vice versa. Performance of a good antenna depends on input impedance matching, radiation pattern and directivity of the radiated beam, antenna efficiency, gain, EM signal polarization, and operating frequency bandwidth. These parameters are responsible for maximum RF power transmission and reception, which is defined as "the ratio of the available power at the terminals of a receiving antenna to the power flux density of a plane wave incident on the antenna from the direction of maximum radiation intensity". If P_{in} is the maximum received or transmitting power of an antenna, then it is directly proportional to the effective aperture of antenna A_{em} [6].

$$P_{in} = A_{em} W_i \tag{16.4}$$

where W_i is the incident RF power density. Therefore, the relation of effective aperture area for a receiving antenna can be expressed as [7]

$$A_{em} = e_{cd}\left(1 - |``|^2\right)\left(\frac{\lambda}{4\pi}\right)^2 D_0 |\hat{\rho}_w.\hat{\rho}_a|^2 \tag{16.5}$$

where λ is incident RF wavelength, e_{cd} is incident RF radiation efficiency, $\left(1 - |``|^2\right)$ and $|\hat{\rho}_w.\hat{\rho}_a|^2$ is responsible for associated losses due to impedance and polarization mismatch, D_0 is directivity depending on the radiation pattern of the antenna or array of antennas.

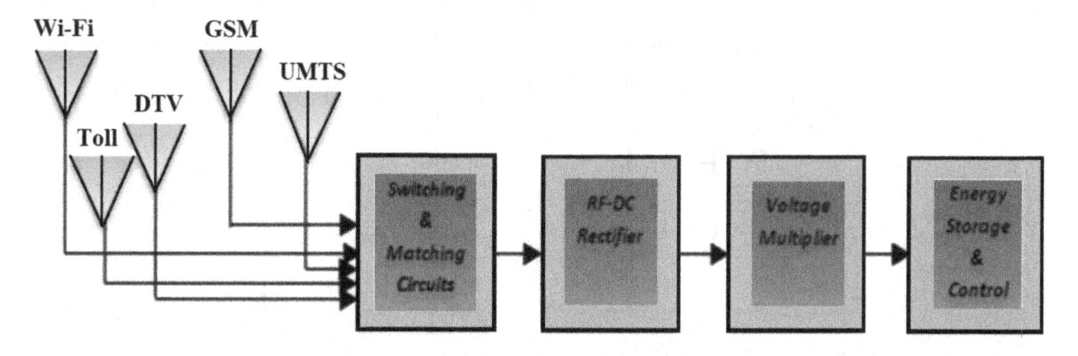

FIGURE 16.2 Block diagram for microwave/RF energy harvesting.

16.2.2 RF to DC Conversion Module

Voltage-doubler circuit is required to convert incident RF energy to usable DC voltage (Figure 16.3) [8–9]. Here, multi- (seven-) stage voltage-doubler circuit using semiconductor diode (schottky diode, 1N6263) is described and the circuit is simulated using SPICE software, given in Figure 16.4. Here each voltage-doubler circuit with internal resistance R_0 and output voltage V_0 is considered. Then, the output voltage V_{out} can be presented as [10]

$$V_{out} = \frac{V_0}{R_0 + R_L} R_L \tag{16.6}$$

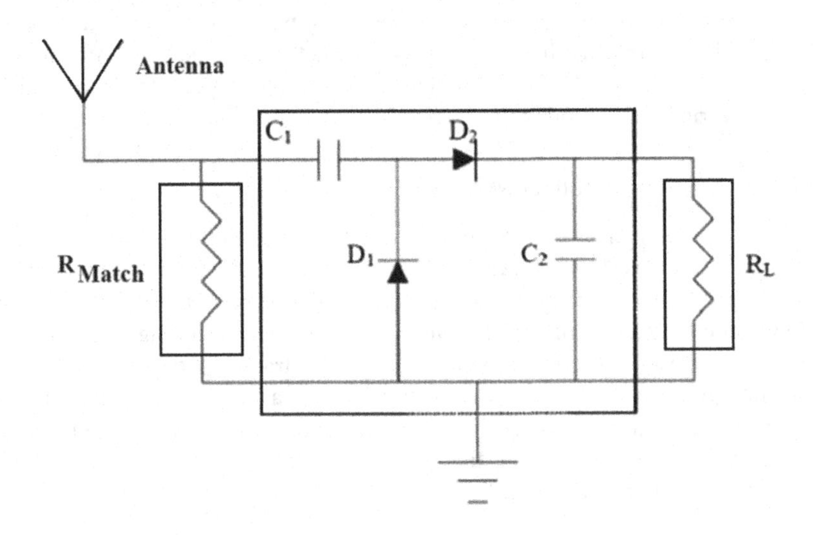

FIGURE 16.3 Single-stage RF power harvesting voltage-doubler circuit.

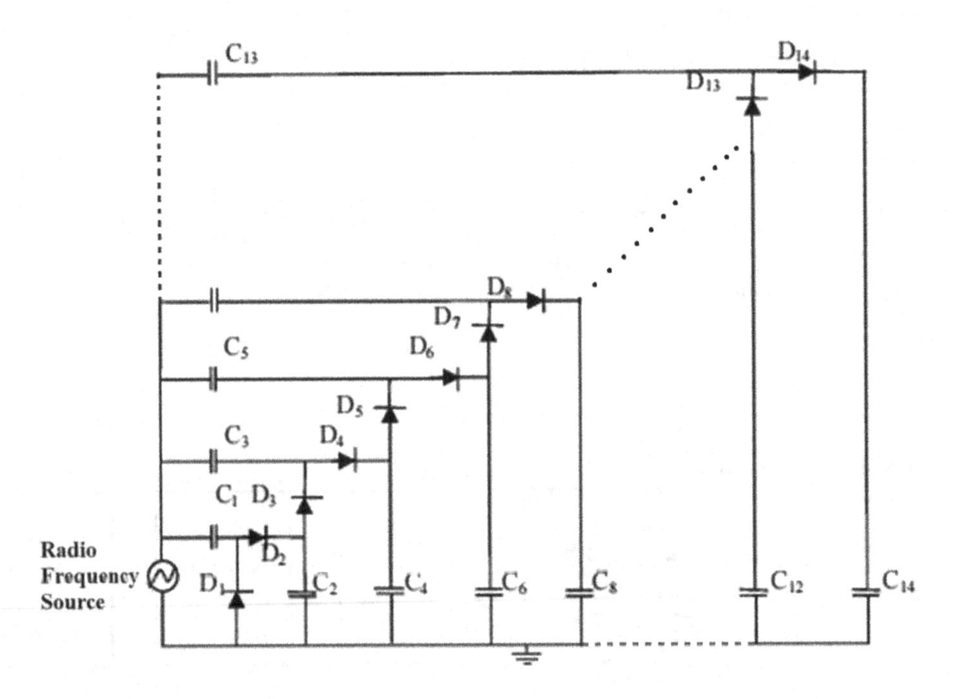

FIGURE 16.4 Seven-stage voltage-doubler circuit.

for n stages, the voltage doubler connected to the load R_L can be expressed as

$$V_{\text{out}} = \frac{nV_0}{nR_0 + R_L} R_L = V_0 \frac{1}{\frac{R_0}{R_L} + \frac{1}{n}} \tag{16.7}$$

To get the maximum output voltage, the circuit has to be optimized through multiple iterations.

16.2.3 Matching Network

A suitably designed and optimized matching network is required between the source and the complex load impedance (DC converter). Here, pi network is considered between the antenna and the RF–DC converter. For easy fabrication and compatibility, mostly microstrip type structures are used for matching networks [11].

$$\frac{W}{h} < 1$$

$$\varepsilon_{reff} = \frac{\varepsilon_r + 1}{2} + \frac{\varepsilon_r - 1}{2}\left[\left(1 + 12\frac{h}{W}\right)^{-\frac{1}{2}} + 0.4\left(1 - \frac{W}{h}\right)^2\right]$$

$$Z_0 = \frac{60}{\sqrt{\varepsilon_{reff}}} \ln\left(\frac{8h}{W} + \frac{W}{4h}\right) \tag{16.8}$$

RF energy harvesting and optimized RF power conversion efficiency is stringently dependent on conditions like different types of polarization and low incident power densities. Received RF power from various radial distances of BTS towers for GSM band is calculated using the Friis transmission equation [12].

$$\frac{P_R}{P_T} = G_T G_R \left[\lambda / (4\pi l)\right]^2 \tag{16.9}$$

where

P_R = received RF power
P_T = transmitted RF power
G_T = effective gain of the transmitting antenna
G_R = effective gain of the receiving antenna
λ = operating wavelength
f = frequency
d = radial distance between transmitter and receiver (i.e. antennas).

Friis power transmission equation in decibel becomes:

$$10\log_{10}\left(\frac{P_R}{P_T}\right) = G_{T,\text{dB}} + G_{R,\text{dB}} - 20\log_{10} f - 20\log_{10} d + 147.56 \tag{16.10}$$

Here it has been observed that nearly 2 V of output voltage may be achieved for a distance of 50 m from the GSM-BTS tower (refer to Figures 16.5 and 16.6). Moreover, the output voltage is enough to recharge the battery and may be used to power the WSNs [13].

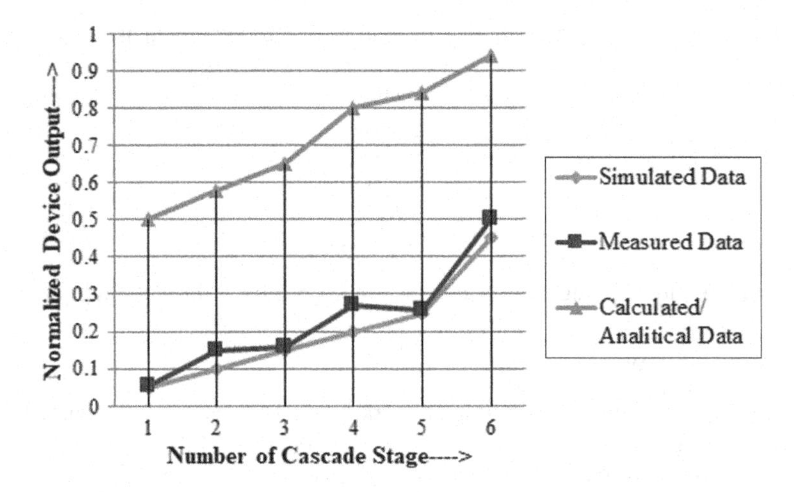

FIGURE 16.5 Normalized output for seven-stage voltage doubler versus the number of stages. [8]

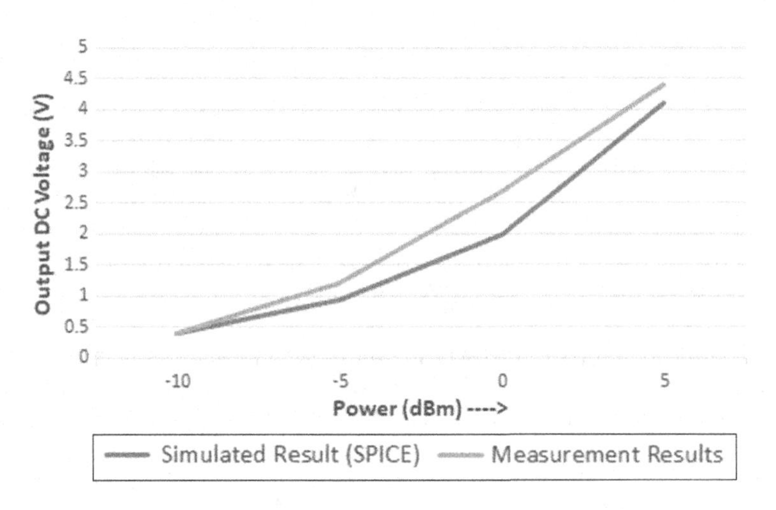

FIGURE 16.6 Output DC voltage (final stage) versus input power for the seven-stage voltage doubler. [8]

16.3 DIFFERENT ANTENNAS USED FOR RF ENERGY HARVESTING

Microwave and RF power harvesting from different open-air sources is a process where microwave and radio frequency (RF) energy radiated by sources such as analogue or digital TV signals, radio/FM networks, different satellites and GSM phone towers is gathered using adequate electronic circuitry. The antenna is an indispensable component for the power-receiving circuit, so the received power quantity mainly depends on antenna gain, efficiency and frequency bandwidth. Here, different types of antennas and array of antennas with high gain and frequency bandwidth for receiving higher RF power are presented, which can be converted into usable DC voltage.

16.3.1 ANTENNA1

The most commonly used RF power harvesting frequency band is the GSM band. Here the proposed antenna is designed, simulated optimized and tested in the GSM frequency band. This antenna is suitable for dual-band operation i.e., 788–936 MHz frequency band (16.5% bandwidth) for lower GSM range and 1.12–1.48 GHz frequency band (28% bandwidth) for higher GSM range [14]. Loading with inductive posts and capacitive-coupled slots produces dual-band operation with the trans-receiving power of circular polarized EM radiation. In addition, this proposed antenna

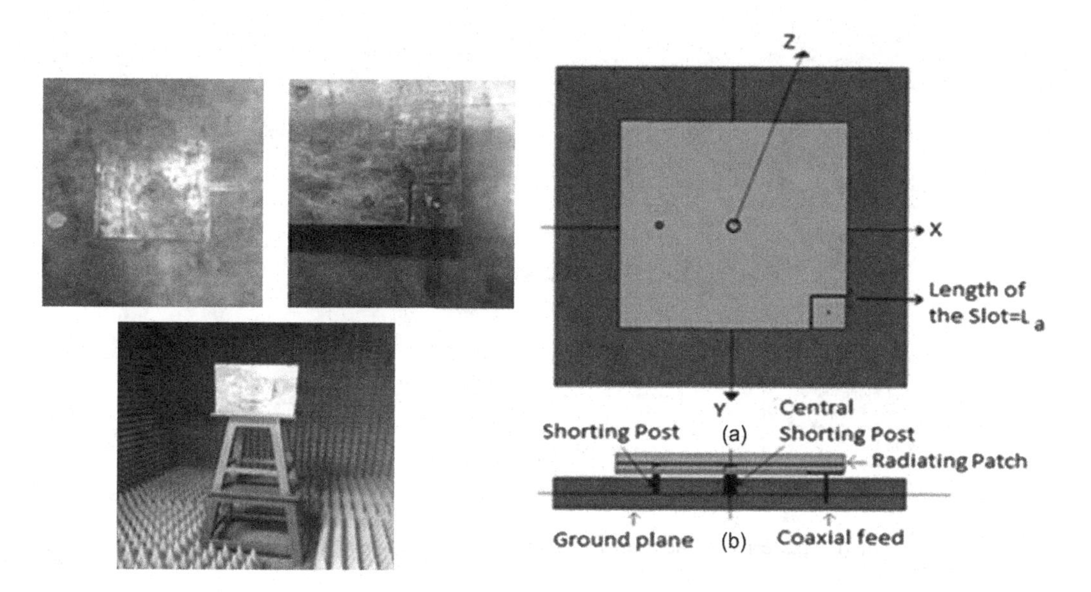

FIGURE 16.7 (a) Top view of antenna and ground plane; (b) schematic of feed position and shorting pin load; (c) antenna with the measurement system.

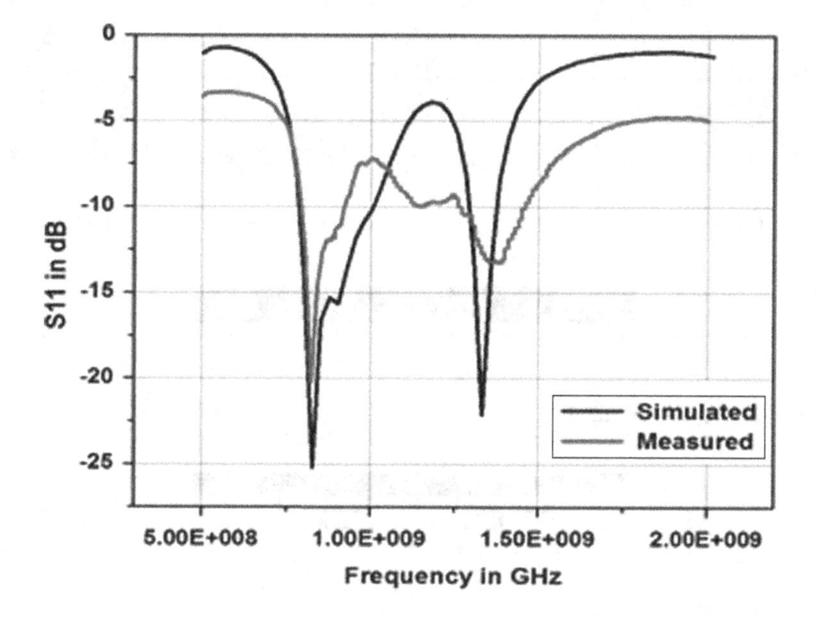

FIGURE 16.8 Comparison of simulated and experimental results of return loss.

produces a high gain. Due to these characteristics, this antenna is extremely suitable for RF power harvesting of GSM and GPS bands without any loss incurred for polarization mismatch. Results are shown in Figures 16.7 and 16.8.

Simulated and measured radiation patterns with the corresponding surface current distribution of this extremely efficient RF power harvesting antenna are given in Figures 16.9 and 16.10.

16.3.2 Antenna2

To maximize the production of RF power in a particular direction, the directive gain of the antenna must be high enough. For this purpose, arraying of multiple antennas is essential, as a single

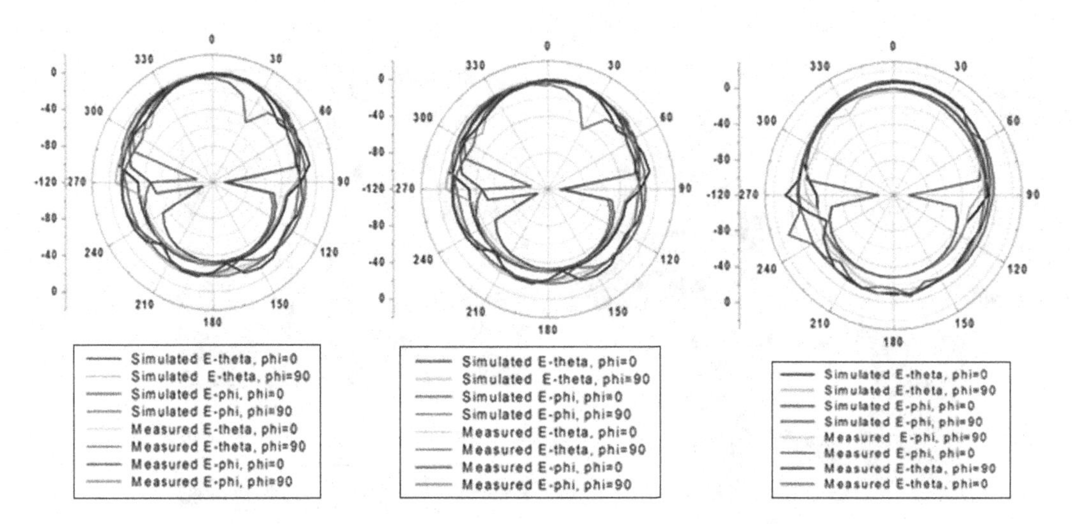

FIGURE 16.9 Radiation patterns for the proposed antenna at (a) 800 MHz, (b) 900 MHz and (c) 1170 MHz.

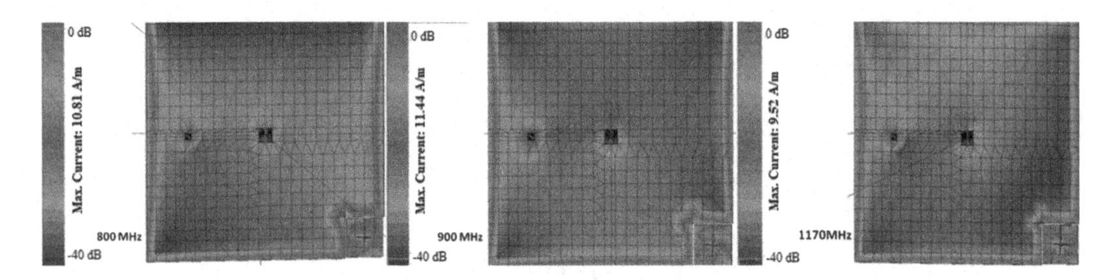

FIGURE 16.10 Current distribution of the proposed antenna at (a) 800 MHz, (b) 900 MHz and (c) 1170 MHz.

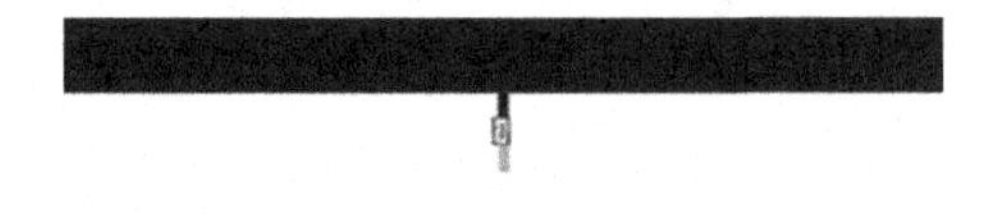

FIGURE 16.11 Single-feed excitation

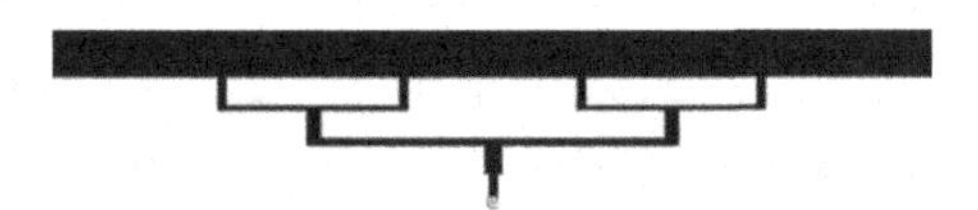

FIGURE 16.12 Four feeds excitation

microstrip antenna suffers from a limited directive gain. Further, in portable IoT-based devices, physical space limitation is a major issue hence continuous aperture microstrip antenna may be a good solution to overcome this problem [15]. For receiving GSM mobile base station RF power, consider a continuous microstrip aperture array antenna with $\varepsilon_r=4.4$, $fr=1.8$ GHz and $h=1.6$ mm, respectively, with multiple corporate feed techniques. Here aperture patch length is 52.515 mm, and with different excitation current weights for eight elements, SLL of –25dB is achieved.

Here this proposed continuous aperture array antenna is simulated (Zeland IE3D) and experimentally verified, which gives more than a 10 dBi directive gain instead of the 5–6 dBi gain in a single-patch antenna with considerable compactness in size. It is also observed that an increase in the number of feed excitation (Figures 16.11–16.13) increases the directive gain; results are shown in Figures 16.14–16.17.

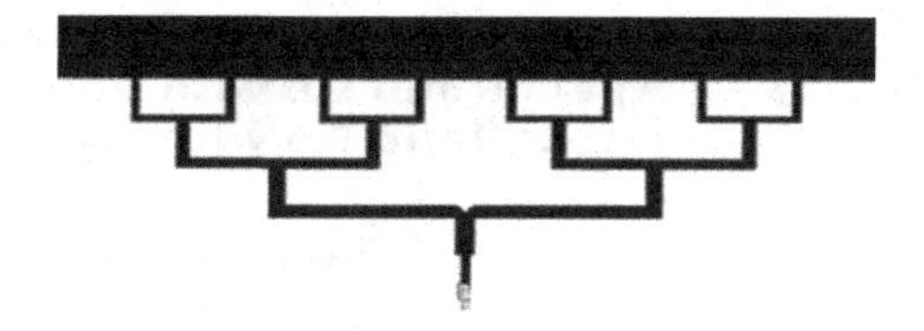

FIGURE 16.13 Eight feeds excitation

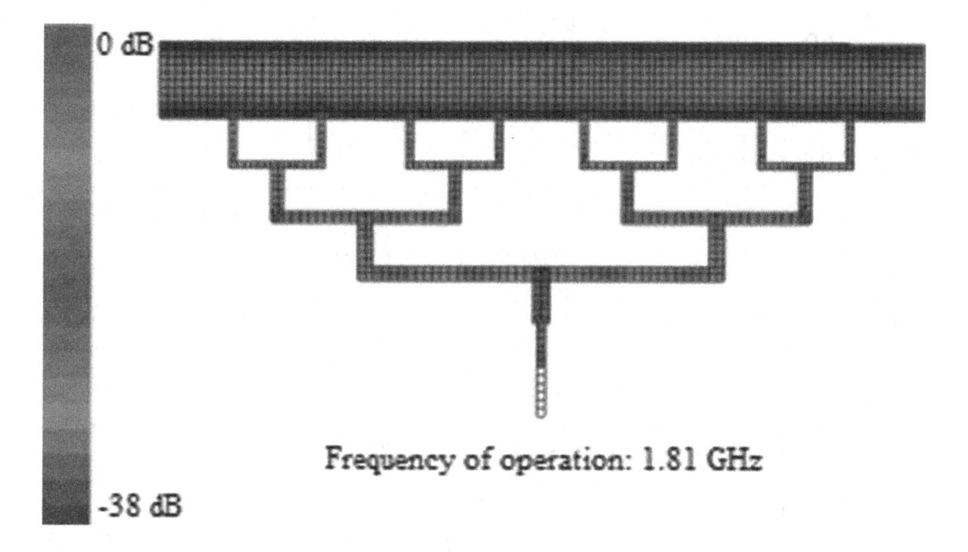

FIGURE 16.14 Excitation current distribution of eight feeds continuous aperture antenna.

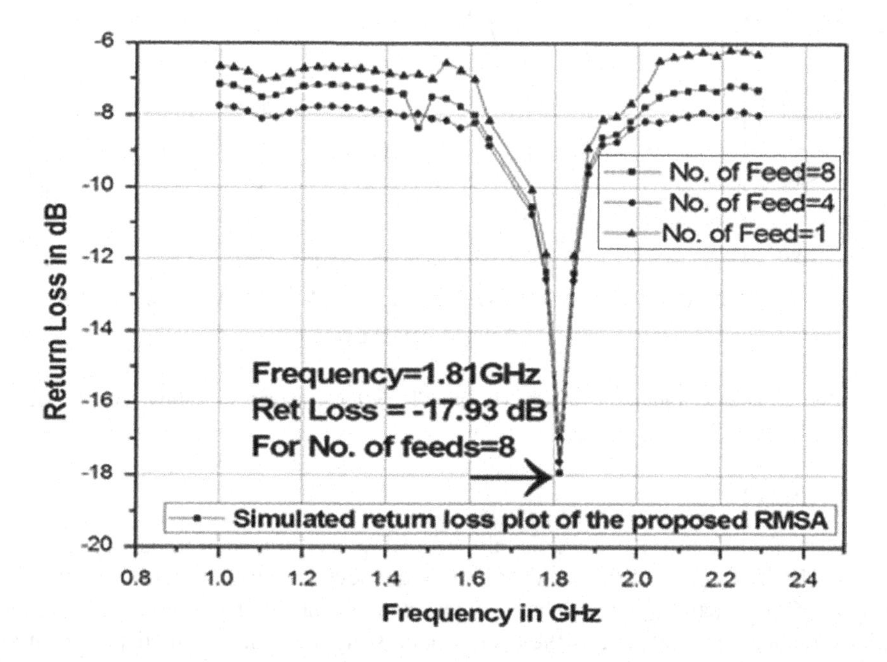

FIGURE 16.15 Simulated return loss of continuous aperture antenna with multiple feeds.

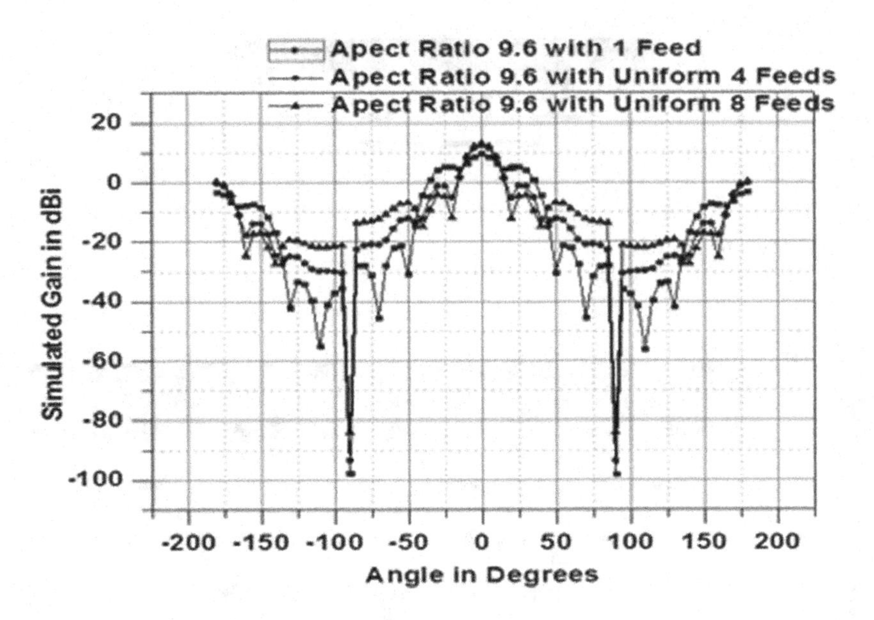

FIGURE 16.16 Simulated radiation patterns and directive gain for continuous aperture antenna with multiple feeds.

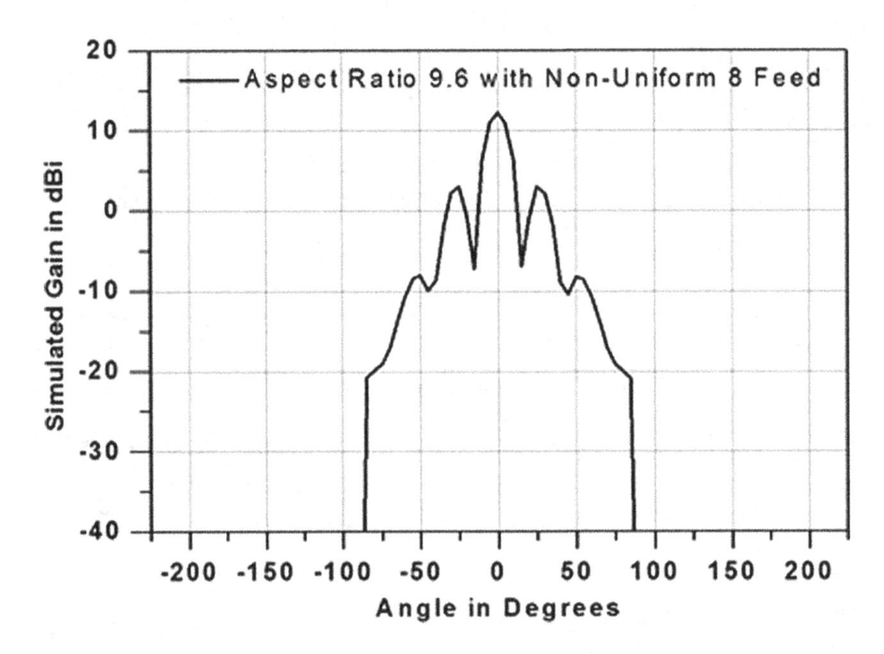

FIGURE 16.17 Simulated radiation pattern (Dolph-Chebyshev current excitation) continuous aperture antenna with eight feeds [15].

16.3.3 Antenna3

Another aspect of harvesting RF power is taking in RF power in a wide frequency spectrum. For this purpose, UWB-RF (Ultra Wide Band-Radio Frequency) energy harvesting is also an essential aspect. Here a C to X band RF power harvesting antenna is shown particularly for satellite communications applications. Further, as the energy harvesting antenna may be deployed in an open environment, a corrosion-free Ultra Wide Band Dielectric Antenna [16] is an excellent solution for the same, which also provides low-cost fabrication. Here an ultrawide band log-periodic dielectric antenna is presented, which offers an ultrawide 3:1 VSWR bandwidth of about 6.48 GHz (from 6.1752 GHz to 12.66 GHz). Simulated and experimental results are shown in Figures 16.18–16.22. In all four principal planes, the radiation patterns are almost regular and abundantly useful for omnidirectional RF power harvesting from satellite transponders (Figures 16.18–16.22).

16.4 CONCLUSION

In this chapter, the authors have presented different types of antenna systems for RF and microwave energy harvesting, which may be widely used in self-sustainable IoT devices, as investigated by

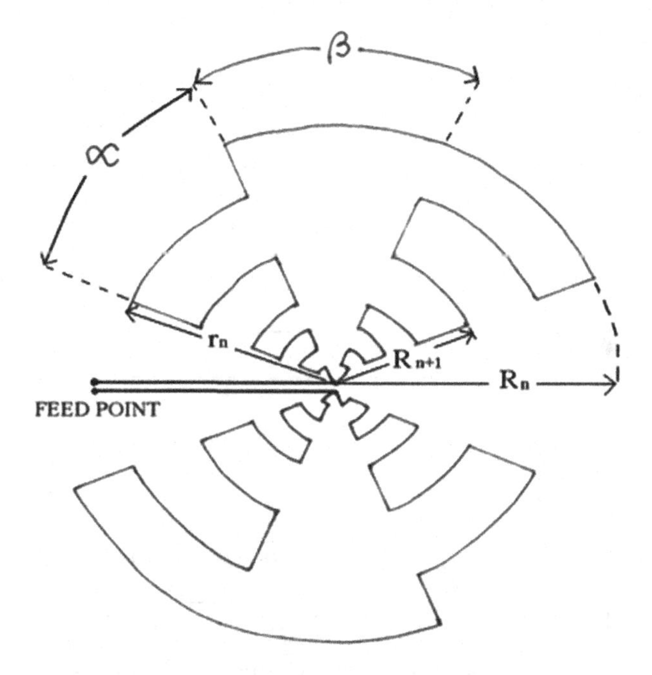

FIGURE 16.18 Top view of dielectric log-periodic antenna with (R3 = 0.78 cm, r3 = 0.719 cm, R2 = 0.92 cm, r2 = 0.848 cm, R1 = 1.08 cm, rl = 0.996 cm).

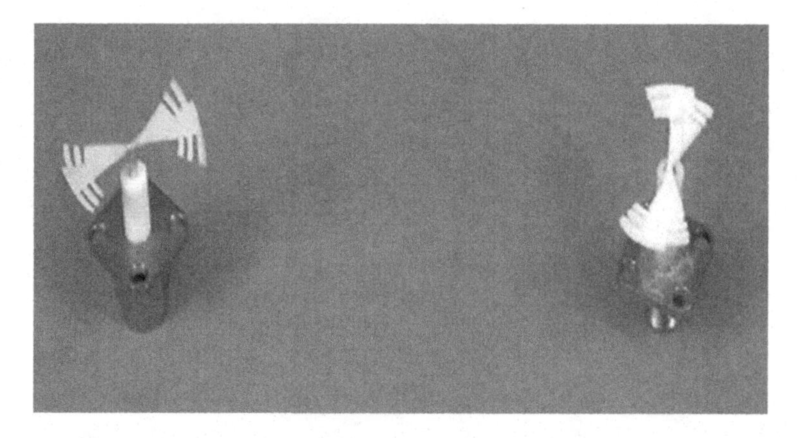

FIGURE 16.19 Fabricated dielectric log-periodic antenna with dielectric material (teflon) with dielectric constant $(\varepsilon_r) = 2.4$.

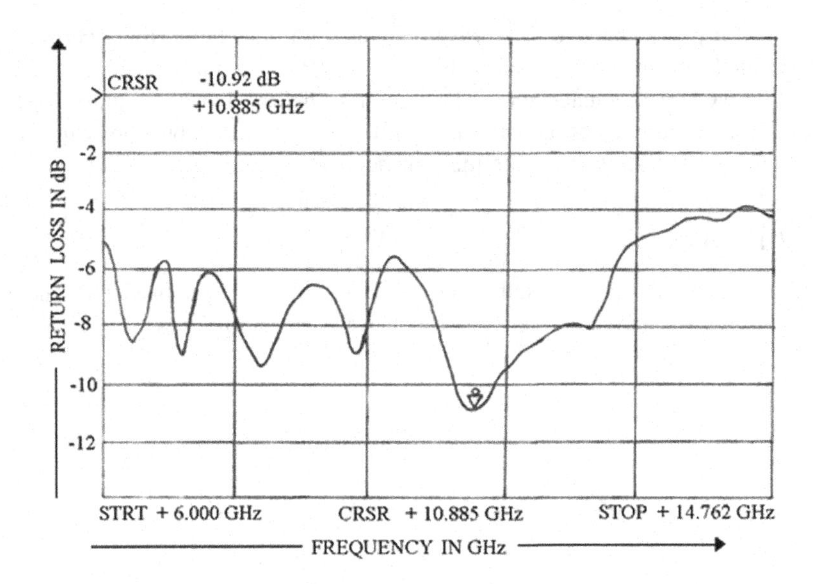

FIGURE 16.20 Measured return loss vs. frequency plot for dielectric log-periodic antenna.

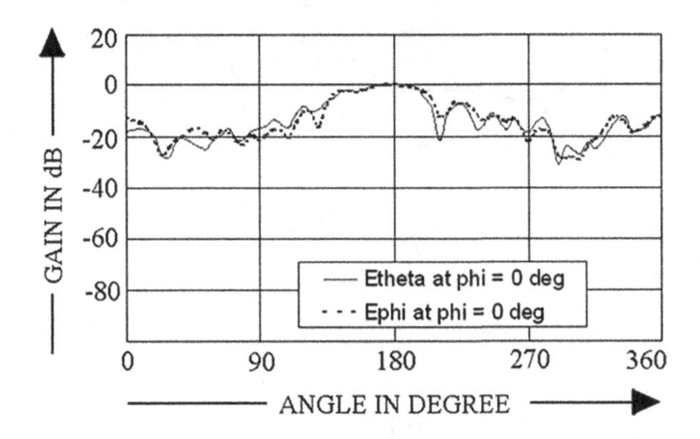

FIGURE 16.21 Measured radiation patterns for E_{theta} and E_{phi} vs. theta at phi = 0 deg.

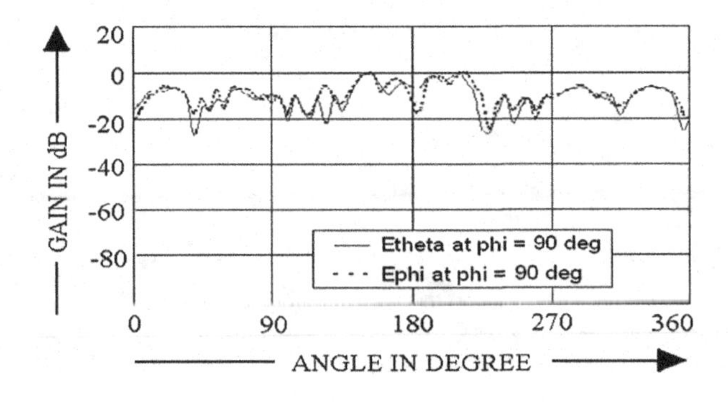

FIGURE 16.22 Measure radiation patterns for $E_{theta}$and E_{phi} vs. theta at phi = 90 deg.

the authors. Here, all the above discussions were carried out considering significantly low incident power densities, highly efficient radiators operating at different frequencies and most importantly exhibiting polarization agility with omni-directional or hemispherical radiation patterns etc. Moreover, the energy harvesting process (conversion from RF to DC power) for self-sustainable IoT devices in relevant commercial applications has been discussed.

REFERENCES

1. W. C. Brown, "The history of power transmission by radio waves," *IEEE Transactions on Microwave Theory and Techniques*, vol. 32, pp. 1230–1242, 1984.
2. .C Mikeka and H. Arai, "Design issues in radio frequency energy harvesting system," in *Sustainable Energy Harvesting Technologies - Past, Present and Future*, ed. Yen Kheng Tan, InTech, 2011, http://www.intechopen.com/books/sustainable-energy-harvestingtechnologies-past-present-and-future/design-issues-in-radio-frequency-energy-harvesting-system.
3. C. R. Valentaand and G. D. Durgin, "Harvesting wireless power: survey of energy-harvester conversion efficiency in far-field, wireless power transfer systems," *IEEE Microwave Magazine*, vol. 15, no. 4, pp. 108–120, 2014.
4. T. Keisuke, Y. Kawahara, and T. Asami, "RF energy intensity survey in Tokyo," in *2009 IEICE*, B-20-3, Matsuyama-shi, 2009.
5. C. Mikeka and H. Arai, *Dual-Band RF Energy-Harvesting Circuit for Range Enhancement in Passive Tags*, EuCAP, Rome, 2011.
6. M. Mi, *Analysis, Design, and Optimization of Antennas on CMOS Integrated Circuits for Energy Harvesting Applications*, Doctoral dissertation, Department of Electrical Engineering, University of Pittsburgh, 2003, http://d-scholarship.pitt.edu/8782/.
7. C. A. Balanis, *Antenna Theory: Analysis and Design*, John Wiley & Sons, 1997, https://www.wiley.com/en-us/Antenna+Theory%3A+Analysis+and+Design%2C+4th+Edition-p-9781118642061.
8. S. Ghosh, S. K. Ghosh, and A. Chakrabarty, "Design of RF energy harvesting system for wireless sensor node using circularly polarized monopole antenna: RF energy harvesting system for WSN node using circularly polarized antenna," in *Proceedings of the 9th International Conference on Industrial and Information Systems (ICIIS '14)*, pp. 1–6, IEEE, Gwalior, December 2014.
9. M. Arrawatia, M. S. Baghini, and G. Kumar, "RF energy harvesting system at 2.67 and 5.8 GHz," in *Proceedings of Asia-Pacific Microwave Conference*, pp. 900–903, 2010.
10. D. W. Harrist, "Wireless battery charging system using radio frequency energy harvesting," BS Thesis, University of Pittsburgh, July 13–15, 2004.
11. N. M. Din, C. K. Chakrabarty, A. Bin Ismail, K. K. A. Devi, and W.-Y. Chen, "Design of RF energy harvesting system for energizing low power devices," *Progress in Electromagnetics Research*, vol. 132, pp. 49–69, 2012. https://www.jpier.org/PIER/pier.php?paper=12072002.
12. Clayton R. Paul, *Introduction to Electromagnetic Compatibility*, 2nd Edition, Wiley-Interscience, 2006, https://www.wiley.com/en-us/Introduction+to+Electromagnetic+Compatibility%2C+2nd+Edition-p-9780471755005.
13. Hubregt J. Visser and Ruud J. M. Vullers, "RF energy harvesting and transport for wireless sensor network applications: Principles and requirements," *Proceedings of the IEEE*, vol. 101, no. 6, pp. 1410–1423, 2013.
14. Ayona Chakraborty, Samik Chakraborty, and Bhaskar Gupta, "Dual band polarization agile compact planar antenna for enhanced bandwidth and gain," *Microwave Review, MTT-IEEE*, vol. 25, no. 2, pp. 15–20, 2019.
15. Ayona Chakraborty, Samik Chakraborty, and Bhaskar Gupta, "Multi-feed rectangular microstrip antenna for enhancement of gain," *International Journal of Electrical Electronics & Computer Science Engineering*, vol. 4, no. 5, pp. 83–88, 2017.
16. Samik Chakraborty, Bhaskar Gupta, and D. R. Poddar, "Ultra wide band dielectric antennas for polarization independent omni directional applications," *Indian Journal of Physics*, vol. 80, pp. 753–755, 2006.

17 An Extremely Compact and Low-Cost Antenna Sensor Designed for IoT-Integrated Biomedical Applications

Ankan Bhattacharya and Souvik Pal

CONTENTS

17.1 INTRODUCTION

This chapter focuses on how devices are utilized and how the world interacts with the current healthcare system; without question, Internet of Things (IoT) is bringing a revolutionary change to the healthcare business. This has a broad field of use, including but not limited to hospitals, patients, insurance companies, and families. Here, we'll discuss how, in contrast to traditional approaches, IoT-based strategies are transforming the healthcare industry.

To create a dependable IoT-enabled health care ecosystem and execute cyber-physical ubiquitous infrastructure solutions, this part employs data and network engineering, as well as intelligent decision support system-by-design concepts. This part will take readers on a trip that begins with an understanding of the health care monitoring paradigm in IoT-enabled technologies, as well as how it may be applied to various aspects and applications. It guides readers through real-time difficulties and helps them create a secure infrastructure for IoT-based health care. This section assists researchers and practitioners in comprehending the IoT-enabled e-health care architecture and the current state of IoT countermeasures.

The rise of healthcare-specific IoT goods creates a plethora of possibilities. The enormous volume of data created by these linked gadgets has the potential to revolutionize healthcare.

Internet of Things features a four-step architecture, which are essentially steps in a process. All four phases are linked together in such a way that data is captured or processed at one level and then passed on to the next. Integrating values into the process generates insights and opens up new business opportunities.

Step 1: The deployment of interconnected devices, such as sensors, actuators, monitors, detectors, and video systems, is the first step. The data is collected by these devices.

Step 2: Data from sensors and other devices is typically in analogue format, which must be gathered and transformed into digital format for further processing.

Step 3: After the data has been digitized and aggregated, it is pre-processed, standardized, and sent to a data centre or the cloud.

DOI: 10.1201/9781003217398-17

Step 4: At the required level, the final data is managed and examined. When applied to this data, advanced analytics provides actionable business insights for better decision-making.

According to studies, healthcare is poised to become one of the fastest-growing IoT markets, with a projected value of $158 billion by 2022. By enabling remote monitoring, IoT in healthcare is assisting businesses and individuals in reducing hospital stays, re-admissions, and treatment expenses.

Internet of Things (IoT) is changing the healthcare business in more ways than merely remote monitoring. It provides fast and frequent real-time access to data and information to patients, experts, and health insurers.

Through the enormous number of applications that are already available and being developed, IoT is steadily making its way into our lives. Different healthcare applications are implantable glucose monitoring systems, activity trackers during cancer treatment, heart monitors with reporting, medical alert systems, ingestible sensors, medication dispensers, trackable inhalers, Bio-sensors antenna etc. In this chapter, we will particularly focus on the role of Bio-sensors antenna in the healthcare industry.

An Bio-sensor antenna has huge applicability in the biomedical industry. It can be used for real-time detection of materials, preferably bio-samples, without any effort like physical or chemical alteration, labelling etc. Hence, an Bio-sensor antenna is gradually gaining popularity in the biomedical industry [1–5]. The Bio-sensor antenna, however, should be compact and planar in configuration so that it can be easily integrated into printed circuit boards (PCBs). Such bio-sensing devices should also have the scope of Internet of Things (IoT) integration so that transmission of data could be performed using the internet, forming a smart bio-sensing device. Many compact microstrip antennas have been designed by researchers for wireless transmission of data [6–9]. A miniaturized, planar microstrip patch antenna with slotted patch and feed has been designed and presented here, which would work as a bio-sensor. It is able to detect the nature of the samples by virtue of the change in antenna responses like return loss, Voltage Standing Wave Ratio (VSWR), gain, radiation pattern etc.

This chapter is categorically organized as follows. Section 17.2 explains the method of analysis and design procedure of the patch antenna. Section 17.3 elaborates on the simulation results and parametric analysis of the proposed antenna sensor. Section 17.4 deals with the conclusion part, where the applicability and the future scope of the proposed bio-sensor have been discussed.

17.2 METHOD OF ANALYSIS AND DESIGN PROCEDURE OF THE BIO-SENSOR ANTENNA

The method of analysis of Bio-sensor antenna is based on the theory of microstrip transmission line. In a microstrip transmission line, most of the energy remains concentrated between the ground plane and the microstrip line. A slot has been created at the rear side of the antenna to provide an electric flux, which is necessary to detect the nature of the bio-samples put in the cavity. And on the other side, the flux is shielded by the copper patch (Figure 17.1).

Figure 17.2 depicts the proposed design of the Bio-sensor antenna. The patch, as well as the feed, consists of slotted sections. The feed line width has approximately been matched to 50.0 Ω. FR-4, having an effective permittivity (ε_{eff}) of 4.4 and loss tangent ($\tan\delta = 00.02$), has been used as a material for the substrate. A rectangular slot has been etched from the ground plane, where the bio-sample (specimen) is to be kept. The various dimensions of the proposed Bio-sensor antenna are as follows: $W = 10.00$ mm, $L = 20.00$ mm, $l1 = 08.60$ mm, $l2 = 05.50$ mm, $l3 = 02.00$ mm, $Fw = 03.00$ mm, $Sw = 08.00$ mm, $Sl = 04.00$ mm.

The resonant frequency of the Bio-sensor antenna can be calculated using the following equation:

$$f_r = \frac{1}{2\pi\sqrt{LC}} \tag{17.1}$$

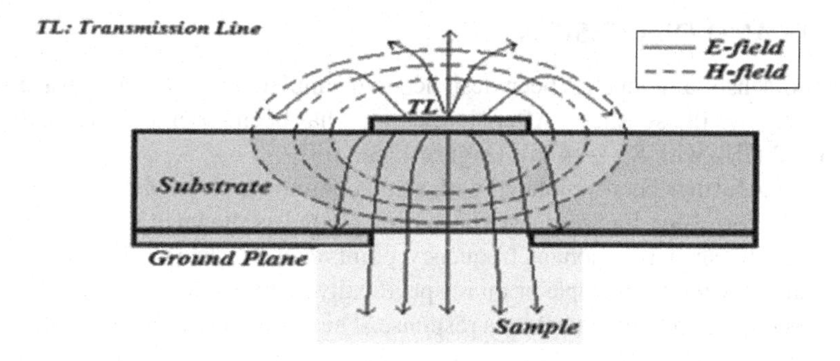

FIGURE 17.1 Distribution of E-field and H-field on either side of the device.

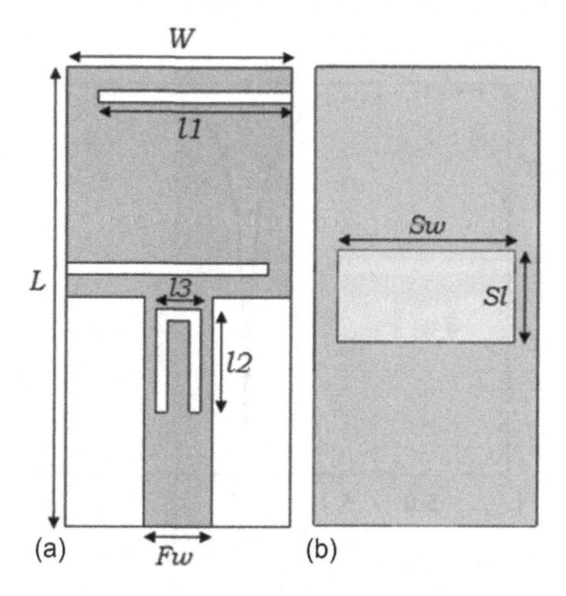

FIGURE 17.2 Bio-sensor antenna: (a) front-side view; (b) reverse-side view.

where the system capacitance is given as,

$$C = \varepsilon_{\text{eff}} \frac{A}{d} \tag{17.2}$$

ε_{eff} is the effective permittivity and the inductance L is introduced via the feeding section. A is the effective area of the substrate and d is the substrate thickness.

The effective permittivity can be expressed in terms of real and imaginary components as

$$\varepsilon_{\text{eff}} = \varepsilon_{\text{eff}}' - j\varepsilon_{\text{eff}}'' \tag{17.3}$$

The ratio of $\varepsilon_{\text{eff}}''$ to $\varepsilon_{\text{eff}}'$ is defined as the loss tangent, which gives a measure of the loss of electromagnetic energy [10].

$$\tan\delta \sim \frac{\varepsilon_{\text{eff}}''}{\varepsilon_{\text{eff}}'} \tag{17.4}$$

17.3 RESULTS AND DISCUSSION

The proposed Bio-sensor antenna has been designed and simulated in CST Microwave Studio with FR-4 as the material for the substrate. After simulation, it has been observed that the antenna resonates exactly at 5.2 GHz with $S_{11} \sim -40$ dB (Figure 17.3).

The structure has further been simulated with some common bio-samples like fat, bone, blood, and muscle, and the corresponding responses have been plotted as shown in Figure 17.4. The change in return loss and the shift in resonant frequency points can be clearly observed in the figure. Change in the nature of the bio-sample or more specifically due to changes in the effective permittivity, there has been a change in the antenna response. The dielectric properties of the various bio-samples have been provided in Table 17.1.

Figure 17.5 shows the VSWR of the bio-sensor device for different bio-samples. The change in VSWR characteristics is due to a change in the nature of the various bio-samples under test.

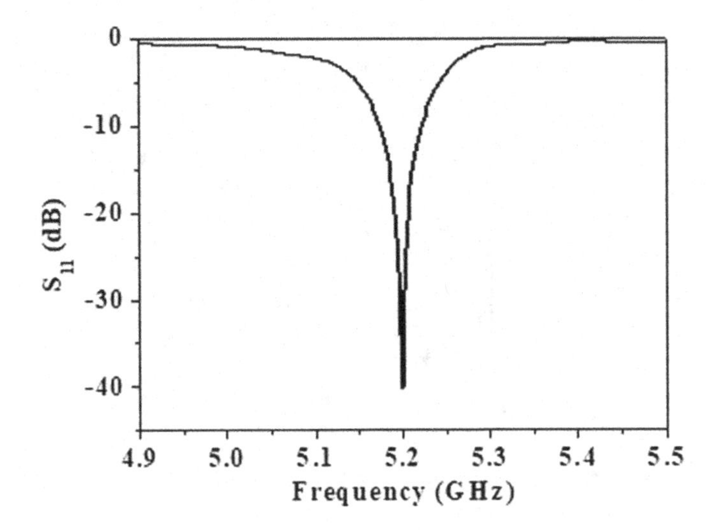

FIGURE 17.3 Frequency response characteristics (with air sample).

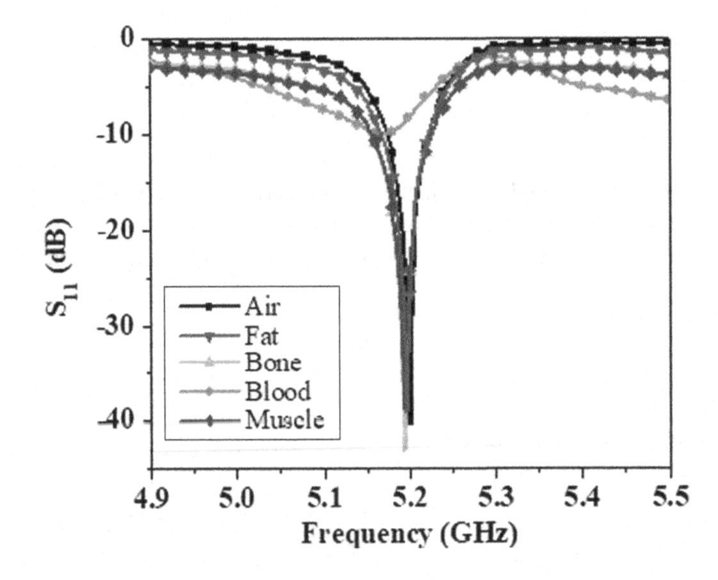

FIGURE 17.4 Frequency response characteristics of proposed Bio-sensor antenna with various bio-samples.

TABLE 17.1
Dielectric Properties of Different Bio-Samples

Nature of Sample	Density (kg/m³)	Relative Permittivity ($\varepsilon/\varepsilon_0$)	Loss Tangent tan δ	Conductivity (S/m)
Fat	909.4	5.24	0.147	0.119
Bone	1750	11.18	0.266	0.46
Blood	1060	57.7	0.318	2.858
Muscle	1059.9	52.31	0.244	1.981

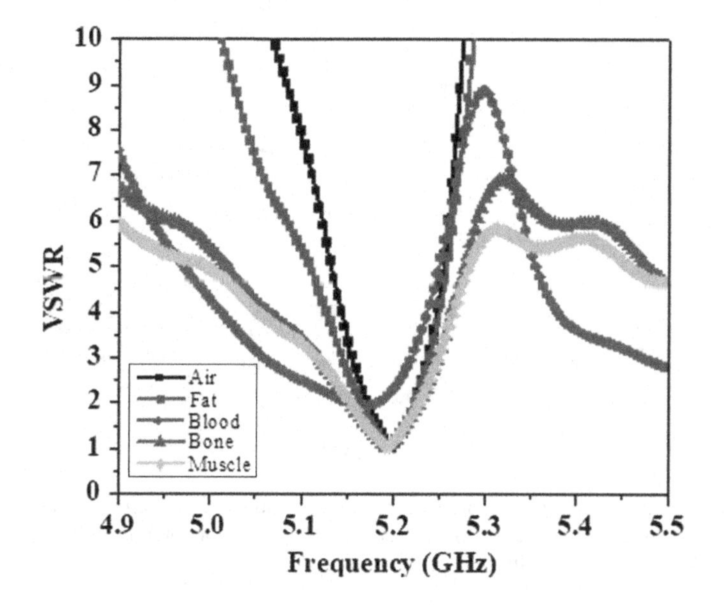

FIGURE 17.5 VSWR of proposed Bio-sensor antenna with different bio-samples.

TABLE 17.2
Gain of the Proposed Bio-Sensor with Different Bio-Samples

Bio-Samples	Max. Realized Gain (dBi)
Fat	3.67
Bone	3.71
Blood	3.89
Muscle	3.66

Table 17.2 shows the realized gain of the bio-sensor antenna under test with various bio-samples at 5.2 GHz. Figure 17.6(a)–(d) shows the 3D radiation pattern of the bio-sensor antenna for various bio-samples like fat, bone, blood, and muscle.

17.4 CONCLUSION

In this work, we have proposed a miniaturized, slotted microstrip bio-sensor antenna. The antenna has been simulated with some common bio-samples. In each and every case, the frequency response characteristics of the bio-sensor antenna differed from each other. This occurs due to the difference in the dielectric properties of separate bio-samples. Variation has also been observed in return loss,

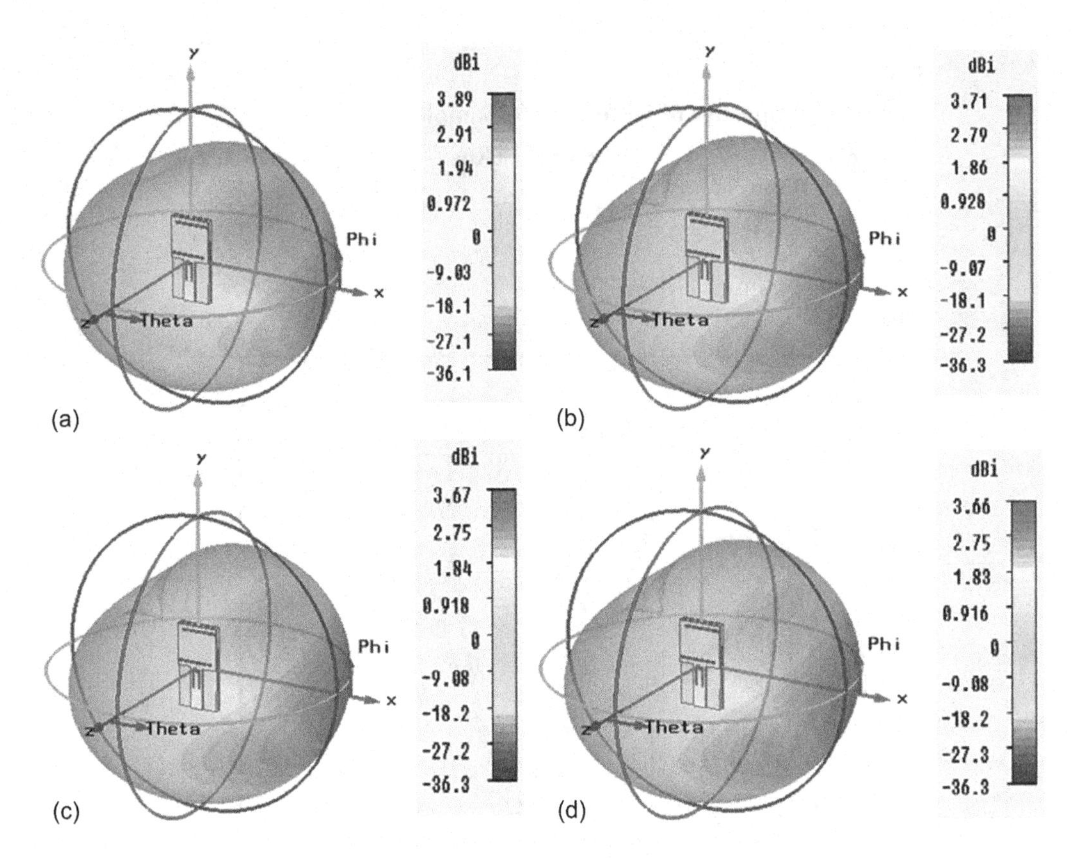

FIGURE 17.6 (a). Realized gain of bio-sensor antenna with blood as a bio-sample; (b) realized gain of bio-sensor antenna with bone as a bio-sample; (c) realized gain of bio-sensor antenna with fat as a bio-sample; (d) realized gain of bio-sensor antenna with muscle as a bio-sample.

VSWR, radiation pattern, and realized gain. The variation in frequency response characteristics of the bio-sensing device helps us detect the nature of the bio-samples. It is able to provide easy and quick detection of bio-samples. The device can also be IoT integrated for wireless interconnectivity and data transmission. The proposed bio-sensor antenna, therefore, demands huge applicability in IoT-integrated biomedical applications.

REFERENCES

1. Khadase RB and Anil N (2018). Antenna as a biosensor. *Recent Trends in Sensor Research & Technology*, 5(1), 1–13.
2. Cui Y (2017). Wireless biological elect. *Sensors. Sensors (Basel, Switzerland)*, 17(10), 2289.
3. Afroz S, Thomas SW, Mumcu G, and Saddow SE (2013). Implantable SiC based RF antenna biosensor for glucose monitoring. *SENSORS*, IEEE, Baltimore, pp. 1–4.
4. Pal A, Mehta A, Marhic ME, Chan KC, and Teng KS (2011). Micro resonator antenna for biosensing applications. *Micro & Nano Letters, IET*, 6, 665–667.
5. Kim B, Uno S, and Nakazato K (2011). Miniature on-chip spiral inductor RFID tag antenna of standard CMOS process for biosensor applications. In *2011 IEEE-APS Topical Conference on Antennas and Propagation in Wireless Communications*, pp. 925–928, doi: 10.1109/APWC.2011.6046817.
6. Bhattacharya A, Roy B, and Bhattacharjee AK (2021). Compact, isolation enhanced, band-notched SWB–MIMO antenna suited for wireless personal communications. *Wireless Personal Communications*, 116, 1575–1592.
7. Bhattacharya A and Roy B (2020). Investigations on an extremely compact MIMO antenna with enhanced isolation and bandwidth. *Microwave and Optical Technology Letters*, 62, 845–851.

8. Bhattacharya A, Roy B, Caldeirinha R, and Bhattacharjee A (2019). Low-profile, extremely wideband, dual-band-notched MIMO antenna for UWB applications. *International Journal of Microwave and Wireless Technologies*, 11(7), 719–728.
9. Bhattacharya A, Roy B, Chowdhury SK, and Bhattacharjee AK (2019). An isolation enhanced, printed, low-profile UWB-MIMO antenna with unique dual band-notching features for WLAN and WiMAX. *IETE Journal of Research*, Taylor & Francis Online.
10. Taylor KM and Weide DW (2005). Ultra-sensitive detection of protein thermal unfolding and refolding using near-zone microwaves. *Microwave Theory and Techniques*, 53, 1576–1586.

Index

Printed in the United States
by Baker & Taylor Publisher Services